BIRTH
Centres

For Books for Midwives:

Senior Commissioning Editor: Mary Seager
Development Editor: Catharine Steers
Project Manager: Morven Dean
Design: George Ajayi
Illustration Manager: Bruce Hogarth

BIRTH
Centres

A Social Model
for Maternity Care

EDITED BY

Mavis Kirkham PhD, MA, BA CERT ED, RM, RN
Professor of Midwifery, University of Sheffield, UK

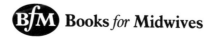 **Books** *for* **Midwives**

BOOKS FOR MIDWIVES
An Imprint of Elsevier Science Limited

First published 2003

ISBN 0 7506 5497 X

British Library Cataloguing in Publication Data
A catalogue record for this book is available from the British Library

Library of Congress Cataloging in Publication Data
A catalog record for this book is available from the Library of Congress

Note
Medical Knowledge is constantly changing. Standard safety precautions must be followed, but as new research and clinical experience broaden our knowledge, changes in treatment and drug therapy may become necessary or appropriate. Readers are advised to check the most current product information provided by the manufacturer of each drug to be administered to verify the recommended dose, the method and duration of administration, and contraindications. It is the responsibility of the practitioner, relying on experience and knowledge of the patient, to determine dosages and the best treatment for each individual patient. Neither the publisher nor the editor assumes any liability for any injury and/or damage to persons or property arising from this publication.
The Publisher

The
Publisher's
policy is to use
**paper manufactured
from sustainable forests**
II

Printed in China

Contents

Foreword

'Pregnancy is a long and very special journey for a woman. It is a journey of dramatic physical, psychological and social change; of becoming a mother, of redefining family relationships and taking on the long-term responsibility for caring and cherishing a new born child. Generations of women have travelled the same route, but each journey is unique'–and that surely is the point. The experience for every woman is unique. Every birth is unique and that is why it is so important to give a woman choice: choice of place of birth, choice of style of care, and choice of professional who is going to accompany her in this unique and very special journey.

In the ten years since I wrote the words in quotation marks (DoH 1993) much has changed. More young women are entering into further education, more women are entering the professions, more women are from ethnic minorities and more women are the sole bread-winners. The birth rate is declining and the teenage pregnancy rate increasing, and yet those words are as true today as they were a decade ago; they are as relevant to those who are less articulate and who struggle to make ends meet as they are to those who have an easier and more comfortable life.

Encouragingly, as this book illustrates, some maternity services have re-shaped their style of care, giving choice and organising their services 'in a way which does not jeopardise safety, yet is kinder, more welcoming and more supportive to the women whose needs it is designed to meet' (DoH 1993). Others have been valiant but have been defeated by the resistance they have encountered. But they deserve our praise and thanks for trying. Women want choice, continuity and control over their pregnancy and birth, but rigid Trust policies, the might of the medical model and a lack of insight and trust all work against them.

One of the very encouraging developments has been the number of Birth Centres that have been established. It is important to distinguish between those which embrace the philosophy of a true Birth Centre and those which parade as such. Sadly many have grown out of a politically untenable position with a related threatened closure. In pockets, midwife-led units have emerged with a high level of appreciation from those who use them. Case-load midwifery has attracted the most committed of midwives and they give women an outstanding service.

I delight and rejoice in the increasing variety of provision. If every journey is unique, women should be given a choice of how to travel. It is useful to listen to other experienced travellers when embarking on a journey. This book charts some of the travels undertaken by those seeking to guide and provide women with a different and kinder service. I hope it will encourage other health professionals who seek a new approach and search for radical solutions, while pointing out the pitfalls which can occur. It certainly makes a useful and an interesting contribution.

Baroness Cumberlege
Lewes,
East Sussex, 2003

References
Changing Childbirth. DoH, 1993

Preface

Birth centres are important to me, both in practice and in theory. I work in a birth centre, at Darley Dale in Derbyshire, though my academic job allows me only four weeks clinical work there each year. I am also a member of a group lobbying for a birth centre in Sheffield. Long ago, when I was a student midwife, this city had three maternity hospitals and a number of small maternity homes around its edge. Now Sheffield has one maternity hospital and we speak the rhetoric of maternal choice. Many cities in the UK are similarly served. I had the privilege of doing research in GP maternity units over twenty years ago. Our recent research is mainly in large units and enables us to examine the dilemmas posed by their culture. I am aware that the proudly proclaimed aims of midwifery care often remain as rhetoric in hospitals–but that they can be achieved in birth centres. The editing of this book has therefore brought many issues together for me.

This is a book that grew. Jane Walker, who was then at Edgware Birth Centre, asked me if I would edit a book about that unit. That original proposal forms Part 2 of this book. As I considered the book, it became clear to me that Edgware Birth Centre is interesting because it has been so thoroughly evaluated, but that evaluation is only important because of its relevance to, and links with, the wider context. Part 1 of the book seeks to provide a picture of the wider context for this country–historically, politically and geographically. Part 3 aims to describe this context for some other countries. Part 2 sits as a case study in the middle of the book. I have endeavoured to pull together the key themes from the whole book in Chapter 23.

Birth centres are defined differently in different places and some of the birth settings described in this book have other names. Julie Hall (Ch. 1) describes 'free-standing low-risk maternity units' which are defined by their position on a separate site from a consultant maternity unit. A small minority of the units she studied had specialist obstetric, paediatric or anaesthetic involvement. There is a similar range of involvement in US birth centres (Ch. 18). There used to be many GP units in the UK but, with the decline in GP involvement in birth, these have become midwife-led units or birth centres. The Wiltshire model (Ch. 3) refers to 'community-based centres'. In New Zealand they are called 'primary care facilities' (Ch. 21).

In Australia the majority of the facilities called 'birth centres' are within large maternity hospitals (Ch. 20). Helen Shallow (Ch. 2) describes birth centres in the UK which are either 'stand alone' or 'alongside' a consultant maternity unit. For her the term 'birth centre' represents 'a set of values and beliefs about birth, without which it has little meaning'. This philosophy is 'centred on the concept of midwifery being at the heart of a social [rather than a medical] model of care' in which midwives give skilled support 'within which women can achieve normal, physiological birth'. This philosophy appears, with different wording, throughout this book and is articulated by many groups now working to set up new birth centres or to protect existing ones.

The web sites of birth centre groups may be of interest to readers of this book: for the UK (http://groups.yahoo.com/groups/birthcentres); Europe (www.birthcenter-europe.net); and the USA (http://www.birthcenters.org).

Despite the growth of the philosophy of birth centres, the collection of chapters in this book is deliberately eclectic. I learnt many years ago that midwives practise differently in isolated settings without immediate medical support. I have therefore included chapters about small units without a clearly articulated philosophy as well as those which identify themselves as birth centres. (Because of the wide variations in the units described I have not used capital letters for the words birth centre, though some chapter authors have chosen to do this.) The authors of this book are similarly wide-ranging. Most are midwives, as befits the subject. Several are members of groups which represent childbearing families. There is a consultant obstetrician, a GP and a professor of public health, as well as researchers who evaluate services. The birth centres described are all different and the writers address their topics very differently. In this they reflect the diversity of birth centres, within very different social and health care settings, as well as the factors they have in common.

I am very aware that there are omissions. Some of the chapters originally planned did not come to fruition–for instance, one author produced her third baby (in a birth centre) but not her chapter. I only became aware of some of the areas that should have been covered when the book was nearly complete. The International Confederation of Midwives conference in April 2002 was a scene of great learning and great frustration for me as I learnt of new birth centres when it was too late to include them as chapters in the book. So the chapter subjects are not wholly representative of the world's birth centres. I would have liked to include chapters on birth centres in Africa, South America and Japan, but this did not prove possible here and could form a future project. It was only when writing the last chapter that I identified one of my inspirations for the book–the midwives of the township units in Capetown.

This is a first attempt to write a book about birth centres. It addresses key themes in modern maternity services and should serve to furnish debates about the scale of those services and about the roles, skills and relationships needed to pursue excellence in their provision. I feel the time is right for such a book and I hope that it will stimulate debate.

M. K.

Acknowledgements

This has been a complicated book to edit because of the number of authors and the need for translation of some contributions. I would like to thank all involved for their patience and perseverance.

I would like to thank my colleagues at Darley Maternity Unit, who have supported me in expanding my knowledge and skill there. I thank the families I have known there for keeping me grounded in their realities. I thank the colleagues who stretch my thinking, especially Helen Stapleton, Penny Curtis, Anna Fielder, and the midwives of the Association of Radical Midwives. I thank all the contributors to this book, especially Jane Walker for the original idea, Ulla Waldenström for producing her chapter despite her illness, and Andrea McGlynn for filling one gap in this book at very short notice. Marianne Mead, Nicky Leap and Sara Wickham used their extensive midwifery networks to provide me with links which led to chapters in this book and I appreciate their help and generosity. I am grateful to Janet Rodriguez Martinez for her support at the beginning of the editing process. Last, and most, I thank Jane Flint who has collected data, translated, and written a chapter for this book, as well as supporting its production throughout. Without her this book would not have been completed.

M. K.

Contributors

Linda Arnold, LM, DM, CPM
Founder, Administrator and Clinical Director of
Casa de Nacimiento El Paso, Texas, USA

Jean Beney, MRCS (Eng.), LRCP (Lond.), MB, BS,
DRCOG
Senior Partner, Oak Lodge Medical Centre,
member of Edgware Birth Centre Management
Group, member of Barnet Local Medical
Committee, UK

Mary Boulton, BA, PhD, HomMFPHM
Professor of Sociology, Social Sciences and Law,
Oxford Brookes University, Oxford, UK

Jean Chapple, MBChB, MCommH, FFPHM, FRCP,
DRCOG, DCH, MFFP
Consultant in Perinatal Epidemiology,
Westminster PCT, Honary Senior Lecturer,
Imperial College, London

Susan Dolman, MSc, RN, RM, DMS
Formerly Head of Midwifery, Northwick Park
and St. Marks NHS Trust, UK

Stephen Farrow, MD, FRCP, FFPHM
Visiting Professor of Public Health, Middlesex
University, UK

Jane Flint, BA (Hons)
Research Administrator, WICH Research Group,
School of Nursing and Midwifery, University of
Sheffield, UK

Diane Fraser, PhD, MPhil, B.Ed, MTD, RM, RGN
Professor of Midwifery, Head of the Academic
Division of Midwifery, School of Human
Development, University of Nottingham, UK

Kate Griew, RN, CM, Dip Hom, MSc-HIV
Clinical Midwifery Educator, New South Wales,
Australia

Elisabeth Groh, RM
West Sussex, UK

Karen Guilliland, RM, RGON, ADN, MA, MNZM
CEO, New Zealand College of Midwives,
Director, PHARMAC, Deputy Chair Person,
New Zealand Health Workforce Advisory
Committee

Julie Hall, MB, BS, MPH, MFPHM
Specialist Registrar in Public Health,
West Yorkshire, UK

Richard Hallett, BSc (Hons), MA, MIoD
Former Chair, Crowborough Hospital Maternity
Unit Monitoring Group, Chair Eastbourne
Maternity Services Liaison Committee, East
Sussex, UK

Marion Hunter, RGON, RM, ADN, BA (Massey
University), MA (First Class Honours, Midwifery,
Massey University)
Senior Lecturer, Auckland University of
Technology, School of Midwifery, New Zealand

Olive Jones, RN, RM, ADM, PgCertSOM, Mphil
Supervisor, Midwives Supporting NHS and
Private Maternity Services, London, UK, Former
Project Leader, Edgware Birth Centre, UK

Elizabeth Manero
Lay Representative, Chair, London Health Link,
Member of Barnet Community Health Council,
Member of ECB Management Group,
London, UK

Andrea Gregor McGlynn, BSN, RN, CNM
Staff Nurse-midwife, Alivio Medical Centre,
Chicago, IL, USA

Fehmidah Munir, BSC, PhD, CPsychol
Lecturer in Applied Psychology, Institute of
Work, Health and Organisations, University of
Nottingham, UK

Sally Pairman, RGON, RM, BA, MA (Midwifery)
Head of School of Midwifery, Otago
Polytechnic, Dunedin, New Zealand,
Education Consultant to New Zealand College
of Midwives, Past President, New Zealand
College of Midwives, New Zealand

Rick Porter FRCOG
Consultant Obstetrician and Gynaecologist,
Royal United Hospital, Weston, Bath, UK

Julie Ratcliffe, MSC Health Economics, PhD Economics
Senior Resident Fellow in Health Economics,
Sheffield Health Economics Group, University
of Sheffield, Sheffield, UK

Dawn Saunders, RN, RM, MSc
Public Health Specialist, Surrey, UK

Verena Schmid
Independent Midwife, Scuola Elementale di
Arte Ostetrica (Elemental School of Midwifery
Art), Florence, Italy

Helen Shallow, M.MEDSci, RM, RGN, ADM,
PGCEA
Midwife Consultant, Southern Derbyshire
Acute Hospitals NHS Trust, UK

Vicky Tinsley, RN, RM, BSc (Midwifery),
MA Industrial Relations
Maternity Services Manager, West Wiltshire
Primary Care Trust, Wiltshire, UK

Linda Turner
Member of Barnet Community Health Council,
Barnet, Enfield and Harringey Maternity
Services, Liaison Committee, Lay Member of
Midwifery Committee of Nursing and
Midwifery Council, Trustee, National
Childbirth Trust, Chair of the Management
Committee, Edgware Birth Centre,
London, UK

Ulla Waldenström, RN, RM, BA, PhD
Professor of Nursing, Midwifery,
Department of Nursing, Karolinska Institutet,
Stockholm, Sweden

Jane Walker, SCM, PGCEA, MA
Consultant Midwife, Homerton
University Hospital, Hackney, North East
London, Former Project Leader, Edgware
Birth Centre, UK

Kim Watts, RN, RM, MSc, PGCAP
Midwife Lecturer, Academic Division of
Midwifery, School of Human Development,
University of Nottingham, UK

Judith Wolf
Currently writing a doctorate thesis in
ethnology, Ecole des Hautes Etudes en Sciences
Sociales, Paris, France

Introduction

PART I: BIRTH CENTRES IN ENGLAND

Julie Hall starts this part of the book with an overview, and an introduction to her 'Directory of Free-standing Low-Risk Maternity Units in England'. This is in keeping with my own experience, that a social model of birth can flourish where the unit is small and low-tech, even without a clear philosophy. An explicit philosophy of nurturing a social model of birth is an advantage and midwives certainly benefit from support in developing and extending the skills associated with such a model. In Chapter 2 Helen Shallow describes the work to ensure this in planning a new birth centre: this birth centre is now open.

The Chapters which follow concern a number of units with very different histories and settings. Some were called 'birth centres' when they were set up and some predate that title. They are described from different viewpoints: an initial plan (Ch. 2), a formal evaluation (Ch. 4), a description of units across a county (Ch. 3) and the story of one unit (Ch. 5).

PART 2: EDGWARE BIRTH CENTRE

The Edgware Birth Centre is taken as a case study because it is relatively new and it has been very thoroughly evaluated. Chapters 6–11 tell the story of that birth centre from different viewpoints, the first of which is that of service users. The need for partnership is addressed in Chapter 9. I am aware of the different terms used in these chapters to describe what I am told should be called the 'steering group'. However, I have not changed these terms as I think it says much for the flexibility of a group which can be seen as either 'advisor' or 'steering'.

Chapter 11 examines new developments in the role of midwifery assistants. Chapters 12 and 13 outline the evaluation of the birth centre at Edgware.

PART 3: BIRTH CENTRES IN THE WIDER WORLD

The social model of birth is approached in very different ways in different contexts. Most chapters in this part of the book address a particular country, some supportive of birth centres, such as New Zealand (Ch. 21), and many where there is considerable hostility. Definitions vary too – most of the birth centres described are free-standing but some, such as those in Australia (Ch. 20), are integrated within large hospitals. Economic models differ greatly too, ranging from birth centres that exist within a variety of state-funded systems of care to a system in which midwives work as entrepreneurs.

The two case studies of birth centres are very different: Chapter 16 describes what is now the only birth centre in France and Chapter 19 tells the story of a birth centre in Texas. In Chapter 14 Ulla Waldenström brings together the ten studies that evaluated the birth centre in Stockholm.

In Chapter 22 Marion Hunter reports her research on the skills that midwives identify as requirements for birth centre practice. Her study was undertaken in New Zealand but her analysis has implications for midwifery education everywhere. In Chapter 23 I seek to bring the key issues together.

Birth centres in England

1

Free-standing maternity units in England

Julie Hall

INTRODUCTION

The place in which the majority of women give birth has changed considerably over the past 100 years. At the turn of the twentieth century the majority of births occurred at home (Macfarlane & Campbell 1994). In the 1920s, however, concern about infant mortality and 'unsanitary conditions' led to a rise in the number of births occurring in institutions, most commonly maternity and lying-in homes (William 1904).

During the 1950s and 1960s giving birth increasingly became seen as a 'surgical procedure' (Bonney 1919). The Peel Report, published in 1970 (Standing Maternity and Midwifery Advisory Committee 1970), concluded that the hospital was the safest place for women to give birth. By the early 1990s over 95% of all births took place in a hospital and between 1970 and 1990 there was a rapid decline in the number of maternity homes and general practitioner assisted deliveries (Zander & Chamberlain 1999).

However, choice of place of delivery has become increasingly important over the past 20 years and the need to ensure that women are offered a range of options was the basis for a key recommendation in *Changing Childbirth* (Department of Health 1993). Despite the predominance of hospital-based deliveries, four very different birth settings exist in England: consultant-led obstetric units, adjacent low-risk maternity units, home and free-standing maternity units.

'Consultant-led obstetric units' (CLUs) are staffed by midwives and obstetricians and care for both high- and low-risk patients. Women are usually admitted under the care of a consultant obstetrician, although in some units women thought to be at low risk of developing complications during labour may choose a midwife or a general practitioner to be their lead clinician. The full range of obstetric interventions is usually available on site and there should be no need to travel to another unit during labour.

'Adjacent low-risk maternity units' are situated in the same hospital as a consultant-led unit. They cater for low risk and are run either solely by midwives or jointly by midwives and general practitioners. Women are admitted under the care of a 'lead clinician'–either a midwife or a general practitioner. Obstetricians are only involved in a patient's care at the request of the lead clinician or of the woman herself. Care from an obstetrician and the full range of obstetric interventions are available within the same institution.

Home offers an alternative to delivery within an institution. Women who book for a home delivery are usually, though not always, classed as 'low risk'. They are cared for by a lead clinician, who can be either a midwife or a general practitioner. Obstetricians are only involved in the patient's care at the request of the lead clinician or of the woman herself. The home, however, is geographically separated from a consultant-led obstetric unit. If complications occur that cannot be managed within the home environment the woman and/or her baby must be transferred by ambulance to the nearest hospital-based consultant unit.

The fourth type of birth setting, the 'free-standing maternity unit' (FMU), aims to provide a 'home-like' environment within an institutional setting. Free-standing units are similar to adjacent low-risk maternity units in that they cater for low-risk women and are run by midwives or/and general practitioners with limited involvement from obstetricians.

The key difference between free-standing units and adjacent units is that free-standing units are geographically separated from a consultant unit and based in a separate institution: if the woman or her baby require an intervention that is not available in the free-standing unit they must travel by ambulance to receive care.

In recent years there has been growing interest in free-standing maternity units (Zander and Chamberlain 1999). The concentration of high-risk obstetric services, public demand for more accessible and personalised care, and midwives' desire for increased professional autonomy have all contributed to the need to explore alternative means of providing high-quality care to low-risk women. This chapter describes the findings of a survey of all the free-standing maternity units that were operational in 1998 in England and provides previously unavailable information on the structure and activity of such units.

OVERVIEW OF THE FREE-STANDING MATERNITY UNITS IN ENGLAND

A free-standing maternity unit is defined as a unit that provides intrapartum care in an institution geographically separated from a consultant-led obstetric unit. Using this definition, 55 operational free-standing maternity units were identified in England in 1998.

Although free-standing units exist throughout the country, access to such a unit was found to be patchy, with the majority of units located in the south of England. The ratio of the number of free-standing maternity units to the number of women of childbearing age ranged from 15.8 units per million women in the South West NHS region to less than one unit per million women of childbearing age in the London and Eastern NHS regions (Table 1.1).

There were few free-standing maternity units in isolated parts of the country. Three-quarters of all free-standing maternity units in England were less than 20 miles from the nearest consultant-led obstetric unit; the most isolated unit was just over 50 miles from a hospital unit.

Three models of free-standing maternity units were identified from the data provided by the survey–midwife-led units, general practitioner

Table 1.1 Regional distribution of free-standing maternity units in England

NHS region (based on 1998 boundaries)	Number of free-standing maternity units	Number of free-standing maternity units/ million women aged 15–44
South West	15	15.8
South East	13	5.7
Northern and Yorkshire	8	6.2
West Midlands	6	5.6
North West	6	4.7
Trent	5	4.8
Eastern	1	0.9
London	1	0.6

units and units with resident middle-grade obstetricians. Twenty-nine of the 55 free-standing maternity units in England in 1998 were run by midwives with no on-site involvement from general practitioners or obstetricians (midwife-led or M-FMUs). Fourteen of the units were run jointly by general practitioners and midwives (general practitioner units or GP-FMUs). In three units intrapartum care was managed jointly by midwives and a middle-grade obstetrician (staff grade or registrar) who was resident in the unit 24 hours a day (O-FMUs).

Around a half of the midwife-led units and two-thirds of the units with resident middle-grade obstetricians opened within the last 5 years, possibly indicating a rise in demand for this type of care. However, no historical data is available for comparison.

Cavenagh reported that there were over a hundred free-standing general practitioner obstetric units in England and Wales in 1982 (Cavenagh et al 1984). As only 14 GP-FMUs were found in this survey and only one opened recently, it appears that this type of unit is in decline.

On average, each free-standing maternity unit delivered around 200 babies a year (191 babies per unit) in 1998 but this ranged from less than 10 deliveries a year in some units to a maximum of 450 deliveries a year in the midwife and general practice units and over 1000 deliveries a year in the units with resident middle-grade obstetricians.

CARE PROVIDED IN THE DIFFERENT MODELS OF FREE-STANDING MATERNITY UNITS

Antenatal care programmes were similar in all three models of free-standing maternity unit. Most units offered a choice of midwife-only antenatal care (41/46 units), shared midwife and general practitioner care (41/46 units) or shared midwife and consultant care (37/46 units).

The range of intra- and postpartum interventions available differed considerably between the different models. Midwife-led units generally catered for normal deliveries and provided no on-site medical interventions, although in a small number of units midwives were able to perform Ventouse deliveries. Most general practitioner units were able to perform instrumental deliveries on site. Units with resident middle-grade obstetricians had facilities to provide virtually all pre-, intra- and postpartum interventions (Table 1.2).

Only one unit had access to a blood gas analyser despite recommendations that continuous electronic monitoring should only be used when this type of equipment is available (RCOG/RCM 1999). Few units could perform emergency caesarean sections on site and only one unit provided epidural anaesthesia.

Average journey times from the FMU to the CLU were only available for a small number of units. However, distance was available for the majority of units. The conclusion was that 10 miles would be the furthest that could be travelled in 30 minutes, based on average journey times and the assumptions that:

• the ambulance would take no more than 10 minutes to arrive at the FMU
• the patient would be fully prepared for travel the moment the ambulance arrived
• in the case of the caesarean section standard, operating theatres at the CLU would be ready to receive the patient on arrival.

Based on the assumption that 10 miles would be the furthest that could be travelled in 30 minutes, only one in six of the midwife-led free-standing units and a similar proportion of

Table 1.2 Interventions available on site in free-standing maternity units

	Midwife-led units (M-FMUs) (n=29)	General practitioner units (GP-FMUs) (n=14)	Units with resident middle-grade obstetricians (O-FMUs) (n=3)
Elective caesarean section	0	0	2
Induction of labour	0	2	2
Continuous electronic fetal monitoring	16	8	3
Instrumental delivery	3	11	3
Emergency caesarean section	1	2	3
Augmentation of labour	0	2	3
Epidural	0	0	1
Repair of third/fourth-degree perineal damage	0	1	3
Removal of retained placenta	0	2	3

the general practitioner units would meet the standard outlined in *Towards Safer Childbirth* (RCOG/RCM 1999) which requires access to emergency caesarean section and epidural anaesthesia within half an hour of a request being made.

STAFFING LEVELS IN THE FREE-STANDING MATERNITY UNITS

The availability of other medical staff correlated closely with the on-site availability of medical staff with obstetric experience. Few of the midwife-led or general practitioner units had access to on-site paediatricians or anaesthetists, unlike most of the units with resident middle-grade obstetricians (Tables 1.3, 1.4).

Units without 24-hour availability of on-site paediatricians relied on in-house training to ensure that staff could deal with neonatal emergencies. Less than half of all the free-standing maternity units had at least one member of staff with an Advanced Obstetric Lifesaving or Advanced Neonatal Resuscitation qualification.

All of the free-standing units responding to the questionnaire claimed to meet the midwifery staffing levels recommended in *Changing Childbirth* (Department of Health 1993). A random sample of 22 FMUs and their affiliated consultant-led units showed that, on average, midwives working in free-standing units each delivered less

than a third of the number of babies delivered annually by midwives working in consultant-led units (8 babies a year per free-standing unit midwife compared with 27 babies a year for midwives working in a consultant-led unit).

RATE OF TRANSFER FROM FREE-STANDING MATERNITY UNITS TO CONSULTANT-LED UNITS

Four different rates of transfer from free-standing maternity units to a consultant-led unit were measured for the year 1998–the intrapartum transfer rate, the maternal postpartum transfer rate, the neonatal transfer rate and the total transfer rate. The *intrapartum transfer rate* was defined as the percentage of women admitted in labour to a free-standing maternity unit who were transferred to a consultant-led unit during labour. The *maternal postpartum transfer rate* is the percentage of women who gave birth in a free-standing maternity unit who, for maternal reasons, were subsequently transferred to a consultant-led unit. The *neonatal transfer rate* describes the percentage of babies born in a free-standing maternity unit who needed to be transferred to a neonatal unit during the postpartum period. The *total transfer rate* is the percentage of admissions to a free-standing unit subsequently transferred to a consultant-led unit during the intra- and postpartum period.

Table 1.3 Availability of paediatricians in free-standing maternity units (FMUs)

Type of free-standing maternity unit	Phone advice only	Neonatal flying squad available 24 hours a day	On site during working hours; phone advice only out of hours	On site 24 hours a day
M-FMU (n=29)	28	0	1	0
GP-FMU (n=14)	11	2	1	0
O-FMU (n=3)	1	1	0	1

Table 1.4 Availability of anaesthetists in free-standing maternity units (FMUs)

Type of free-standing maternity unit	Phone advice only	On site during working hours; phone advice out of hours	On site during working hours; formal on-call arrangements to cover out of hours	On site 24 hours a day
M-FMU (n=29)	27	0	0	2
GP-FMU (n=14)	12	1	0	1
O-FMU (n=3)	0	0	3	0

Intrapartum, postpartum and total transfer rates for the calendar year 1998 are shown in Table 1.5. Nearly one in five (18.3%) of all patients admitted in labour to a free-standing maternity unit were transferred to a consultant unit during the intrapartum or postpartum periods. Midwife-led and general practitioner units had similar total transfer rates ($P=0.862$), intrapartum transfer rates ($P=0.923$), and rates of transfers during the postpartum period for maternal reasons ($P=0.890$). Postpartum transfers for neonatal reasons were, however, significantly lower in general practitioner units than in the midwife-led units ($P=0.031$).

The small number of units with resident middle-grade obstetricians means that drawing statistically valid conclusions is difficult. However, there appears to be a trend towards lower transfer rates in these types of free-standing units when compared with free-standing midwife-led and general practitioner units. This may reflect the increased availability of on-site intervention in O-FMUs.

Overall, there was considerable variation in the intrapartum transfer rates between units, with rates ranging from 0% to over 30%. However, no relationship was found between the rate at which women were transferred to the consultant unit and the size of unit[1], the length of time the free-standing maternity unit had been operational[2], the number of admission criteria used by the unit[3], the distance to the nearest consultant-led unit[4] or the availability of on-site interventions[5].

Previous studies have suggested that units delivering more than 200 babies a year have significantly lower intrapartum transfer rates than smaller units and that there is a trend towards lower intrapartum rates transfer in older units. A number of studies have also suggested that the proportion of primiparous women admitted to a free-standing maternity unit can have a significant impact on the intrapartum transfer rate. Units treating large numbers of primiparous women are likely to have significantly higher intrapartum transfer rates than units which exclude primiparous women (Holz et al 1989, Fullerton et al 1997). Inability to control for parity during this study of free-standing units in England may have affected the likelihood of detecting a relationship

[1]Pearson's test of correlation, $r=-0.088$; $P=0.57$
[2]Pearson's test of correlation, $r=0.0001$; $P=0.99$
[3]Pearson's test of correlation, $r=0.072$; $P=0.65$
[4]Pearson's test of correlation, $r=0.16$; $P=0.36$
[5]Spearman's test of correlation, $r=-0.052$; $P=0.78$

Table 1.5   Transfer rates from free-standing maternity units to consultant-led units

		All free-standing units	M-FMUs	GP-FMUs	O-FMUs
Intrapartum transfer rate	mean	15.8	16.3	15.5	12.5
	range	0–31.1	4–30	0–31.1	4.6–17
	n	46	29	13	4
Postpartum transfer for maternal reasons	mean	1.64	1.92	1.44	0
	range	0–7.4	0–7.4	0–4	0
	n	24	16	6	2
Postpartum transfer for neonatal reasons	mean	1.56	1.83	0.82	2.1
	range	0–3.96	0–3.96	0–2.7	1–3.2
	n	28	18	8	2
Total transfer rate (intrapartum plus all postpartum transfers)	mean	18.3	18.2	20.3	10.3
	range	4.9–33.9	4.9–27.3	12.6–33.9	7.6–16.3
	n	20	12	6	2

between the intrapartum transfer rate and factors such as the size of the unit.

ADMISSION POLICIES

All of the free-standing units admitted only low-risk women in labour. However, no common definition of 'low risk' was found and individual unit's admission criteria differed considerably. Table 1.6 summarises the different exclusion criteria that were used by the free-standing maternity units in 1998. There was no consistency in the criteria that were applied by different models of free-standing units and no trend towards 'stricter' criteria was found in midwife-led units compared with the other types of free-standing maternity units[6].

The considerable variation in admission criteria and interpretation of what is meant by 'low risk' may be due to a lack of agreement on the type of risk that is being assessed. Some of the individual units' admission criteria seemed to be based on risk scoring systems whose criteria lack relevance to free-standing units (e.g. the risk of premature delivery). The risk that should be

assessed is the risk that the woman and/or her baby may require a form of treatment during or shortly after labour that is not available in the free-standing unit. Only two such risk scoring systems specifically designed to assess this type of risk have been reported in the literature (Koong et al 1997, Marshall 1989). Neither system has very high predictive power despite classifying up to half of all pregnant women as low risk (Table 1.7).

The sensitivity and specificity of the various admission criteria used by free-standing maternity units could not be assessed from the data provided in the survey. However, the positive predictive power of the criteria common to over 90% of all units was estimated to be approximately 0.8. Compared with the scoring systems used in the Koong and Marshall studies, the criteria common to over 90% of all units appear to have a significantly higher positive predictive value. Confounding factors associated with patients' self-selection of free-standing units and the possible exclusion of a large proportion of the eligible population may have biased this finding.

SUMMARY

The description of the structure and activity of the free-standing maternity units that were operational in 1998 in England in this chapter was

---

[6]Mean number of exclusion criteria tested against increasing levels of obstetric availability using Pearson's test for correlation: $r = 0.072$; $P = 0.65$.

Table 1.6 Percentage of units excluding women with certain conditions

Percentage	Condition
100%	*Past history of:* diabetes significant medical problems Rhesus disease severe pregnancy-induced hypertension/eclampsia <16 or >40 years[1] *Current pregnancy:* malpresentation pregnancy <36 weeks gestational diabetes hypertension
90–99%	*Past history of:* caesarean section uterine inversion shoulder dystocia placental abruption *Current pregnancy:* unstable lie polyhydramnios multiple pregnancy intra-uterine growth retardation antepartum haemorrhage
80–89%	*Past history of:* baby weighing >4.5 kg retained placenta perinatal death *Current pregnancy:* parity >3 known significant fetal abnormality
60%	Previous forceps delivery
20%	Maternal height <152 cm
One unit	Primiparity

[1]All units operated some kind of age exclusion. These differed considerably and many units had separate and more restrictive policies for primiparas. As a broad generalisation, women under 16 years of age and those over 40 years of age were excluded from all free-standing maternity units.

Table 1.7 Risk scoring systems for admission to free-standing maternity units

Study	Type of unit	Applied at	Number of variables	PPV	Percentage low risk
Koong et al 1997	M-FMU GP-FMU	36 weeks	23	0.51 0.82	54 84
Marshall 1989	M-FMU	37 weeks	64	0.38	—
Survey of English FMUs	All FMUs M-FMUs GP-FMUs	Onset of labour	20 variables common to >89% of FMUs (see Table 17)	0.81 0.82 0.79	9

PPV = positive predictive value. False positive defined as 'any transfer' after admission in labour.
Percentage low risk = percentage of all pregnant women classed as 'low risk'. Survey data–estimated by comparing the number of deliveries occurring in FMUs with the number occurring in affiliated CLUs.

based on information gathered in the first comprehensive survey of these types of units ever undertaken. A considerable number of the maternity units in England are geographically separated from a consultant-led service and a significant number of these units have opened recently. Although all the units considered in this chapter were described as 'free-standing maternity units', the survey revealed considerable diversity in staffing levels, admission criteria, transfer rates and size of the units. An attempt was made to classify the different units on the basis of the availability of medical staff with obstetric experience. However, further work would be required to confirm adequate intra-group homogeneity and inter-group heterogeneity before these definitions could be used more widely.

The findings raise a number of issues, most notably the considerable variation in admission criteria and transfer rates. Further research is needed into the factors that affect transfer rates, including the development of a better understanding of the sensitivity and specificity of different exclusion criteria.

REFERENCES

Bonney V 1919 An address on the continued high maternal mortality of childbirth. The reason and the remedy. Lancet I: 775–776

Cavenagh A et al 1984 Contribution of isolated general practitioner maternity units. British Medical Journal 288: 1438–1441

Department of Health 1993 Changing Childbirth. The Stationery Office Books London

Fullerton J 1997 Transfer rates from free-standing Birth Centres–a comparison with the National Birth Center Study. Journal of nurse-midwifery 42 (1): 9–16

Holz K et al 1989 Outcomes of mature primiparas in an out-of hospital birth centre. Journal of nurse-midwifery 34 (4): 185–189

Koong D et al 1997 A scoring system for the prediction of successful delivery in low-risk birthing units. Obstetrics and Gynaecology 89 (5): 654–659

Macfarlane A, Campbell R 1994 Where to be born? The debate and the evidence. 2nd edn. National Perinatal Epidemiology Unit, Oxford

Marshall V 1989 A comparison of two obstetric risk assessment tools. Journal of nurse-midwifery 34 (1): 3–7

Royal College of Obstetricians and Gynaecologists and Royal College of Midwives 1999 Report of the Joint Working Party. Towards Safer Childbirth: minimum standards for the organisation of labour wards. RCOG, London

Standing Maternity and Midwifery Advisory Committee (Chairman J. Peel) 1970 Domiciliary midwifery and maternity bed needs. The Stationery Office Books London

William W 1904 Deaths in childbed, a preventable mortality. H K Lewis, London

Zander L, Chamberlain G 1999 ABC of labour care: place of birth. British Medical Journal 318: 721–723

2

The birth centre project

Helen Shallow

PROLOGUE

Late in the summer of 2000 I heard that 'somewhere' in Northern England there were plans to open a Birth Centre. It transpired that the area's Health Authority were seeking a suitable person to undertake a 6-month secondment to look into and to help set up a maternity facility for local women that would be led and run by midwives.

Any midwife who is interested in the principles outlined in *Changing Childbirth* (Department of Health 1993) and in pursuing a social model of midwifery (J Rosser, 2001) would jump at such an opportunity, as indeed I did. However, I had several hurdles to overcome, not least of which were securing a secondment from my workplace and preparing for the interview. My secondment was secured thanks to the support of my then Head of Midwifery. During the week prior to the interview, as I tramped the mountains of France, I mulled over my presentation and, with nothing to lose, gave free rein to my passion for all things midwifery. At the interview I waxed lyrical about the potential of midwifery-led care in the Birth Centre setting. My enthusiasm and belief paid off. On November 7th (incidentally my birthday) I found myself sitting at a desk at the Health Authority. New colleagues kindly welcomed me as I stared blankly at the computer screen–and promptly left, saying that if I needed anything I should schedule an appointment!

What the reader must understand is that I had never worked in any office before, let alone a Health Authority one. I am a practising midwife. I currently work in a hospital on a labour ward. I had no experience of computerised diaries and scheduling electronic appointments. My ignorance of office procedure and protocol resulted in several gaffes and blunders. It was assumed that I knew what everyone else knew about the intricacies of computer networking. All I knew was how to switch a computer to Microsoft Word. After what seemed like an eternity and a rising feeling of panic, I pulled myself together and recalled what I had said I would do at interview. I set about fulfilling my commitment to get to know and include local people in the project. My first call was to the Head of Midwifery, followed by contact with members of the local Community Health Council (CHC). I scheduled appointments (in my *paper* diary!) and felt somewhat cheered that at last I was on my way.

INTRODUCTION

I believe that the term 'Birth Centre' is more than mere bricks and mortar–it represents a set of values and beliefs about birth. In view of this I have used capital letters for it in the hope and belief that one day the concept of Birth Centres will be protected by registration, safeguarding the values and principles that brought the term into existence.

In this chapter I will take the reader through the major aspects of the Birth Centre project, including the background to the project. I will outline a broad definition of what Birth Centres are, how they are managed and staffed, and what their potential could be. This information is based on features common to many Birth Centres. For more specific details I recommend the reader seek out *The Birth Centre Report* (Shallow 2001). For the sake of clarity I have included some thoughts on terminology.

This particular story is ongoing and I have brought it up to date by adding a postscript. I have not revealed the identity of this particular Birth Centre in order to depersonalise the issues that are raised. I am sure that many of the difficulties I encountered will be familiar to the reader however. This story and its postscript will, I hope, help others to recognise the pitfalls and challenges that face us as midwives and as women when tackling an organisation such as the National Health Service, which is steeped in a long tradition of patriarchal and utilitarian rule. I commenced the project with a wealth of midwifery knowledge and a dearth of managerial and political experience. My naivety was nevertheless an asset at times as I was able to ask the most basic of questions which often cut to the very heart of the matter. I'm not sure if I ever want to develop the language of the politicians and the NHS bureaucrats as therein lies the danger of losing sight of what this is all about–reclaiming birth and restoring midwifery practices.

BACKGROUND TO THE PROJECT

Centralisation of services and Trust mergers have been occurring all over the country and this area was no different. Two maternity units, 9 miles apart, serving their own unique catchment populations were to unite, leaving one area with no inpatient maternity facility. In total, both units provide a maternity service for 3600 women a year. Midwives and members of the public in the area about to lose their local unit had fought the impending closure for years. They were very concerned about the merger and had fought a long campaign to keep their unit open. Nevertheless, from September 2001 the inpatient maternity services were to merge. The merger was seen as an interim measure, providing services until the opening of a new acute hospital with an incorporated obstetric unit at 'some time' in the future.

In order to continue to provide women with a local maternity service and (more significantly) to achieve agreement for the future service configuration, the local Health Authority proposed to open a midwifery-led unit. The remit of the project manager was to research how such a centre could be set up; what it would cost, both to staff and to run; and to explore potential models and possible sites.

There were several terms of reference attached to the post, the first being to review midwifery-led models elsewhere in the country. By examining the strengths and weaknesses of the existing models I was to recommend an appropriate model for the area. A crucial part of this analysis was to consider what impact midwifery-led care would have on the local midwives and how they might adapt to the autonomous style of practice required of Birth Centre midwives. Up to this time the local midwives had either worked as hospital midwives or were based in the community. The Trust insisted that midwifery-led care was something they were already familiar with. However, midwives throughout the whole area continued to be governed (as they are in most Trusts) by medicalised obstetric-led practice and guidelines. At this time the Trust were proposing to 'roll out' team midwifery across the 'patch' and concerns were very quickly raised about where the staff would come from to run the Birth Centre.

THE BIRTH CENTRE CONCEPT

TERMINOLOGY

When I commenced the project it became clear that terms were being muddled. The proposed midwifery-led unit was also referred to as the 'midwifery-run unit'. It was evident that few had a real understanding of the meaning of 'midwifery-led'–in that midwives would work autonomously: they would not be governed by obstetricians but instead would work in partnership with them. I found the term 'midwifery-led unit' cumbersome and it said little about how the centre would function. As I was already aware of Birth Centre principles as outlined by J Rosser (2001), I determined to refer to the project as the 'Birth Centre Project'. With the benefit of hindsight I see that understanding terminology has become an imperative as the concept

that underpins the term 'Birth Centre' is in danger of being hijacked by those who want to provide an out-of-hospital facility for women without adopting and embracing Birth Centre principles and practice. The safety and best interests of women and their babies may not be well served in such facilities and they could ultimately discredit the Birth Centre philosophy of care.

WHAT IS THE BIRTH CENTRE PHILOSOPHY?

The Birth Centre philosophy is based on the concept of midwifery being at the heart of a social (rather than medical) model of care. Such a philosophy has evolved to enable women and their families to experience a positive start to parenthood. This philosophy has at its core the underlying belief that a woman's body is designed to nurture and grow her baby during pregnancy, birth her baby through her own efforts, and care for her baby in the immediate postnatal period. Interventions are kept to a minimum and only used to support labour and birth when complications arise. There is also a belief that social support provided by midwives is the optimum framework within which women can achieve normal physiological birth (N Edwards, Childbirth Educator (Edinburgh), personal communication, 2002).

Birth Centres are facilities that provide individualised and family-centred maternity care with a strong emphasis on skilled, sensitive and respectful midwifery care. They provide a relaxed and informal environment where women are encouraged to move through their labours at their own pace. Birth Centres seek to promote normal physiological childbirth by recognising, respecting and safeguarding normal birth processes.

MANAGING BIRTH CENTRES

Birth Centres are managed, staffed and run by midwives skilled in supporting women through birth. They liaise and work closely with all the relevant local health and social care agencies, such as primary care groups, acute trusts, GPs, health visitors, the community psychiatric team, schools, voluntary groups and social services. Some centres offer placements to student midwives as an integral part of their training (O'Dell & Hallett 2000).

Birth Centre care is underpinned by evidence-based guidelines that are midwifery-led and jointly agreed with obstetricians and paediatricians (Jones 2000). Evaluation is continuous, rigorous and collaborative. Midwives working in Birth Centres are encouraged to develop their whole range of professional skills and to share their knowledge with others.

THE SIZE OF BIRTH CENTRES

The size of the Birth Centre depends on location, demand and regional variation. However, based on maximum annual caseload capacity of 30–35 women per midwife as a guide (Flint 1993, Royal College of Midwives, 1987), a workable number could be between 500 and 600 births per year. It is thought that the success of Birth Centres (O'Dell & Hallett 2000, Saunders et al 2000) rests not only on the philosophy of care but also on the size of the facility–they are special partly because of their intimate and home-like surroundings. As demand for Birth Centre care increases there may be detrimental effects on quality, and standards therefore need to be protected. The size of the centre also depends on what other facilities are provided on the same site, such as:

- antenatal clinics
- drop-in facilities
- birth preparation, parenting and health education classes
- visiting consultant clinics (for high-risk women, to save them travelling to hospital)
- postnatal care (intermediate care for post-caesarean women)
- other interrelated services along the lines of 'one-stop centres' (Department of Health 2000).

Birth Centres may be either 'stand alone' or 'alongside': stand-alone Birth Centres are geographically separate from the acute hospital; 'alongside' facilities are often attached to, or within the grounds of, the main hospital where there are also acute obstetric and paediatric facilities. In either case the Birth Centre should have distinct and dedicated staff who sign up to and understand Birth Centre principles. They should have their own management structure that promotes and supports a collaborative and facilitative working environment and they should have a clearly defined philosophy of care which promotes normality and accessibility, in line with other Birth Centres.

THE CLIENT GROUP

A Birth Centre provides maternity care for women who may be seeking an alternative to an obstetric unit and for whom home birth, for a variety of reasons, is not an option. Birth Centres are designed not to replace the home birth option but rather to offer an alternative to medicalised birth in a conventional obstetric unit. Clients are therefore likely to be women expected to give birth without intervention and who are at low risk of developing complications. The Birth Centre option provides increased choice of where some women can give birth and gives all women access to a locally situated, supportive, woman-friendly service both before and after the birth.

WAYS OF SUPPORTING WOMEN

Epidural anaesthesia is not available, though pethidine and entonox generally are. Birth Centre midwives, however, should be skilled in other, non-pharmacological approaches to supporting women in labour, such as massage and the use of water, and enabling women to find their own ways of working through their pain in a proactive and constructive way. Women's own choice of birth partner(s) would be welcomed. Antenatal active birth preparation classes would be a crucial part of the midwife's role in enabling women and their partners to prepare for their active participation in the birth process. Without this preparation and the skilled support of appropriately trained midwives it has been suggested that Birth Centres (and, more importantly, the women who use them) will be destined to fail (J Frohlich, midwife and Editor of MIDIRS *Midwifery Digest*, personal communication, 2002). Culturally, we are steeped in a model of caring that emphasises compliance, control and conformity, rather than facilitation, empowerment and personal growth (Davis-Floyd & Sargent 1997). Birth preparation and changing expectations are therefore integral aspects of the partnership between midwife and woman that is at the heart of a social model of care (Guilliland & Pairman 1995).

CARE IN AN EMERGENCY

Midwives working in a Birth Centre should be skilled in advanced life support techniques, such as neonatal and adult resuscitation, intravenous cannulation, and the management of obstetric emergencies. It is recommended that all Birth Centre midwives regularly attend courses in obstetric emergencies, such as the Advanced Life Support in Obstetrics (ALSO) course or an equivalent. By doing this the midwife enhances her ability to anticipate and react to potentially difficult situations with confidence and skill. Clear lines of referral would enable midwives to transfer women to the acute unit if necessary, using the paramedic ambulance service according to pre-agreed transfer protocols.

Midwives should also network with other midwives who are experienced in out-of-hospital birth, creating an environment of shared learning through peer assessment, reflective practice and the exchanging of birth stories and experience.

THE POTENTIAL OF BIRTH CENTRES

1. To reduce health inequalities by offering an out-of-hospital service to women who would otherwise have no choice but to access conventional hospital services.
2. To address social exclusion by creating an open-door, flexible and accessible non-judgemental approach to care.
3. To build communities by forging links with parallel agencies.
4. To support and empower young women in pregnancy to fulfil their potential and to avoid further (possibly unwanted) pregnancies.
5. To lower caesarean section rates and reduce morbidity (Saunders et al 2000).
6. To enhance recruitment and retention of midwives by increasing job satisfaction.
7. To realise *The NHS Plan* (Department of Health 2000) by providing appropriate care in the appropriate place by the appropriate professionals.
8. To encourage partnerships and multidisciplinary working by working in the heart of the community.
9. To reducing the cost of maternity care through a reduction in interventions.

Adapted from guidelines produced by the Birth Centre Network 2000.

THE BIRTH CENTRE PROJECT

THE FIELDWORK

Visits to three stand-alone midwifery-led Birth Centres were organised and all interested stakeholders were invited, either to accompany us or to provide questions for us to ask during the visits. I was given one question to ask by a paediatrician but had no response from obstetricians. Trust management declined to attend. However, one local midwife joined us, as did two members of the CHC. The Head of Nursing and Clinical Governance (herself a trained midwife) from the Health Authority and a representative from the Health Authority's finance department also accompanied us.

The Birth Centres visited were chosen for their diversity. We visited Grantham in Lincolnshire, Darley Dale in Derbyshire and Trowbridge and Bath in Wiltshire. Goole in East Yorkshire was later included as it is has a closed midwifery suite which is only opened when a woman is in labour – after the birth, once she is ready to go home (usually after 2–3 hours), it is closed again

(Smethurst 1998). I was also privy to information from 52 Birth Centres throughout England. As a result I was able to make direct contact with many of the centres to glean information about practice and models of care. Throughout this investigative process I became convinced of the value and worth of a 24-hour open service run by midwives and supported by midwifery assistants as opposed to a closed option. It became clear to me that the essence of Birth Centre care went well beyond a place in which to give birth, that it reflected a social model of midwifery that could have far-reaching positive repercussions for all women. However, the burning questions posed by the antagonists were, 'Would there be sufficient demand? and 'Who would use such a service given the low numbers of home births in the area?'

IDENTIFYING LOCAL NEED AND POTENTIAL DEMANDS FOR A BIRTH CENTRE

The Health Authority had already projected that up to 350 women a year would be eligible to give birth in an out-of-hospital facility (Wight 2000). This figure had been challenged by the Trust on numerous occasions as they felt this to be an overestimate. I therefore carried out a survey in collaboration with members of the CHC, which clearly demonstrated that there was indeed a demand for a locally situated Birth Centre. It also showed that if there were no such facility in the area local women would not necessarily go to the merged unit 9 miles away–over two-thirds of women questioned stated that they would in fact go elsewhere. The geographical location meant that there were other options for women in the surrounding districts that were no more difficult to access despite being in different Trusts. This finding therefore contradicted the Trust assumptions about demand for such a service and showed that there could be negative financial implications with The Trust losing 'critical mass' out of the area. Despite these findings the Trust continued to challenge the Health Authority's projections. With the help of my colleague from the finance

department we looked at figures in existing Birth Centres and were able to show how numbers could build from year one to year three. Indeed, as a result of this exercise we were able to show that not only was the original projection realistic but that it was more likely to be an underestimate than an overestimate.

CHANGING THE WAY MIDWIVES WORK

Midwives' roles are and have been changing markedly since the publication of *Changing Childbirth* (Department of Health 1993). In many areas midwives have integrated their practice so that they can work both in and out of hospital. Integration came about as a result of a widespread move to create teams of midwives who could provide more continuity of care for women (Green et al 1998). However, in the area I was studying midwives were still working within the traditional model of either community or hospital practice. The move to roll out team midwifery across the Trust was not being welcomed by local midwives, especially in the light of evidence that was beginning to emerge that cast doubt on whether in fact team midwifery does achieve continuity of care or carer (Shallow 2001a–d). The local midwives wanted instead to explore the possibility of developing small group practices and in my view this would have fitted well with Birth Centre practice.

It was clear from many of the midwives' comments to me, however, that their views were not being heard. I sensed an atmosphere of dejection and helplessness, which seemed to reflect the uncertainty under which the midwives had worked for so long. Having grieved the passing of their maternity unit, the midwives were beginning to embrace the idea of the Birth Centre and realised that they would need to develop and enhance some of their skills in order to be able to offer a safe and effective service for local women.

Over the months I sensed a change in atmosphere as some (notably community) midwives started attending the ALSO course and arranged for Andrea Robertson (active birth educator) to work with them in preparation for autonomous practice. They were beginning to show enthusiasm and readiness for the Birth Centre and had taken the initiative despite getting little or no encouragement from senior (non-midwifery) management.

THE STAKEHOLDERS

The NHS Plan (Department of Health 2000) advocated interprofessional partnership working and urged professionals to break down the barriers that inhibit creative and best practice. It also advocated more consumer involvement. I felt that making myself known to professional and consumer groups alike and encouraging their involvement would add strength and cohesion to the project in that these groups would have a greater sense of ownership and say in how the project developed. I maintained that the success of the project depended on taking into account the views of *all* interested parties. Integral to this, service users who wished to become involved in the ongoing work of the project were welcomed.

I worked closely with members of the CHC and their support and commitment gave me great strength. I made contact with the local women's consortia and attended two general meetings, first to introduce the Birth Centre concept and proposals and then to update them on progress. Members of the consortia helped to distribute our survey to local women as we were keen to access the broadest cohort of women possible in order to elicit public opinion regarding the Birth Centre. Members of the women's consortia also offered to write letters in support of the project and were generally keen to help in any way they could. I met and spoke with representatives of the local branch of the National Childbirth Trust (NCT) and they too lent their support and were keen to get involved. As a result of my meetings with the NCT they published an article about the proposed Birth Centre in their local newsletter which reached members throughout the area.

At interview I had identified how I would take the project forward by including key stakeholders, and how I would address their concerns

and attempt to allay their fears. With some this proved most difficult to achieve. I wrote, emailed and telephoned obstetricians and paediatricians and offered to talk to them about the Birth Centre proposal. Two months into the project I had a wealth of information and evidence to share. My offers were neither acknowledged nor taken up. I heard from senior Trust management that some obstetricians thought the whole idea was 'bonkers'. As a result, I was unable to discuss in detail with them either their views or my findings regarding the Birth Centre concept. One obstetrician had tentatively but openly supported the Birth Centre 'in principle' at an open meeting. I tried to make contact with him. I received no reply to my emails or phone calls. It is possible, therefore, that any concerns or misconceptions that those particular obstetricians may have had about Birth Centre care may well continue to this day.

It was almost as difficult to meet the Trust midwives and I had to resort to imaginative methods in order to gain access to them. On one occasion (arising from a formal invitation by the midwives themselves) I was told by a senior Trust manager that all information to midwives should be channelled through him and not sent directly to midwives. He did not want 'his' midwives receiving 'mixed messages'. I found this restriction of freedom to discuss midwifery issues with midwives both sinister and threatening and it explained why it appeared that the midwives (and possibly the doctors) were reluctant to talk to me.

Nevertheless, I did have opportunities to discuss the Birth Centre with midwives. In my other life as a practising midwife I lead workshops on how to use the birth ball in pregnancy and labour (Johnston 1997). I offered my services directly to the hospital and community staff. As a result I led several workshops with midwives in hospital and in the community where I was also able to talk to midwives as well as to local women about the Birth Centre Project. It was apparent to me that midwives were unclear about what the future held for them and they seemed hungry for information. When I expressed my concern that midwives appeared uninformed, senior managers insisted that they already had adequate and effective communication channels for staff. Midwives nevertheless consistently told me that they did not know what was going on.

GPs expressed concern and frustration at not knowing what to tell women about the closure of the local inpatient maternity services. They had not been fully informed and knew little about the Birth Centre other than what they had heard through rumour. I therefore contacted all the local surgeries in the district and offered to present a seminar for them entitled, 'Birth Centres and Primary Care–a cohesive and comprehensive community service'. I detected some scepticism, their main concern centring on what would be expected of them. It was evident that the GPs I met did not want to be clinically involved with the Birth Centre and relaxed visibly when reassured that they would not be. As with the midwives I was surprised by how little they knew, and I felt that I was playing an important part in raising awareness in the area of the potential for a locally based Birth Centre.

Health professionals have a powerful influence over the choices women make regarding where and how they will give birth. The low home-birth rate in the area indicated to me that women were not being fully informed. The evidence that home birth and Birth Centre care are safe options for well women is well established (Tew 1990, Walsh 2000). However, I knew that many women were (and still are) steered away from these options by the cultural beliefs prevalent in our current high-tech, medically dominated culture (Dumit & Davis-Floyd 1998). What is required is a fundamental shift away from the generally held notion that birth is inherently unsafe. There remains much work to be done to counter this undermining belief. My series of seminar presentations was a beginning to this process as I addressed lay and professional groups alike, as well as making myself available to the media for interview. I was mindful that without this consciousness-raising work the Birth Centre would become little more than a paper option as midwives and GPs are the principal gatekeepers.

Communication within the Health Authority was generally not a problem. I was able to speak with personnel at the highest level and all members of the Health Authority were approachable, friendly and very supportive of my work. It was not long before curious colleagues would call into the office and 'have a go' on the birth ball. I heard many birth stories as a result. I did nevertheless become aware that not all departments were working in a cohesive and 'joined up' way in support of the project. For example, decisions were made in the finance department about potential funding for the Birth Centre without informing those most closely involved with the project in the public health department.

Senior Health Authority officials were quickly persuaded of the merits of a Birth Centre. My main frustrations resulted from not being able to convey the Birth Centre concept to senior Trust officials who, it seemed, had information channelled to them through the Head of Nursing, who was openly opposed to the Birth Centre proposal from the outset. On the one occasion when I was present at a top-level Trust/Health Authority meeting, it was clear that senior Trust officials were not conversant with Birth Centre principles or what a social model of midwifery could potentially mean for the community. This gave me cause for concern as it was at this level that crucial decisions were being made about the future of maternity services.

I had a lot to learn about the machinations of high-level discussions. About half-way through the project the Health Authority and the Trust reached an impasse regarding who would fund the Birth Centre–from the outset it had been less than clear where this finance was going to come from. I had been led to believe that there would be savings as a result of merging the two units and that this money would be used. This notion was quickly dispelled when Trust officials advised us that there would be no savings resulting from the merger. I never really understood why this was so. The question of funding was left unanswered and ultimately led to a delay, not only in opening the Birth Centre but also in merging the two units.

The Trust consistently refuted the need for a locally based facility for women and claimed that they could not therefore justify the cost. The Health Authority was in a position to insist that the Trust fund the project but was reluctant to adopt a heavy-handed approach. It took me a while to realise that I was attending meetings where agendas were less than clear and a sort of pseudo-communication existed whereby I was unable to interpret what some people meant despite what they said. On one occasion, after a long and protracted debate between senior Health Authority and Trust officials, the meeting was about to conclude with the tacit agreement that they had reached consensus. I plucked up courage (and believe me, it takes a bit of nerve!) and interrupted, asking if I could outline my interpretation of what had been said. All present agreed I had understood the content of the meeting. My conclusion was that, regardless of all that had been said, we were no further forward and that in fact there was no agreement. There followed an awkward silence and then, as if I hadn't spoken at all, the meeting closed and we withdrew. I began to question the existence of a parallel universe at times like these. I realised that I was witnessing a much bigger game, the rules of which were known to but a few.

COSTING THE BIRTH CENTRE

Part of my remit was to cost the Birth Centre. There is little research or guidance in this area as costings are complex, depending on what is included and excluded as part of that cost. There is cost to the state and costs tied up in buildings and running costs. More importantly, and what is often not considered, are the wider costs of *not* having a Birth Centre, including the cost of increased visits to the GP following interventionist births and the cost to individuals in terms of disempowerment and poor mental or physical health resulting from the ever-increasing incidence of traumatic birth experiences (N Edwards, personal communication, 2002).

At the start of the project I barely knew the difference between capital and revenue, let alone the meaning of capital charges or cost-benefit analysis. My learning curve continued to be steep and meteoric as I grappled with this, the simplest of questions–how much would it all cost?

I met the challenge with some considerable trepidation. I was offered only limited support from the finance department and consequently felt very alone in this part of my work. What became apparent was that such an undertaking was not commonplace and few people were able to help. Initially, I struggled to find a way in. My breakthrough came when I decided on the spur of the moment to call in on a local architects' office. I told them what I needed to know, and why, and they made an immediate and generous offer to draw up plans of a building. I outlined what I thought a Birth Centre would require in terms of rooms and they worked out square footage, building costs and rentals. I had some, albeit limited, experience of hospital design and planning from having been on the planning group for a new hospital-build a couple of years before. At last I had something concrete to work with and within a fortnight I had a set of architectural plans. I was fully aware that these plans were unlikely to become a real building but from them I was able to make a comparison with other private rented property of a similar size. I was also then able to give the Trust's estates department clear information from which they could work out the capital charges for such a facility.

I began to understand what Jane Walker meant when she talked about a 'bottom-up-cost-analysis' (J Walker, consultant midwife, London, personal communication, Edgware Birth Centre Breakfast Seminar, 2000) in that I had to adopt a step-by-step approach, starting with the fundamentals and gradually building up a financial picture that would in some way reflect the overall costs of running, staffing and maintaining the Birth Centre.

In order to furnish, equip and stock the Birth Centre I sat at my computer and did a 'virtual' journey through a maternity unit, mapping out and listing what the centre would need. From this exercise I was able to make lists for specific departments, for example pharmacy, pathology and linen services. Now I was getting somewhere. Slowly but surely a picture began to emerge of how the Birth Centre could come together, what it would require and what it would cost.

If this exercise taught me anything it taught me that when you think others know more than you, do not be so sure, as they probably do not! I was continually astounded by how little appeared to be known about the cost of items purchased within the NHS. What is more worrying is that when it came to costing items of equipment I often found a large variation in prices and it appeared that the Trust was not necessarily always getting the best deal. I did contact many midwives in existing Birth Centres and it was apparent that they too had little knowledge about the overall cost of running the service.

THE SERVICE SPECIFICATION

A major requirement of my role was to produce a service specification by January 2001. Given that I commenced the post in November, had completed the visits by Christmas, and had only just started the costing, the timescale for producing a detailed service specification was very tight indeed. Nevertheless, the draft copy went out for comment in the second week in February. Never having written a service specification before, I asked several colleagues in the department how to do it. The response was not encouraging in that no one was able to lay out a structure for me or provide a template that I could follow. The best I got was a service specification for the provision of wheelchairs! Notwithstanding, I got on with the job, hoping that what I was producing was indeed a service specification. The final document, although detailed and well received, was not then thought to be a service specification! This was somewhat alarming and disappointing as I had asked for guidance earlier in the process. Nevertheless, the information deemed appropriate for a service specification was encompassed in the work that became known as *The Birth Centre Report* (Shallow 2001) and so the draft service specification was then written and submitted. What

went out for public consultation, however, was a reduced version (without my knowledge). I felt this to be a much-diminished version of the original, lacking as it did the essence of Birth Centre principles. The reduced version of my specification was sent out for circulation to members of the Project Board and members of the Trust. One of the first criticisms of this version was that it was 'rather short on detail'! I was nonplussed and frustrated by this and subsequently sent copies of the *Birth Centre Report* to all recipients of the service specification. The report was then read in conjunction with the service specification in order to provide more in-depth information.

On reflection, it would have been useful to have had something more formal in terms of information on 'how to' when it comes to writing official reports–in my case I 'hit the ground running' and learned the hard way. Looking back, I now recognise the disjuncture between different views and different ways of doing things and the bureaucratic systems that tend to favour the status quo and ultimately hamper change (N Edwards, personal communication, 2002). In my naivety I made assumptions about other people and was then surprised to discover that perhaps we were not all working towards the same goal. This most disconcerting discovery left me with a sense of disappointment that I had lost some of the trust (or perhaps it was just innocence) that I had started out with.

THE INTERFACE WITH ACUTE SERVICES

I was asked to consider and make recommendations regarding how the Birth Centre would interface with primary care and hospital-based obstetric and neonatal services. Concerns had been raised about mechanisms for referral, communication between the Birth Centre and the acute unit and appropriate and timely transfer of women in labour. Based on information from the Edgware Birth Centre (J Walker, personal communication, 2000) I knew it would be essential that criteria should be drawn up by joint collaboration of all key parties so that there would be no misunderstanding or confusion. Midwifery-led care and the underpinning philosophy of the Birth Centre model meant that guidelines should be based on the best available evidence. They would be midwifery-led, woman-centred and *not* medically driven. Artificial time constraints imposed by medicalised custom and practice, such as restricting the length of the second stage for example (which is not evidence-based), were to be avoided. Midwives (and women) must be enabled to exercise autonomy in decision making. Nevertheless, I recommended that round-table discussions should include the following key people in order to reach consensus and that this would be crucial to the success and safety of the Birth Centre:

- representatives from the Maternity Services Liaison Committee and the CHC
- Head of Midwifery Practice
- Director of Nursing
- Lead Birth Centre midwife
- Local Supervising Authority (LSA) officer
- Head of Clinical Governance
- obstetric and paediatric representatives, including an advanced neonatal practitioner
- GP representatives
- Head of Ambulance Services.

These key representatives were to be involved in agreeing mechanisms for clear procedural pathways in the event of complications occurring in pregnancy, labour and the postnatal period. It was also recommended that the Birth Centre IT systems should be compatible with the hospital information system so that the transfer of women and babies and the sharing of information between the Birth Centre and the acute unit would be seamless, fast and efficient. In line with clinical governance it was expected that a no-blame and supportive culture would be fostered between obstetric and Birth Centre professionals. It would inevitably take time and commitment on both sides to forge these links and build up a sense of trust and mutual respect which could move maternity services beyond the confines of hospital boundaries towards a service able to embrace maternity care in all settings. Experience in other areas has demonstrated that change is painful but that when it is achieved, new working relationships develop which enrich and enhance all professional practice (O'Dell & Hallett 2000, Saunders et al 2000).

WORKING WITH OPPOSITION

I encountered continued opposition from the Trust throughout the secondment. Meetings were cancelled or Trust members did not turn up, and when they did they were often late. They were nevertheless open about their opposition to the Birth Centre as they felt it was the wrong time and that resources could be better spent. In the end, however, the Trust altered its position and accepted that a Birth Centre would open and that they would fund it, although prior to my leaving the project in May 2001 there was still nothing formal in writing. There had also been no agreement reached regarding the model of service. The Trust intimated that the preferred option would be a closed model but as the project manager I insisted that a closed unit would be an inappropriate model for the area. In Goole where the closed unit is accessed by the Goole team of midwives, the midwives are very experienced in birth out of hospital. The home-birth rate there is around 11% whereas in this area the rate was less than 1%. I therefore concluded that midwives would be unlikely to access a closed unit, say in the middle of the night, on their own, with very little prior experience of attending birth on a regular basis out of hospital. A closed unit was therefore doomed to failure. This was a crucial point that ultimately led to the Trust changing their position and agreeing to have a Birth Centre that would be open 24 hours a day.

CONCLUSION

The 6-month project soon came to a conclusion with much left to be done. However, the ground work had been completed and the foundations laid. I left the project before agreement was reached that the Trust would fund and staff the Birth Centre. This took a further 5 months to achieve and is part of the continuing story.

The title of my post was 'Project Manager', although this turned out to be something of a misnomer as I believe the project had only just begun when I left. I think that perhaps 'Researcher into setting up a Birth Centre' may have been more appropriate. The responsibility I had involved clarifying what Birth Centres are and raising awareness locally. It involved examining the local context, the feasibility of running a Birth Centre for that area and making recommendations about the most appropriate model. *The Birth Centre Report* (Shallow 2001) outlined what kind of Birth Centre would be most appropriate for the area and why.

In this chapter I have reviewed the terms of reference of my post as Project Manager for the Birth Centre. I have also identified some of the difficulties I encountered. It was an enlightening foray into the wider world of public health, strategic development and resource management. My outlook was broadened and I gained a greater understanding of how the world of midwifery, women and childbirth fits, or does not fit, into local agendas of prioritisation, service level agreements, strategic outline case, and service and financial frameworks. I have long held the view that the NHS is something akin to a juggernaut with a momentum of its own that is little influenced by changes in government policy or political party, let alone the individual voices of service users and grassroots staff.

This secondment was nevertheless an opportunity for me to give voice to the concerns of many women and midwives who often feel powerless and silenced. Now and again the forces for change are such that a window of opportunity emerges (Rosser, conference presentation, Lichfield, 2001). I firmly believe this to be a time of possibility and opportunity for change in how maternity care is delivered in this country. This view is gathering momentum and gaining the support of those who have the power to turn the NHS in new directions. I have played a role in this new direction, albeit on a micro level,

in terms of raising awareness and helping to put Birth Centre care and the needs of women high on the local agenda. After 6 months my secondment with the Health Authority ended. I left the area to return to my 'old life' in rural Lincolnshire. Although sad, I was hopeful that the project would continue, and that I had played a part in enabling well women to birth their babies in the heart of the community where they belong.

POSTSCRIPT: A CAUTIONARY TALE

It is now February 2002 and, perhaps symbolically, it is a full 9 months since my secondment ended. The conception was completed and development continued after I left. Last November I heard, with delight, that capital funding had been secured and that the model would be 24-hour opening, run by Birth Centre midwives and supported by midwifery assistants. In addition I heard that the post of Birth Centre Coordinator was soon to be advertised by the Trust. I realised then how much I wanted that job. I wanted to take the Birth Centre forward and make real the principles that are central to Birth Centre practice. I therefore applied for the post and to my delight was offered the job.

I became the Birth Centre Coordinator for one day. In that day several things happened which made me question what in fact the Centre would be. As I stood being measured for my nurse uniform (not even a midwife's uniform) I became increasingly troubled. I had up to this point ignored the grading, which was G for the coordinator and F for the Centre midwives which, incidentally and significantly, would exclude those community midwives who had been preparing themselves for the Birth Centre from applying as they were already G-grade midwives. The proposed grading for staff concerned me and at a pre-interview meeting with management I expressed my views. Based on my findings of centres elsewhere, my report had recommended that the lead midwife should be at least graded as H and that the majority of the Birth Centre staff should be on G grade to reflect the knowledge, skills and experience they would bring to the post. I was clear in my mind that the issue was not about money. It therefore dawned on me that the grading on offer appeared to be a deliberate move *not* to attract the very midwives the Birth Centre needed in order to succeed.

As I learned more, I tried to engage in a dialogue about midwifery-led guidelines and how the Birth Centre, although a part of the Trust, was a new concept, a social model, something new and innovative. My words fell on deaf ears. I was told categorically, for example, that women using the birth pool would have to get out of the water for the birth as this was Trust policy. The conclusion I was rapidly coming to was that this facility was in danger of being little more than a satellite of the acute hospital, without the support that the acute service has available to deal with many of the problems that medicalised practice creates. Over the following days I made phone calls and requested a meeting with the Head of Midwifery, the Head of Nursing and the Senior Community Midwife. I needed to know exactly what the Trust expected of the Birth Centre and those who worked in it.

In essence I realised that although there was to be a facility for local women, as planned, and that it would be called a 'Birth Centre', it would bear little resemblance to the facility I had outlined in my report. It was painfully evident that the philosophy of care that underpins Birth Centre practice was being marginalised and 'dumbed down' to ensure that it would be in line with uniform Trust policy and procedure. In effect, the model looked for all intents and purposes like hospital birth in an out-of-hospital setting. I could see no evidence of a commitment to Birth Centre principles, which are elemental to ensuring safe practice. It is *within* this social model of midwifery that safety lies. Not understanding this fundamental principle is to miss the very *raison d'être* of Birth Centres and to render anything else potentially unsafe and non-viable.

As a result of the meeting (at which, significantly, no other midwife or woman was present) it was clear to me that the coordinator would have very little influence over how the facility would be run. It was evident that this had already been decided. I felt that I would be starting the job not with one hand tied behind my back but with both, firmly secured. The principles of Birth Centre working were to be sidelined from the outset. I made three distinct requests:

1. That I table a set of Birth Centre practice guidelines for consultation and ratification prior to the Birth Centre opening.
2. That the grading be reviewed.
3. That Birth Centre staff should be self-determining in what image they presented to the public and that it would reflect a social rather than a medical model.

The following day I received a call offering me the post again with exactly the same conditions as before. I had been prepared to accept the grade for the post despite a large drop in salary and having to live away from home. I could have accepted the uniform, knowing that in time I could have changed that. However, I knew that these apparently superficial issues were indicative of an underlying malaise that continues to undermine midwifery today and which prevents the profession from moving in directions that empower not only midwives but most importantly the women we care for. I have spent much of my career to date compromising and working round a system that discourages midwives from practising autonomously. On this occasion I felt that to compromise would mean to capitulate, and this I was unwilling to do. I declined the offer because the Trust demonstrated that it was not prepared to meet me even half-way and I instinctively felt that this boded ill for the future.

My hope is that shedding light on these issues will help us all to realise that there *are* different ways of working and being as midwives, and of being with women that truly represent woman-centred care. However, in order to succeed we have to stand up and be counted. We have to learn how to challenge the status quo and the authorities that dominate the NHS today and who undermine and threaten the very future of midwifery.

REFERENCES

Davis-Floyd R, Sargent C F 1997 Introduction: the anthropology of birth. In: Davis-Floyd R, Sargent C F (eds) Childbirth and authoritative knowledge: cross-cultural perspectives. University of California Press, Berkeley, California

Dumit J, Davis-Floyd R 1998 Cyborg Babies. In: Davis-Floyd R, Dumit J (eds) Cyborg babies from techno-sex to techno-tots. Routledge, New York

Department of Health 1993 Changing Childbirth: report of the Expert Maternity Group Part 1. The Stationery Office, London

Department of Health 2000 The NHS Plan. The Stationery Office, London

Flint C 1993 Midwifery teams and caseloads. Butterworth Heinemann, Oxford

Green J et al 1998 Continuing to Care: the organisation of midwifery services in the UK: a structured review of the evidence. Books for Midwives Press, Hale

Guilliland K, Pairman S 1995 The Midwifery Partnership: a model for practice. Department of Nursing and Midwifery, Monograph series 95/1, Victoria University of Wellington ISBN 0-475-20050-0, New Zealand

Johnston J 1997 Birth balls MIDIRS Midwifery Digest 8 (1) March

Jones O 2000 Supervision in a midwife-managed birth centre In: Kirkham M (ed) Developments in the Supervision of Midwives. Books for Midwives Press, Hale, 149–168

O'Dell H, Hallett R 2000 Crowborough birthing centre: A Midwife-Led Maternity Unit. Contact H O'Dell, Eastbourne General Hospital, Sussex

Rosser J 2001 Birth Centres–the key to modernising the maternity services. MIDIRS Midwifery Digest 11 (3) Suppl 2: 23–26

Royal College of Midwives 1987 Towards a healthy nation: a policy for the maternity services. RCM publications, London

Saunders D et al 2000 Evaluation of the Edgware Birth Centre. Barnet Health Authority, London

Shallow H 2001 Part 1 Integrating into teams: the midwife's experience. British Journal of Midwifery 9 (1): 53–57

Shallow H 2001 Part 2 Connection and disconnection: experiences of integration. British Journal of Midwifery 9 (2): 115–121

Shallow, H 2001 Part 3 Teams and the marginalisation of midwifery knowledge. British Journal of Midwifery 9 (3): 167–171

Shallow H 2001 part 4 Competence and confidence: working in a climate of fear. British Journal of Midwifery 9 (4): 237–244

Shallow, H 2001 The Birth Centre Report. Copies available: email: *helen.shallow@btinternet.com*

Smethurst G 1998 Goole Midwifery Suite: an audit of transfers July 1996–1998 inclusive. Practising Midwife 1 (10): 21–23

Tew M 1990 Safer Childbirth? a critical history of maternity care. Chapman and Hall, London

Walsh D 2000 Evidence-based care series 2: free-standing birth centres. British Journal of Midwifery 8 (6) June: 351–355

Wight J 2000 Short-term changes in maternity services and gynaecology. Local Health Authority. Copies available: email *helen.shallow@btinternet.com*

3

The Wiltshire model

Rick Porter
Vicky Tinsley

INTRODUCTION

Smith & Jewell (1991) suggest that complete obstetric care (antenatal, intrapartum and postnatal) used to be an essential part of British general practice. The norm now is for General Practitioners (GPs) to provide only antenatal and postnatal care. The Royal Colleges reported that the number of women giving birth under the care of their GP had decreased steadily from more than 85% in 1927, to 50% in 1946, and to about 15% in 1975 (RCOG and RCGP, 1981). Marsh et al (1985) argued that there has been an increase in institutional birth. The decline in intrapartum care by GPs is not confined to the UK–over the past 30 years there have been marked reductions in the provision of intrapartum care by GPs in many countries.

Various factors have been proposed to explain the reluctance of GPs to be involved in intrapartum care. These factors have included fear of litigation, the high cost of medical insurance premiums, declining clinical competence, lack of training, interference with lifestyle, medico-political pressure, practice type, lack of an appropriate role model, lack of time and training, inadequate remuneration, and lack of role definition. Young (1991) and Smith & Jewell (1991) suggest that it is not known which of these have most impact on the declining provision of intrapartum care by GPs, but given the number and range of reasons it is not surprising that there has been a very major reduction. The current picture locally appears to be of a small number of enthusiasts keen to continue this work if at all possible, but these too seem to be declining.

A significant change in emphasis was signalled in 1992 with the publication of the House of Commons Health Committee report on maternity services. The report considered evidence which supported the view that home confinements or deliveries in lower technology units were not detrimental to the health of either the mother or the baby in low-risk pregnancies. The report supported the encouragement of less medically orientated maternity care, the provision of more choice for women regarding their intended place of delivery and the offer of the facility for home confinement as a valid option. This change in direction was supported by the 1993 Department of Health report *Changing Childbirth*, which advocated greater choice for women on how and where they could give birth.

Many GPs, however, were reluctant to take up the challenge and gradually the community units known as 'GP units' have become known as 'midwife-led units' or 'birth centres'. In reality, midwives had always provided most of the intrapartum care in most GP units, but called in local GPs to perform instrumental deliveries. In parallel with this, midwives have moved through a process of change and re-evaluation and are now the main providers of antenatal care as well as intrapartum and postnatal care for women.

Midwives locally have combined their skills and experience so that they can work equally well both in and out of the hospital setting. They have become recognised specialists in the care of low-risk women and also possess the skills to recognise and deal with medical emergencies when the situation arises.

The maternity service managed by West Wiltshire Primary Care Trust is located in seven community-based centres and at the Princess Anne Wing (PAW), where women with more complicated pregnancies may choose to give birth. The community-based service aims to provide antenatal, intrapartum and postpartum care to low-risk mothers and their babies as well as antenatal care to women who live in their geographical catchment area. The stand-alone birth centres are at Malmesbury, Chippenham, Devizes, Trowbridge, Frome, Shepton Mallet and Paulton. Since 1995 all these units have been in various stages of development towards becoming midwifery-led birth centres. The West Wiltshire Primary Care Trust delivers approximately 5200 women a year with 1800 deliveries (37% of the total) being conducted either in the community units or at home. Trust-wide, the overall normal delivery rate is 68%. The transfer-in-labour time from the community birth centres to the consultant unit is approximately 1 hour.

These birth centres are all stand-alone facilities, situated between 12 and 24 miles from consultant obstetric services (Table 3.1). They are midwifery-managed, with no medical input and they extend the choice for women who meet the acceptance criteria for birth without active intervention in a home-from-home setting. The philosophy of care is one of empowerment of women and maternity carers and reflects the principles of *Changing Childbirth* (Department of

Table 3.1 Distance from birth centres to the consultant unit (West Wiltshire Primary Care Trust)

Community birth centre	Distance from consultant unit (miles)	Number of delivery beds	Number of postnatal beds	Waterbirth facilities
Malmesbury	24	2	5	Yes
Chippenham	15.5	2	10	Yes
Devizes	21.5	1	5	Yes
Trowbridge	14	3	13	Yes
Frome	17	2	7	Yes
Shepton Mallet	22	1	7	Yes
Paulton	12	2	9	Yes

Health 1993) in terms of choice, continuity and control of women. In practice, this has evolved into a concept of family-centred care as partners, children and grandparents immediately share in this major life event. The midwives seek to facilitate informed choice and foster a non-intrusive, non-interventionist approach to birth. Such a philosophy has evolved to enable women and their families to experience a positive start to parenthood. Each of the birth centres has developed and evolved in its own unique way, shaped by local circumstances. The West Wiltshire Primary Care Trust birth centres are all a variation on a theme.

SAFETY

The Steering Group of Birth Centres UK (2001) has suggested that the issue of safety for births occurring outside an acute unit is no longer the major concern it once was. Although it might seem reasonable to assume that the safest place for birth would be a large maternity hospital, the evidence does not support this belief. Over the past 20 years a large body of research evidence has accumulated which consistently demonstrates the safety of community-based intrapartum care for healthy women with a normal pregnancy. Studies have consistently demonstrated that maternal and infant outcomes associated with birth centre care (mortality and morbidity) are equal or better than those achieved on traditional labour wards for women of similar low-risk status.

Waldenstrom & Nilsson (1997) reported a similar pattern of outcomes over a 10-year period by comparable birth centres in the United States. Albers & Katz (1991) found that these freestanding birth centres present 'advantages for low-risk women as compared with traditional hospital settings: lower cost of maternity care and lower use of maternity procedures without significant differences in perinatal mortality'. Rooks et al (1992) has published the largest study to date, of over 1200 women giving birth in 84 birth centres. This study found that women who gave birth in birth centres had fewer medical interventions in labour, and that maternal and neonatal mortality and morbidity rates were no different from those of large conventional hospitals. This is supported by similar findings from birth centres in Germany, Australia and Scandinavia.

Generally speaking, women who fulfil the criteria for a home confinement would be appropriate candidates to deliver in birth centres. A guideline principle is that nothing will be undertaken in a birth centre unless it can be done with confidence in the woman's own home. In the event of complications arising, transfer is arranged to the consultant unit by ambulance with paramedic support. There is no evidence locally that primigravidas should be excluded from delivering in birth centres. What is more significant is women's understanding of what birth centres do and do not offer. There is now considerable evidence of a variety of benefits of normal birth for women, their families and the midwives in all birth centres. There is substantial evidence that many consultant delivery units are detrimental to normal birth and that they disempower both midwives and women. The question of whether there is an ethical obligation for maternity staff to inform women about the possible adverse effects of delivering in many consultant units needs to be addressed.

In 1993 the Third Annual Confidential Enquiry into the Sudden Death of Infants (CESDI) Report looked at the intrapartum issues associated with home birth and neonatal mortality. Of the 21 babies born at home who then died, 12 were unplanned home births. Nevertheless, concerns were raised about the following issues:

- delay in expediting the birth
- insufficient skills of the attending professional
- post risk-recognition procedure

Guidelines for managing emergency situations are essential, especially in isolated practice settings. There must be immediate recourse to medical back-up and it is imperative that midwives know how to, and are able to, act safely and effectively to preserve the life and well-being of mothers and babies. The Fourth CESDI report (Department of Health 1997) was critical of carers ignoring established guidelines. Guidelines and protocols are integral to risk management and recommendations from this report and subsequent reports need to be addressed through a local action plan. As a result, the West Wiltshire Primary Care Trust have embarked on a variety of initiatives, including the improvement and upgrading of midwives' skills by regular in-service training and attendance at more specialised courses.

CARE IN AN EMERGENCY SITUATION

All staff working in birth centres must be skilled in advance life support techniques, infant resuscitation, intravenous cannulation, perineal suturing and the management of obstetric emergencies. It is mandatory locally for all birth centre midwives to attend the Advanced Life Support in Obstetrics (ALSO) course. This is a 2-day intensive multiprofessional course of practical workshops and lectures. At the end of the course there is a multiple-choice exam and a practical scenario of the 'delivery from hell' for the candidates to work through in a systematic way. The *workshops* cover:

- basic life support/postpartum haemorrhage
- adult resuscitation
- infant resuscitation
- shoulder dystocia
- forceps/vacuum extraction
- CTG interpretation
- malpresentation (OP, face, brow, breech presentations).

The *lectures* now include:

- normal mechanisms of labour
- dysfunctional labour
- neonatal resuscitation
- antepartum haemorrhage
- third-stage emergencies (primary postpartum haemorrhage and uterine inversion)
- maternal resuscitation
- communication issues
- management of cord prolapse

- venous thrombo-embolism and amniotic fluid embolism
- trends in maternity mortality in the UK
- review of CESDI reports
- severe hypertension, eclampsia.

In addition to this, skill drills have been introduced to ensure that the midwives are able to respond in line with CESDI requirements. The West Wiltshire Primary Care Trust midwives have been actively involved with the ALSO initiative since its introduction in 1995/6 and there is now a growing number of ALSO instructors and advisory board members working within the birth centres. In all the birth centres there are manikins which are used to practice the skill drills, particularly shoulder dystocia and breech deliveries. There are currently plans to ensure that all birth centre midwives are taken through bimanual compression in the case of a massive postpartum haemorrhage and the practical management of cord prolapse.

In the event of a baby requiring resuscitation the midwife would, until appropriate medical assistance arrives, 'bag and mask'. The midwives are not expected to intubate the baby. This has been clearly documented in the Trust's care-in-labour policy and agreement has been reached between the midwives, obstetricians, GPs and paediatricians. The reasoning behind the decision was that effective basic resuscitation skills were thought to be more effective in emergency situations than training several midwives in more advanced intubation skills. It would also be difficult to ensure that all midwives remained competent in a skill that may be needed only on an occasional basis.

The midwives' back-up in these emergency situations would be paramedic support via the ambulance service. There are no obstetric and neonatal flying squads currently operating within this maternity service (they were disbanded about 5 years ago). When complications or emergencies arise it is preferable, whenever possible, to transfer women and their babies to the consultant unit, usually the Princess Anne Wing of the Royal United Hospital in Bath. Midwives may telephone to seek advice from senior obstetricians and paediatricians at any time. Occasionally a paediatrician will prefer to stabilise a baby's condition prior to transfer. This is known as the 'neonatal retrieval' service and is coordinated by Neonatal Intensive Care Unit (NICU) in Bath along with Avon Ambulance Services.

Midwifery practice in an isolated setting necessitated midwives learning new skills and refreshing old ones. Midwives regularly undertake self-analysis as part of their annual supervisory review to identify their educational needs and these have been addressed in a number of ways. Updating in the consultant unit has been arranged when required. Specialist practitioners and medical staff have contributed to programmes of clinical teaching on, for example, adult/infant resuscitation, intravenous cannulation and perineal repair. Modules appropriate to addressing those identified needs have been accessed through the local universities, for example midwife Ventouse practitioner, examination of the newborn, waterbirth, and active birthing workshops. The midwifery tutors from Bournemouth University have been particularly proactive and visionary in developing evidence-based training, delivered locally, to meet these identified service developments. A proactive interface between supervisors of midwives and providers of education is essential in commissioning education to meet local training needs.

PROTOCOLS

Protocols are an indispensable security net which ensures that all professional groups are confident that the roles undertaken by each group are appropriate. The nature and scope of the protocols are locally determined and cover issues such as the criteria for referral to an obstetrician at booking; antepartum complications (e.g. when to refer in cases of hypertension or malpresentation); intrapartum problems (e.g. the criteria for changing care to the obstetrician); as well as issues that are common to all care groups (e.g. postpartum haemorrhage).

All protocols have been written by multidisciplinary groups and are based on research findings where available (e.g. the Cochrane Pregnancy and Childbirth Database) and on consensus opinion on effectiveness. In this, as in many other areas of multidisciplinary interaction, one of the strengths is that the protocols are the same throughout all the maternity services sites and are readily available in all the clinical areas. They are all fully evidence-based and are referenced with a review date for revalidation.

Any member of staff (or professional group) may put forward a draft protocol, which will be open for discussion throughout the professional groups prior to being tabled at the Maternity Services Liaison Committee. A key issue throughout the development of any protocol is the importance of ongoing local consultation in order to offer and encourage ownership of the finished product and to increase the likelihood of its use. Midwifery supervision, with its primary function of protecting the public from unsafe practice, cannot be separated from risk management and the supervisor has an important role in developing and implementing protocols and guidelines for practice locally.

The booking policy is one of the cornerstones in the running of the birth centres and we therefore make no apology for reproducing our policy here in full.

WEST WILTSHIRE PRIMARY CARE TRUST: BOOKING POLICY FOR BIRTH CENTRES

Group 1—women who do not need to see a consultant

Women not classified in groups 2 or 3.

Notes

1. Women in group 1 do *not* need to be seen in a consultant clinic.
2. Photocopies of pages 1 and 3 of the maternity pack should be sent with the booking form to the consultant if ratification is desired.
3. This ratification will *not* result in the woman being booked under consultant care.

4. Please specify on the booking form that a consultant appointment is *not* required.

5. Clients with special needs must be identified.

Group 2—women for whom a consultant review is desirable

- women >35 years at 14 weeks pregnant (to discuss prenatal diagnosis)
- small stature (e.g. <150 cm)
- previous 3° tear
- previous stillbirth
- previous prolonged labour
- previous perinatal death
- a past history of pre-term labour (<37 completed weeks)
- any previous anaesthetic problem
- previous IUGR
- P4+.

Current pregnancy

- hypertension
- suspected IUGR
- excessive maternal weight gain
- maternal weight >100 kg or <50 kg (or body mass index <19 or >30)
- proteinuria
- anaemia (haemoglobin <9 g/dL)
- failure of engagement of fetal head near term (particularly primiparas)
- malpresentation
- any psychiatric illness.

Group 3—women who should be delivered under consultant care

- multiple pregnancy
- diabetes
- hypertension (non-pregnant BP >150 systolic and/or >90 diastolic)
- significant medical conditions (e.g. cardiac, renal, respiratory, deep vein thrombosis, embolism and blood dyscrasias)
- known active or suspected maternal herpes simplex genitalis infection
- known Hepatitis B antigen positive or HIV screen positive
- known intravenous drug abuser

- epilepsy or treatment for epilepsy
- myasthenia gravis
- thyrotoxicosis (even if not underactive following treatment).

Past obstetric history

- rhesus isoimmunisation
- severe pre-eclampsia or eclampsia
- severe abruption
- caesarean section
- primary postpartum haemorrhage (>1 litre)
- morbidly adherent placenta
- inverted uterus
- shoulder dystocia
- forceps/Ventouse (other than 'lift-out').

Current pregnancy

- antepartum haemorrhage (other than trivial amounts)
- 'proven' IUGR (<10th centile)
- large baby (>4.5 kg)
- polyhydramnios (still present at delivery).

Past gynaecological surgery

- major gynaecological surgery
- uterine abnormality (e.g. fibroids).

Fetal conditions

- bilateral renal abnormality detected by ultrasound
- other significant congenital abnormalities diagnosed antenatally
- less than 37 weeks gestation
- social–child to go into care (unless alternative arrangements agreed with paediatricians).

The following are not indications for delivery at The Princess Anne Wing:

- ABO antibodies without a history of severe jaundice (refer if early jaundice develops after birth)
- unilateral fetal renal anomalies (refer after birth).

Please note this list is not exhaustive.

HOW THE BIRTH CENTRES WORK

All the midwives are based in the birth centres and are divided into teams, which provide an integrated midwifery service into the local communities (Fig. 3.1). The composition and numbers of the teams varies across the community units. There is a small core team of midwives and maternity assistants who provide 24-hour cover in the birth centres. The teams are encouraged to be self-managing within

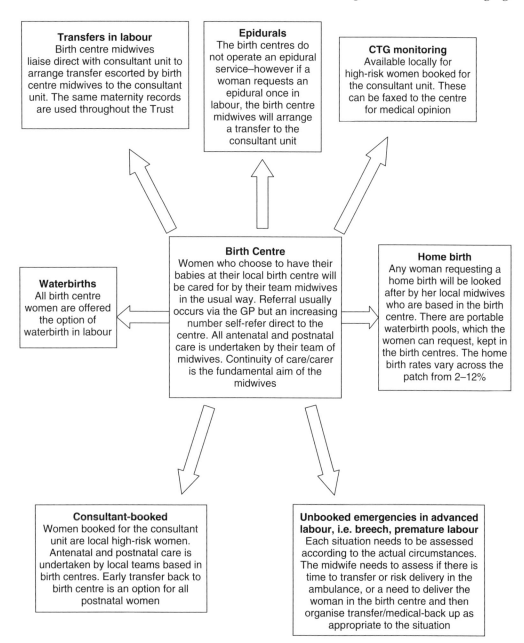

Transfers in labour
Birth centre midwives liaise direct with consultant unit to arrange transfer escorted by birth centre midwives to the consultant unit. The same maternity records are used throughout the Trust

Epidurals
The birth centres do not operate an epidural service–however if a woman requests an epidural once in labour, the birth centre midwives will arrange a transfer to the consultant unit

CTG monitoring
Available locally for high-risk women booked for the consultant unit. These can be faxed to the centre for medical opinion

Birth Centre
Women who choose to have their babies at their local birth centre will be cared for by their team midwives in the usual way. Referral usually occurs via the GP but an increasing number self-refer direct to the centre. All antenatal and postnatal care is undertaken by their team of midwives. Continuity of care/carer is the fundamental aim of the midwives

Waterbirths
All birth centre women are offered the option of waterbirth in labour

Home birth
Any woman requesting a home birth will be looked after by her local midwives who are based in the birth centre. There are portable waterbirth pools, which the women can request, kept in the birth centres. The home birth rates vary across the patch from 2–12%

Consultant-booked
Women booked for the consultant unit are local high-risk women. Antenatal and postnatal care is undertaken by local teams based in birth centres. Early transfer back to birth centre is an option for all postnatal women

Unbooked emergencies in advanced labour, i.e. breech, premature labour
Each situation needs to be assessed according to the actual circumstances. The midwife needs to assess if there is time to transfer or risk delivery in the ambulance, or a need to deliver the woman in the birth centre and then organise transfer/medical-back up as appropriate to the situation

Figure 3.1 West Wiltshire Primary Care Trust birth centres–how the system works in principle. Reproduced, with permission, by West Wiltshire Primary Care Trust Annual Statistics.

predetermined boundaries. Should a woman wish to have a home confinement this would be provided by her local team of midwives, working out of the birth centres. There are portable waterbirth pools which are used from the birth centres for women wishing to have a waterbirth at home.

Midwives undertake the antenatal care for women booked to deliver in the community units but also for women who are booked to deliver in the consultant unit. In addition, the community birth centres are the first point of contact for pregnant, labouring and postnatal women across the maternity services as they are open 24 hours a day. All telephone calls are logged by the member of staff taking the call for medicolegal reasons and because of the amount of time that they can spend on the telephone. All the birth centres have an attached consultant who visits each of the birth centres for a consultant clinic on a monthly basis.

WORKING WITH WOMEN'S PAIN

Epidural anaesthesia is not available in the community units. The midwives actively encourage non-pharmacological labour care methods, such as massage (and in some areas reflexology and aromatherapy) and the use of water (hydrotherapy units are available in some of the birth centres), enabling women to find their own ways of working through their labour in an active and positive way. Experience to date in the birth centres is that very few women choose to give birth on a bed–the majority, given the choice, opt to use water or adopt vertical birthing positions.

As permanent water-birth facilities have become available in the birth centres so there has been a steady rise in the water-birth delivery rate. At Greenways at Chippenham Hospital for example, the water-birth rate has risen from 11% in 1999 to 41% in 2001 as women and midwives become more confident. In the delivery rooms, when it is practically possible, the bed has been pushed away from the centre so that it is not the focus point of the room. There are birthing platforms and birthing mattresses in most of the delivery rooms. Transcutaneous Electrical Nerve

Stimulation (TENS), pethidine and Entonox are available. Should a woman decide on epidural anaesthesia she can be transferred to the consultant unit by the midwives. The West Wiltshire Primary Care Trust maintains the professional standard of having two midwives available at deliveries both in the birth centres and at home confinements.

MONITORING IN LABOUR

Although cardiotocograph (CTG) machines are available in the birth centres, for women who are healthy and have an uncomplicated pregnancy intermittent auscultation via 'Dopplex' or Pinnard is the norm. The West Wiltshire Primary Care Trust care in labour policy (2001) clearly states that the 'current evidence does not support the use of the admission CTG in low-risk pregnancy' and it is therefore not recommended in the birth centres for low-risk women. However, if there are any concerns during the labour the CTG monitor is available and it is left to the individual practitioners' professional judgement to decide whether to use electronic monitoring. The CTG machines should not normally be kept in the delivery rooms. If the midwives perform a CTG tracing locally for women delivering in the consultant unit (or low-risk women delivering in a birth centre) there is a fax machine which is linked directly to the consultant unit should a medical opinion be required.

TRANSFERS IN LABOUR

Information has been gathered since 1997 to monitor reasons for transfer of care from the birth centres to the acute maternity service. Midwives generate this information by completing transfer forms. The information is then cross-referenced with the monthly maternity statistics compiled by each of the birth centres. Once the forms have been reviewed by the clinical audit midwives the results are entered into a database for summary and comparison, enabling maternity managers and individual centres to look at emerging trends and consider the safety of the care which they provide (Table 3.2).

Table 3.2 Comparison of birth centre transfer rates at West Wiltshire Primary Care Trust birth centres 1997–2000

		Total number of deliveries	Number of intrapartum transfers	Percentage of intrapartum transfers[1]	Number of neonatal transfers	Percentage of neonatal transfers[2]	Number of postpartum transfers	Percentage of postpartum transfers[3]	Number of other transfers	Total number of transfers
Trowbridge	2000	407	70	15	10	2	9	2	7	96
	1999	450	85	16	5	1	16	3	—	—
	1998	446	89	17	5	1	8	2	—	—
	1997	400	114	22	6	1	17	4	—	—
Frome	2000	306	40	12	1	0	16	5	2	59
	1999	302	38	11	4	1	5	2	—	—
	1998	245	46	16	2	1	4	2	—	—
	1997	266	50	16	4	1	10	4	—	—
Chippenham	2000	295	51	15	9	3	11	4	5	76
	1999	267	75	22	3	1	5	2	—	—
	1998	275	56	17	8	3	8	3	—	—
	1997	234	46	16	14	6	7	3	—	—
Paulton	2000	159	44	22	8	5	11	6	8	71
	1999	171	23	12	0	0	4	2	—	—
	1998	188	40	18	7	4	9	5	—	—
	1997	183	30	14	4	2	11	6	—	—
Devizes	2000	154	31	17	4	3	2	1	1	38
	1999	162	30	16	1	1	7	4	—	—
	1998	142	36	20	1	1	7	5	—	—
	1997	162	39	19	9	5	2	1	—	—
Malmesbury	2000	133	30	18	6	4	3	2	2	41
	1999	109	32	23	0	0	4	4	—	—
	1998	110	37	25	2	2	1	1	—	—
	1997	112	15	12	4	3	2	2	—	—
Shepton Mallet	2000	107	31	22	4	4	2	2	1	38
	1999	114	27	19	5	4	6	5	—	—
	1998	118	35	23	5	4	7	6	—	—
	1997	115	34	23	1	1	4	3	—	—

[1]Number of intrapartum transfers as a percentage of intrapartum transfers + total deliveries
[2]Number of neonatal transfers as a percentage of neonatal transfers + total deliveries
[3]Number of postpartum transfers as a percentage of postpartum transfers + total deliveries

Over the past 3 years the data collected has varied according to agreed objectives. These audits have included intrapartum escorts, acute antenatal transfers, ambulance transfer times and failure to progress in the second stage.

It is interesting to note that both Malmesbury's and St Peter's at Shepton Mallet Hospital intrapartum transfers average at about 23%. Given that they are approximately 23 miles away from the consultant unit, it may be that their transfers-in-labour tolerance levels may be lower than those of the other birth centres. However, when trying to address rising transfer rates or trends, it must be taken into consideration that any pressure placed on midwives not to transfer may have a detrimental effect on the safety of birth centres.

On a practical note, once the decision is made by the midwife to transfer a woman in labour to the consultant unit, she immediately changes from low-risk to high-risk category. The midwives in the birth centres would then give the woman cimetidine (a hydrochloric acid suppressant) prior to transfer. The midwives would also take any relevant blood samples prior to transfer (such as group and save, haemoglobin). The bloods would accompany the woman into the consultant unit and be handed over at transfer.

It is perhaps the biggest weakness in the maternity services as a whole that the birthing centre midwife is usually unable to stay with the mother once she has been transferred. This is due to staffing arrangements, on-call cover and often the practicalities of arranging transport back to the birthing centres for the accompanying midwife.

MIDWIFE VENTOUSE PRACTITIONERS IN BIRTH CENTRES

Table 3.3 shows the birth outcomes in 2000 in the West Wiltshire Primary Care Trust when there was failure to progress in the second stage of labour. Until the introduction of midwife Ventouse practitioners (MVPs), if a woman had a prolonged second stage of labour or if fetal distress occurred and there was no GP available or willing to perform an instrumental delivery, she would need to undergo an ambulance journey to a consultant unit in the second stage of labour for an instrumental delivery. This can be extremely traumatic for all concerned and midwives felt that they were failing to give quality care to women at a time when they were most vulnerable. It is also apparent that these women demonstrated a sense of loss when transferred to another unit, a loss not only of continuity and support from a familiar face but also of choice and control.

Midwifery practice should remain sensitive, relevant and responsive to the needs of individual women and it was felt that this was achievable in

Table 3.3 Failure to progress in the second stage: birth outcomes in the West Wiltshire Primary Care Trust in 2000

	Number of births	Normal delivery	Ventouse delivery	Caesarean section	Forceps delivery	Total FTP in second stage
Trowbridge	407	1	—	1	3 (KF) 1 (NB)	6
Frome	306	1	1	2	—	4
Chippenham	295	1	1	2	2 (NB)	6
Paulton	159	4	4	1	1 (WF) 1 (KF)	11
Devizes	154	—	2	1	1 (NB)	4
Malmesbury	133	1	4	1	2 (NB)	8
Shepton Mallet	107	1	2	3	—	6
All centres	1561	9	14	11	11	45

KF = Khelland's forceps
FTP = Failure to progress
NB = Neville—Barnes forceps
WF = Wrigley's forceps

this situation if midwives become competent in performing Ventouse deliveries. *The Scope of Professional Practice* (UKCC 1997) confirmed that midwives may go outside traditional parameters to improve care, provided that they are trained appropriately and have the support of both managers and supervisors of midwives. Diamond (1999) argues that there is no limit placed by legislation on the activities of a midwife provided she has the skill, training and competency in the procedure. Midwives should not be frightened of considering radical changes to the way that they work. It could also be argued that clinging emotionally to specific activities rather than providing a holistic service to women presents a danger to the midwifery profession.

The vision here is for 18 midwives in the community units to be trained as MVPs. At present, 12 community-based MVPs have completed the training and others are currently in training. Planning began in 1995 with the development of policy relating to Ventouse deliveries by midwives. This took much discussion and interprofessional collaboration in all areas of the Trust. A protocol was developed and has been indispensable as a guide and a support as the midwives have extended the scope and boundaries of their role within the maternity service. MVPs work within the guidelines that a midwife may only perform a Ventouse delivery when specific criteria have been satisfied and only after undertaking training and receiving a certificate.

Recruitment of midwife Ventouse practitioners

An internal Trust advertisement was placed for experienced midwives who wished to undertake this training, using an employee specification for the required competencies. The midwives needed to be competent in intravenous cannulation, CTG interpretation and perineal suturing. They also needed to have excellent presentation and communication skills and to be able to demonstrate a clearly defined philosophy of midwifery care. Each applicant was interviewed and asked to make a case presentation as part of the selection process. At the same time, obstetricians who would act as mentors and trainers for the midwives were identified and a local programme of theoretical and practical training was developed collaboratively. The midwives who were successful with their application came from both the consultant unit and from the birth centres. In the first group five midwives were trained. Training as it now exists then began in 1996.

Training and practice procedures

Discussions throughout the Trust at all levels were as inclusive and consultative as possible and involved all key stakeholders. Trainees were to witness three Ventouse deliveries, after which they would undertake a minimum of 10 Ventouse deliveries under supervision. After a final assessment, midwives were verified as competent to perform Ventouse extraction following the agreed policy (see Box 3.1). The course is predominantly practice-based and is taught in conjunction with David Walker, a lead consultant at the Central Delivery Suite (CDS) at PAW in Bath. The training programme also includes lectures, video guidance and simulated practice using models. All the trainees have also completed their ALSO® course. The length of time for training has varied from 4 months to 12 months with the average of 6–8 months. A recent trainee who worked part-time (22 hours a week), however, took over 12 months to complete her training.

All the MVP deliveries are part of an ongoing audit programme. All the MVPs complete a logbook of all the cases they are involved with and this also includes the Ventouse deliveries that are unsuccessful. More recently, the MVPs working in the community have also been keeping a record in a separate logbook of all cases that they are called to assess but in which they decide not to undertake a Ventouse. These can then be shared with the group as a case discussion which encourages individual and collective learning. Table 3.4 shows the reasons for midwife Ventouse deliveries since 1996, although there are, of course, often more than one indication for the Ventouse delivery.

Box 3.1 Indications and criteria for midwife Ventouse practitioners (West Wiltshire Primary Care Trust)

Indications
- Maternal exhaustion
- Failure to progress. The failure rate for Ventouse deliveries is higher if the 7-centile to 10-centile has been longer than 3 hours. If this is the case, the client should be transferred to Princess Anne Wing for assessment by a registrar/consultant.
- Fetal Distress. (In Princess Anne Wing–it must be discussed with a registrar who will make a personal assessment as he feels it appropriate.) The midwife should note in the maternity pack and logbook the reason they considered it to be fetal distress, i.e. suboptimal cardiotocograph, meconium liquor

NB: Fetal distress is not used as a criteria for MVPs under training

Criteria
- Term pregnancy (37 completed weeks)
- Cephalic presentation
- Singleton
- Vertex (fully engaged with no fifths palpable)
- Occipito-anterior position
- Vertex 1 cm below the ischial spines
- Vertex well flexed
- No asynclitism
- The cervix should be fully dilated

Table 3.4 Midwife Ventouse deliveries since November 1996 in West Wiltshire Primary Care Trust

Reason	Number
Failure to progress	105
Maternal exhaustion	30
Fetal distress	17
Other	1
Length of second stage	
More than 30 minutes	20 (14.8%)
More than 1 hour	56 (41.4%)
More than 2 hours	28 (20.7%)
More than 3 hours	30 (22.2%)
More than 5 hours	1 (0.74%)
OP Ventouse delivery	5
Shoulder dystocia	5
Primips	112 (82.9%)
Multips	23 (17.3%)
Prevention of transfer to CDS	135
Episiotomy	70 (51.85%)
Number of failed Ventouse	6

What have the benefits been?

One of the unforeseen but important advantages has been the close links that have become established between the midwives and their medical colleagues, working together collaboratively in both the community birth centres and in the consultant units. This has led to a greater understanding of each other's roles, greater competence and enhanced clinical decision-making. The MVPs have all reported increased levels of self-confidence in their practice. The short-term successes include the reduced rate of transfers in labour from the birth centres to the consultant unit, (e.g. a 9% decrease as a result of a 24-hour MVP cover at Trowbridge) and an initial 10% increase in deliveries.

The response from women and their partners has also been overwhelming. The high degree of maternal and paternal satisfaction, demonstrated openly to the MVPs, has been extremely rewarding for all concerned.

POSTNATAL CARE

Postnatal care in birth centres also offers the advantages of family-friendly facilities situated in or close to the woman's home and community, with 24-hour breastfeeding support and follow-up care. Women delivering in the consultant units can transfer back to the birth centres for postnatal care straight from the consultant unit delivery suite. Malmesbury, Chippenham, Devizes, Trowbridge, Frome and Shepton Mallet have all achieved the UNICEF breastfeeding global award.

EXAMINATION OF THE NEWBORN

Immediately following birth, either at home or in the birth centres, every baby receives a physical examination by the midwives. In addition, every baby receives a more detailed physical examination, ideally within the first 24 hours. This has traditionally been undertaken by GPs locally. The midwives in the local birth centres have undertaken additional training to enable them to perform these examinations which were previously carried out by the GPs. This initiative has progressed since September 1998 and it is envisaged that all midwives working in the local birth centres will have this qualification as a core competency. There are some local GPs who still wish to undertake the examination of the newborn for their patients whilst in the birth centres but this number appears to be dwindling.

Criteria for midwives' examination of the newborn

- singleton fetus
- term pregnancy, 37 completed weeks, birth weight > 2.5 kg
- normal delivery/midwife Ventouse delivery
- no apparent birth injuries
- no apparent congenital abnormalities at birth
- apgar score not less than 8 at 5 minutes
- ideally performed between 12–24 hours after birth.

Contraindications

- any babies requiring intubation
- maternal condition such as diabetes (whether or not insulin-dependant), hyperthyroidism, drug abuse
- small-for-dates baby (< 2.5 kg).

MIDWIFERY SUPERVISION

The National Health Service Executive (1999) stated that clinical governance would provide a framework through which NHS organisations are accountable for continuously improving the quality of their service and safeguarding high standards of care by creating an environment in which excellence in clinical care will flourish. Midwifery has a well-established existing structure within which to achieve these aims in the

form of supervision of midwives. The aims of supervision mirror those of clinical governance. Jones (2000) reports that effective supervision has clearly demonstrated its inestimable value in the setting up of a birth centre in London. Locally there is a process of peer selection for the nomination of the supervisor of midwives, and only one of the seven birth centres does not have a supervisor who is based and works in the birth centre. Most of the supervisors of midwives supervise groups of midwives in other birth centres to prevent the units from becoming too insular and to allow the supervisor of midwives some degree of independence from any internal politics. The voice of the supervisor has been at the core of the development process, acting as a link across organisational and institutional processes. In this context, the aim of supervision is for midwives to be empowered as autonomous practitioners in providing the care that women want.

Empowerment is about helping midwives to achieve their full potential. It is about expanding knowledge to give midwives confidence in their decision making. Kirkham (1996) applied the parallel processes described by Eckstein and Wallenstein (1958) to midwifery–that as supervisors treat midwives, so midwives treat clients. Warwick (1998) echoed this, stating that to empower women midwives must first themselves be empowered. Experience gained in birth centres has suggested that once the parallel process is initiated it becomes cyclical in nature.

CONCLUSION

As traditional GP units are replaced by the birth centres, any expansion of the midwives' roles and responsibilities cannot be undertaken lightly. There must be extensive preparation and training. There must be supervised practice, clear protocols, ongoing clinical audit and the appropriate equipment made available. Managerial support as well as agreement and support from local obstetricians and GPs are all necessary to ensure that the midwives feel supported in their practice working in birth centres.

The support that midwives require when undertaking new roles and responsibilities presents a significant challenge to all involved throughout the maternity services. *Changing Childbirth* (Department of Health 1993) recommended that the role of the midwife be reviewed and strengthened and argued that the midwives' role is a key one if we are to move away from the inappropriate imposition of a medical model of care. But midwives will only be able to balance the medical model of care with a midwifery model if they have the appropriate status within the policy-making and operational management of maternity services. In addition to this, the model of midwifery practice in birth centres can only emerge in practice if midwives are empowered to use their clinical judgement and to make clinical decisions for which they are responsible and accountable. Any clinical decisions should continue to reflect the unique midwifery philosophy of care, which remains central to midwives' practice at the local level.

ACKNOWLEDGEMENT

Figures and tables are courtesy of West Wiltshire Primary Care Trust Annual Statistics.

REFERENCES

Albers L, Katz V 1991 Birth setting for low-risk pregnancies: an analysis of the current literature. Journal of nurse-midwifery 36: 215–220

Birthing Centres (2001). A briefing paper for the APPG on maternity services. Steering Group of Birth Centres UK, Crowborough

Confidential Enquiry into Stillbirths and Deaths in Infancy (1993). 3rd Annual Report. London: Maternal and Child Health Research Consortium. Department of Health

Department of Health 1993 Changing Childbirth. The report of the Expert Maternity Group. Part 1. The Stationery Office London

Diamond B (1999). The Midwife Consultant and the Law, British Journal of Midwifery, Volume 7, pages 8–10.

Eckstein R, Wallenstein R 1958. The teaching and learning of psychotherapy. Basic Books, New York

House of Commons Health Committee 1992 Second Report Session (1991–92). Maternity services. Volume 1. The Stationery Office Books, London

Jones O 2000. Supervision in a midwife-managed birth centre. In: Kirkham M (ed) Developments in the Supervision of Midwives. Books for Midwives Press, Hale

Kirkham M 1996 Supervision of midwives. Books for Midwives Press, Hale

Marsh G N, Cashman H A, Russell I T 1985 General practitioner obstetrics in the northern region in 1983. British Medical Journal 290: 901–903

Maternal and child health research consortium 1993 Confidential Enquiry into Stillbirths and Deaths in Infancy. Third Annual Report. London

National Health Service Executive 1999 Clinical Governance. NHS Executive, London

Parliamentary Select Committee on Health 1992 Second Report on the Maternity Services. The Stationery Office Books, London

Rooks J, Weatherby N, Ernst E 1992 The National Birth Centre Study. Part II. Intrapartum and immediate postpartum and neonatal care. Journal of nurse-midwifery 37 (5): 301–330

Royal College of Obstetricians and Gynaecologists and Royal College of General Practitioners 1981 Report on training for obstetrics and gynaecology for general practice: a joint working party. RCOG and RCGP, London

Smith L F P, Jewell D 1991 Role of midwives and GPs in hospital intrapartum care, England and Wales 1998. British Medical Journal 303: 1443–1444

Steering Group of Birth Centres UK 2001 Birthing Centres. A briefing paper for the APPG on maternity services. Crowborough, UK

UKCC 1997 The scope of professional practice. UKCC, London

Waldenström U, Nilsson C A 1997 Randomised controlled study of birth centre care versus standard maternity care: effects on women's health. Birth 24: 17–26

Warwick C 1996 Supervision and Practice Change at King's. In Kirkham M (ed) Supervisors of Midwives. Hale Books for Midwifery Press.

Young G L 1991 General practice and the future of obstetric care. British Journal of General Practice 41: 266–267

4

Under the spotlight: Grantham's midwife-managed unit

*Diane Fraser   Kim Watts
Fehmidah Munir*

INTRODUCTION

The factors influencing the establishment of NHS midwife-led birth centres are likely to vary according to the local context. The setting up of the midwife-managed unit (MMU) in Grantham was surrounded by factors which put it in the public and political spotlight. The most significant factor was the effect the conviction of Beverly Allitt (Clothier et al 1994) had on the local hospital and community. The inquiry following the deaths of the babies and children murdered by her led to changes in the management of the local paediatric services. Initially the running of these services was taken over by another NHS Trust and eventually the 24-hour paediatric service at the hospital in Grantham town was lost altogether.

The loss of this service affected the consultant obstetric unit and a decision was subsequently taken to close the maternity unit at Grantham and transfer women booked there to the nearest consultant unit, 25 miles away. The Grantham public were angered by this decision and, after consultation, the Health Authority agreed that for a trial period Grantham should have a midwife-led birth centre. Medical opinion was divided about the safety of such a service and therefore an evaluation study was commissioned to inform future decisions about the maternity services in and around Grantham. This chapter provides an outline of that study and a discussion of some of the key issues that emerged.

THE SETTING UP OF THE MMU

Against a backdrop of intense public, media and political attention, the MMU opened in April 1999. The MMU is located in the former labour ward area of Grantham Hospital and comprises four individual birthing rooms and a 'pool' room. At the time of the evaluation the MMU was served by two teams of midwives. Of the 16 midwives, over half were part-time. Grantham town community midwives were automatically given jobs as MMU midwives and the decision to establish two teams enabled the majority of former Grantham Hospital midwives to be given jobs as well (although they, unlike the community midwives, had to apply for the remaining posts). A number of community midwives from outside the town were also able to use the MMU if it was the choice of women in their caseload.

The number of staff appointed to the teams was based on an anticipated 250 births per year and the need to provide a community midwifery service for all women living in the area, irrespective of their booked place of birth. When criteria were drawn up for MMU bookings a decision was taken to exclude primigravidae. A midwife manager from outside the area was appointed to set up and manage the MMU, the two teams of midwives and health care support workers (HCSWs). HCSWs provide full 24-hour cover on the unit, contacting the midwife on call if a woman is about to arrive in labour or if advice is needed.

By the time the evaluation started, the MMU had been open for 11 months and the manager had left to take up another post elsewhere. As an interim measure, team leaders were identified for the two teams and they were managed by the hospital's Director of Nursing Services. During the course of the evaluation there was a restructuring of the hospital services in Lincolnshire, bringing all three previously separate hospitals with maternity services under one NHS Trust. The findings from the evaluation therefore had to be considered with this changing context and uncertain future in mind.

METHODOLOGY

The study was carried out between March and August 2000. A case study evaluation design was selected as, according to Stake (1995) and Yin (1994), it is able to address the complex process of evaluating effectiveness in a specific context such as that of the MMU in Grantham. Surveys and focus groups were used as well as the major case study data collection methods of interviews (Table 4.1), observation and document analysis.

THE POPULATION SAMPLED
User groups

The study sample drawn from Grantham women who were users of the maternity services had two components:

1. Postal questionnaires to women who had given birth in the first 12 months of the MMU.
2. Face-to-face interviews with women who had given birth in the second year of the MMU.

Health professionals

Four groups of health care professionals were invited to take part in the study. These were:

1. All MMU midwives, midwives from the surrounding areas employed by Grantham NHS Trust, the university's link midwife teacher (who provided the education programmes for Grantham), a Grantham student midwife and a focus group sample of midwives from the 'host' consultant unit.
2. All general practitioners who referred to the former consultant unit at Grantham.
3. Consultant obstetricians.
4. Managers and the Local Supervising Authority Responsible Officer at that time.

Other stakeholder groups

1. The MMU health care support workers.
2. Community Health Council representatives.
3. The Ambulance Liaison Officer for Lincolnshire.

Table 4.1 Evaluation of Grantham's midwife-managed unit: number of face-to-face interviews with different stakeholder groups

Stakeholder group	Number of interviews
MMU midwives	26
Women who had recently birthed at the MMU	8
General practitioners	8
Managers and supervisors of midwives	7
Consultant obstetricians	6
Health care support workers	6
Community Health Council representatives	2
Ambulance Service representative	1
University link tutor	1
Student midwife on placement	1
Total number of interviews	66

One focus group interview was held with a sample of midwives from the 'host' unit. All grades of seniority were represented.

Records

Women's case records were audited as well as the delivery records and transfer forms kept by MMU staff.

ETHICAL ISSUES AND PROBLEMS WITH ACCESS

Access to the MMU was sought from and granted by the Director of Nursing Services at Grantham. Professional staff and other key personnel were then contacted on an individual basis to seek their agreement to participate in the study. All gave their permission to be interviewed.

Ethical approval to contact women who had given birth in Grantham was granted once the questionnaires and semi-structured interview schedules had been approved by one of the Local Research Ethics Committees (LREC). Access to Grantham women who had given birth in the host unit was more problematic. The LREC only agreed to women being contacted through their own hospital staff. When scrutinising the returned questionnaires it became apparent that the sample included women who did

not meet the criteria for the study and hence a number had to be excluded. The research team had no way of establishing for themselves how many of the Grantham women who gave birth at the host unit would have been eligible for the MMU.

FINDINGS OF THE STUDY

The stakeholder groups were found to hold different and complementary perspectives and are therefore presented separately.

THE MANAGEMENT VIEW ON SETTING UP THE MMU

Midwife managers, directors of nursing and supervisors of midwives had been involved in the discussion about establishing a birth centre in Grantham. The original suggestion was that there should be:

...a clean cut...it would be a midwifery-managed model...to serve Grantham and immediate surrounding areas...to be a success story it had to be small, manageable and you have got to be able to monitor it and develop it within a framework, but it would take time...It would be a quality service, get it embedded in the thinking process of the community and the GPs. ...The population of the model was to be by experienced midwives and our recommendation I think was no more than eight. One of them would be a head midwife who would have a smaller caseload than anyone else so that supervision could be upheld...and develop the model with individual midwives....

The location of a midwife-managed unit was also discussed by the group which felt that it should be clear to women that it was '... *home from home, not a hospital, no obstetrician... we talked about a bungalow on site or that type of provision...*'. Another individual added that '... *the worst thing was to make the old maternity ward into a midwifery-managed unit. I mean it just gives the wrong message*'.

The final outcome was to site the MMU in the old maternity unit and to have two teams, not one. The manager appointed did not carry a caseload but had the major task of writing guidelines and protocols for the unit in a short period of time. The managers interviewed were also divided as to whether HCSWs should provide 24-hour cover for the unit as these quotes illustrate:

...I think to have an unqualified member of staff sat there 24 hours a day is a gross waste of manpower. There is nothing to stop that person being located on another ward... I mean you could put an admin grade 2 to take messages for community midwives... I mean it is just crazy....

...basically from the risk management perspective they [HCSWs covering 24 hours] are needed.... Also the fact that the midwife then doesn't have to stay with the lady when really all she needs is sleep and a cup of tea. Maybe the baby needs cuddling for 5 minutes while she goes into the shower or something... it's purely from a risk management point of view....

Although the intense political and media attention on the MMU had not helped in setting it up in a short period of time, the managers expressed an opinion that the MMU is successful 'very much against the odds'. They believed that the good midwife/woman ratio enabled a quality service to be provided in Grantham but concerns were expressed that staff might eventually become bored and lose essential midwifery skills if they did not book more women for MMU birth.

The managers also drew attention to inequities in workloads, both for midwives in the area surrounding Grantham where there had been a sudden increase in home births and for midwives in the host unit because of the increase in births there now that the Grantham consultants had moved there.

Contrasting views were expressed about the issue of primigravida being able to birth at the MMU. Some managers believed that if primigravida could give birth at home they should be given the choice to select the MMU whereas other managers were concerned that there would be an increase in the number of women needing to be transferred to the host unit by 'blue light' ambulance.

VIEWS OF WOMEN USING THE MATERNITY SERVICES

The number of women who returned questionnaires is shown in Table 4.2. When asked why women chose to give birth at the MMU, *'close to home'* was cited as the most important reason. Other reasons included: *'I know the midwives'*, *'I prefer a small unit'* and *'I know the hospital'*. Of those who gave birth at home, six had booked for the MMU initially but when the midwife arrived they decided to stay at home for the birth (an option offered by MMU midwives). Other reasons listed were: *'no time to get to the consultant unit'*, *'I felt more in control and relaxed at home'*, *'I do not like hospitals'* and *'I wanted to stay with my other children'*.

Women in all groups surveyed were asked about methods of pain relief. Entonox was the most commonly used and was the only method used by 53% of MMU women, in 42% of home births and in 33% of host-unit births. Pethidine was only used by four of the MMU women (out of a total of 59), one of the home-birth women

Table 4.2 Evaluation of Grantham's midwife-managed unit: response rates from all groups sent postal questionnaires

Sample groups	Number recruited	Number responding	Response rate
MMU births	91	59	65%
Home births	61	41	67%
Host-unit births (low-risk)	107[1]	54	51%
Host-unit transfers	12	10	83%
GPs	73	55	75%

[1] The research team were not permitted to identify eligible women in this category themselves but were reliant on Trust staff. From the data on the returned questionnaires it became apparent that not all those sent questionnaires were part of an eligible sample. Only 12 of the returned questionnaires were from women who met MMU criteria.

(out of 38) and three of the host-unit women (out of 12). Eight women at the MMU used the pool for pain relief.

The majority of women in both the MMU and home-birth groups knew the midwife who had delivered them. This was because they had seen nearly all the team midwives antenatally. Although there was no significant difference between the two groups in the number of different midwives seen postnatally, women in the home-birth group were more likely to be visited regularly by their 'delivery' midwife than women in the MMU group.

Overall, a high percentage of women in all three groups reported satisfaction with their care (see Table 4.3), with 66% saying that they would not change *anything* about their care. Twenty would recommend a small change: 16 said they would have liked a consultant available on-call for emergencies; three would have liked a longer postnatal stay (they were expected to go home after 6 hours unless this was at night).

Ten women from Grantham who returned questionnaires were transferred by ambulance to the host unit, either from home or from the MMU. One was transferred for induction of labour and the other nine were assessed in labour and transferred: one for caesarean section, four for assistance with the birth, three for retained placenta, and one because of excess blood loss post-delivery. The transfer group of women were not satisfied with aspects of their care even though there had been a safe outcome for them and their babies. In particular, one woman commented that she had had a 20-minute wait for an ambulance *'when the birth started to go wrong'*. Another woman said, 'It was, very traumatic, I was trying to push my baby out all the way, whilst trying to hold on to the stretcher and the midwife. I thought I was going to die along with my baby.' Although one woman said the midwives were great, she still felt insecure having so far to travel by ambulance.

In order to explore women's views in more depth, 10 women who had recently given birth were invited to be interviewed. Eight women responded and were interviewed in their homes when their babies were about 6 weeks old. All the women were very pleased that they had had the opportunity to birth at the MMU and were very satisfied with their care. In particular, they liked the one-to-one care the midwives gave in labour, the homely, relaxed atmosphere of the MMU and the proximity to their homes. Women described the confidence they had in the MMU and the midwives and believed that the choice of place of birth should always be theirs:

... at home [in labour] I was a bit scared... the funny thing was, once I got under the roof, once I knew I were there [the MMU] I lost my fear... I can't even explain it as there's nothing there... except the midwives... I have got so much faith in them... that

Table 4.3 Evaluation of Grantham's midwife-managed unit: level of satisfaction with aspects of care

	Midwife-managed unit (n = 59)		Home births (n = 38)		Host unit (n = 12)	
	n	%	n	%	n	%
Satisfied with care in pregnancy:						
Yes	56	94.9	36	94.7	12	100
No	2	3.4	2	5.3	0	—
Missing reply	1	1.7	0	—	0	—
Satisfied with care in labour:						
Yes	57	96.6	36	94.7	11	91.7
No	2	3.4	1	2.65	1	8.3
Missing reply	0	—	1	2.65	0	—
Satisfied with care after birth:						
Yes	59	100	37	97.35	11	91.7
No	0	—	1	2.65	1	8.3

once I knew they were about I just, that's it, I wasn't frightened anymore ... .

I think they should give the woman the choice, like you say the choice is yours, if you know that there is no consultant there and no pain relief, big relief, and you choose to go there [the MMU] and you end up in an ambulance ... on a blue light then it's all your own fault ... you could sign a form ... if anything goes wrong, then the women take it on themselves ... .

... there was more one to one ... more personal ... they were sort of there for you ... if they went out of the room they would come back straight away ... I would go for the midwife-led again even if the consultant unit came back ... .

A few of the partners present during the interviews interjected that they had been anxious about the MMU as a safe place to give birth but had accepted their partner's decision.

VIEWS OF THE MMU MIDWIVES

A total of 26 individual interviews were carried out with midwives. Before the MMU opened, 12 were community midwives and 14 had been Grantham consultant unit midwives. One of these is now employed by the host unit to work in the antenatal clinic at Grantham to support local women booked to have their baby there. Sixteen (10.5 whole-time equivalent) of the midwives work full- or part-time in the two MMU teams and the remainder are midwives from outside the town but who also offer an MMU birth to their mothers.

From an analysis of the data, six aspects of the MMU system emerged as being important to the MMU midwives: changing ways of working and anxieties about the future; management and leadership; education and training; interprofessional relationships; the effects on childbearing women; and the effects on the health service.

The effects of changes and anxieties about the future

The effects of changes that the midwives mentioned most frequently included:

- anxiety about their role and the future
- the dramatic increase in home births

- changes in work patterns and volume of work
- the increase (for former hospital midwives) and decrease (for former community midwives) in the continuity of care they were personally able to give to women
- the effectiveness of team work
- the increase in autonomy and job satisfaction
- the amount and effectiveness of support and supervision offered and received.

The publicity and feeling 'as though you are in a goldfish bowl' did initially affect the clinical decisions the midwives made–a few commented that this made them overcautious. For all midwives there had been changes to their work patterns. The workload had decreased for all of them, except for those working in the more rural areas where home births had increased dramatically. Former hospital midwives had to get used to working in the community and to being on-call. Former community midwives experienced a decrease in their on-call commitment. This reduced their take-home pay. The rotas were initially very complex but were being revised to bring about improvements and better midwife attachment and continuity for GP practices. The majority of midwives commented on the job satisfaction they gained from working between the MMU and the community. They enjoyed their work and believed that the women were satisfied with the care they received. Where there was less job satisfaction, it related more to lack of an individual caseload, this having been sacrificed as part of creating the teams.

Management and leadership

In relation to management and leadership, the majority of midwives were critical of the decision to bring in a new manager rather than a clinical team leader. They believed there had been an emphasis on getting the structures in place, rather than working on the process, which resulted in a top-down rather than an inclusive approach, with little attention being paid to the management of change. They had not been involved in the drafting of protocols and were resentful about the way some staff had been slotted into MMU teams while others had had to apply for the remaining posts.

Administrative difficulties caused problems for staff, especially in relation to records. This was particularly problematic when women transferred between the MMU and the host unit or vice versa.

Education and training

Good education and training for working as MMU midwives had been provided. They had all been enabled to attend the Advanced Life Support in Obstetrics (ALSO) course. Many midwives had taken the initiative to prepare for a more community-orientated role by shadowing their community midwife colleagues. A number of midwives also attended natural or active birth workshops and these had been particularly beneficial for former consultant unit midwives. A few host-unit midwives, however, were resentful that they had had limited opportunities for attending such courses.

Interprofessional relationships

In terms of interprofessional relationships, the midwives believed that they were now, for the most part, positive. They felt that there had been an initial deterioration in relationships with GPs but there was now a consensus that this had improved since management of the MMU had changed and the team leaders had met with the GPs to discuss the difficulties and their resolution. The two consultants who continued to provide antenatal clinic facilities in Grantham continued to work well with the MMU midwives. One of the consultants was particularly supportive and regularly visited the MMU to meet with the midwives.

Relationships with paediatricians at the host unit appeared to be less positive. Two MMU midwives were setting up neonatal resuscitation skills training sessions for the teams. They had approached a consultant paediatrician for advice but found his response unhelpful.

Effects on childbearing women

Midwives were most concerned about the effects the closure of the consultant unit had on women in Grantham. More than half of the midwives commented on the increase in home births. A sudden rise occurred when there was no birth facility in Grantham, apart from home births, but it still remains well above the national average, even with the provision of the MMU. Part of the increase can be attributed to women who do not meet the very strict criteria for the MMU but who refuse to go to another unit some distance away from their home. As well as booked home births, midwives were aware that the number of unbooked home births had risen:

...I think the primips are realising that they can't deliver at Grantham so they deliver at home.

...it is the criteria...the home confinement rate has gone up probably six-fold from what it used to be because they can have the babies at home and we can't stop them doing that...there's one we've got at the moment...she's adamant she wants a home confinement.... As a supervisor I feel absolutely confident she does understand the issues involved, that she does understand the dangers....

Midwives had different views about whether they were able to provide better continuity of care and carer for women since the MMU opened. The rotas appeared to take priority over providing continuity of carer for women. The team concept meant that many women met most of the team antenatally and hence 'knew' their carer during labour. However, a number of midwives expressed the view that it ought to be possible to have a caseload within the team concept so that one midwife could provide the majority of care for an individual woman but be covered for her time off by team midwives.

A large number of midwives commented on the anxiety expressed by women about the travelling distance to the host unit if they developed a problem in labour. This occasionally resulted in women giving birth in the hospital's accident and emergency (A&E) department (rather than the midwife being able to take them to the MMU) if they were booked for a consultant unit but had stopped at Grantham because they felt that they would not get there in time. They appreciated the reason for rigid protocols for the MMU but would prefer to use their clinical judgement when it seemed in the woman's best interests.

Effects on the health service

The midwives believed that the costs and benefits of providing the MMU service were influenced by political issues in Grantham. They thought that many decisions had been influenced by outside factors, such as the protocols, the number of midwives, the role of HCSWs and the use of A & E. They were particularly conscious of the effect the closure had had on the ambulance service and on the service the GPs were able to provide. Midwives compared home and MMU births and could see no real differences. They were aware, however, that because the MMU is located in hospital premises, a resuscitation team could be called in an emergency, as could a paediatrician on weekdays.

VIEWS OF THE MEDICAL STAFF

The six consultant obstetricians who were interviewed (two originally from Grantham and four from the host unit) were influential in the decisions taken about the restructuring of the maternity services in Grantham. One of them believed Grantham should have been able to retain a low-risk consultant unit, possibly with neonatal-trained midwives covering the 24-hour period. His colleagues did not support this view. The majority were also opposed to the setting up of the MMU as they questioned the safety of an isolated birth centre and also believed that it would be far too expensive to maintain.

All the consultants agreed that their fears about a rise in maternal or perinatal mortality and morbidity had not materialised. They thought this was due to good selection criteria for MMU births and the expertise of the midwives. Only one of the consultants commented that it was paradoxical that primigravidae could have a home birth but were not permitted to give birth at the MMU. The others did not want the criteria to include primigravidae. Most were unaware that the

increase in home births included primigravidae and others deemed unsuitable for an MMU birth.

The majority of GPs surveyed and the eight subsequently interviewed thought that the booking criteria were appropriate. Only 11 of the questionnaire respondents believed that the criteria should include primigravidae. Overall, the GPs believed the closure of the services at Grantham had been a political decision and that their views had not been taken into account sufficiently. None had any involvement in the MMU but were pleased that at least the town had a birth centre so that women's choices could be accommodated.

OTHER STAKEHOLDER VIEWS

Health care support workers

Seven HCSWs are employed to cover the full 24 hours on the MMU. The majority of them had worked on the consultant unit before it was closed. They enjoyed their work although it was different from what they had experienced before. Now they were engaged for most of the time on clerical duties, answering the phone, redirecting enquiries to the midwife on-call, and preparing for women about to arrive in labour. They assisted the midwife as necessary, but normally a second midwife had arrived in time for the actual birth. The part of their job they enjoyed most was the care of women and helping them to look after their babies until they went home. They would like the unit to allow women to stay longer than the recommended 6 hours if the mother needed more rest. The HCSWs found the morning shift busy, but shifts at other times of the day and night were normally quiet. It was noted from the birth records that the majority of the admissions to the MMU took place at night. The HCSWs believed they provided an important service in answering the phone and contacting the midwife as required.

The Community Health Council

The Community Health Council (CHC) representatives had not felt involved in the decision-making process in setting up the MMU but were pleased that some facility had been provided for women to give birth locally. Of particular concern to them was the sharp rise in home births and they would prefer the hospital consultant unit services to be reinstated.

The Ambulance Service

The ambulance service had anticipated an increase in workload and had increased the service by one extra ambulance and an extra crew member for each shift. As well as providing for transfers from the MMU in an emergency they also had to be prepared for the unexpectedly high number of home births, for which emergency transfer might be needed. However, the call upon emergency ambulance services by the maternity services had been minimal. The changes to the paediatric services, in contrast, had had a far greater impact, with far more transfers of babies and children than of pregnant women.

DOCUMENTARY ANALYSIS

The quality of data obtained from case records was variable. Reasons included access problems if written consent was not obtained, differences and changeover in computer systems, and missing sections from notes. One of the explanations for missing notes was that 'hand-held records' had not been filed or were retained by the health professionals at the time of the study. The findings from this limited data set were, however, similar to those of the questionnaire and interview data. In terms of pain relief, women giving birth at the MMU or at home were less likely than host-unit women to have pethidine and were also less likely to have a second-degree laceration of the perineum or episiotomy.

From the register of births per midwife it was noted that of the 27 midwives who use the MMU, the number of births they assisted at ranged from two to 32 per midwife in year one.

DISCUSSION

The findings from this study identify a number of positive and negative aspects of setting up and managing a more isolated birth centre. It is

hoped that lessons may be learned from these which would assist others in such an initiative.

KEY PLAYERS AND POLITICAL ISSUES

Grantham is atypical in that its health services have attracted more than the normal political and media attention. This scrutiny had positive and negative effects on the setting up of a birth centre. The positive effects lay in the way the public vociferously raised their objections to the loss of a maternity unit. One would have thought that the problems associated with Beverly Allitt would have led them to understand why the Health Authority wanted to follow the Royal College guidelines (RCOG & RCM 1999).

Most of the obstetricians and paediatricians believed a viable, safe maternity service could not be provided in a unit as small as that in Grantham. Once the 24-hour paediatric service could no longer be provided an assumption then seemed to be made that 'common sense' would prevail and there would not be objections to the closure. However, Grantham families had found that the maternity unit had provided an excellent service in the past and were opposed to the loss of this service. Accusations were made that it was a cost-cutting exercise and women were not prepared to travel what was, in their view, a long distance to give birth.

The Health Authority listened to the complaints not only from the users of the service but also from midwives and GPs and eventually agreed to the setting up of the MMU. By this time, however, births to Grantham women were very much in the local, and at times, the national spotlight. The midwives felt they were 'working in a goldfish bowl' and the media and Health Authority scrutiny of everything they did created anxieties. It is possible that the decision makers failed to consult adequately and early enough with the users and all providers of the maternity services. Had there been sufficient consultation with key players at the outset a more phased introduction of the MMU might have been possible. The 9-month period between the closure of the maternity unit in Grantham and the opening of the MMU was particularly difficult for women whose babies were due to be born then, the Grantham midwives who were uncertain about their future, and the host-unit staff who were faced with angry mothers and their relatives.

A few respondents believed that the MMU had been set up to fail, although others disputed this assertion. If this was the case, then the intense interest from the media and particularly any adverse media coverage would have been likely to work against those who believed in the value of midwife-led birth centres. Perhaps a lesson to learn from the experience in Grantham is that media involvement and cooperation is needed from the outset in order to foster a culture of responsible rather than sensational local journalism.

STAFFING AND MANAGING A MIDWIFE-LED BIRTH CENTRE

Attempts were made during the course of the evaluation to draw comparisons with birth centres elsewhere. Contextual and geographic variations among those contacted were so great that comparisons proved difficult to make. In the five isolated units contacted, births per annum ranged from six to 250 and they all allowed primigravidae to give birth in the unit. The distance from the nearest consultant unit varied from 12 to 53 miles but the travel time was not necessarily proportional as the quality of the roads and the density of the traffic varied. In four of the units there were GPs who undertook forceps deliveries if necessary. Unlike Grantham, all five units provided 24-hour midwife cover.

The speed with which the MMU in Grantham had been set up had allowed limited time for midwives to visit and learn from other birth centres. It seems surprising that it was decided not to have a midwife present on the MMU on a 24-hour basis as in other centres. The compromise of having HCSWs as core staff does, however, appear to have worked well, although it was not always clear when they were interviewed whether they always referred calls for advice to the on-call midwife or whether they

sometimes gave advice themselves. They may only have given the sort of advice that a mother might give to a daughter, but there remains a possibility that inappropriate advice could be given. Whether this potential for error is justification for midwife cover on the unit is an interesting question and no doubt will form part of a Trust risk management strategy. On the one hand, the midwife's presence could reduce such a risk but, on the other, 'wasted' midwife time could deprive women elsewhere of one-to-one care in labour because of staff shortages. To date there does not appear to have been any adverse outcomes as a consequence of the lack of 24-hour core-midwife cover on the unit.

The managers involved in the discussions about setting up the MMU had initially agreed that a manager with a clinical caseload would be their preferred option. Instead, the manager appointed (although she had left the unit and was not available for interview) appeared to be more involved in setting up systems and organising duty rosters than working clinically. She did, however, provide a midwife presence during most daytime hours. Again, the speed in setting up the unit meant that she wrote most of the guidelines and protocols herself rather than consulting with the MMU midwives who would be using them. At the time of the evaluation the guidelines were being rewritten by the MMU midwives to reflect developments at the MMU and incorporate best available evidence.

Other successful models of staffing MMUs appear to have been based on selecting midwives who have a vision for working in a birth centre and who are enthusiastic about the concept. In contrast, a decision was taken to ring-fence the community midwives' posts already held in Grantham town and to offer preferential interviews to former hospital midwives who had been displaced. This avoided any compulsory redundancies. Initially there was friction in the mixed team of former hospital and community midwives but they soon learned that there were advantages in their complementary skills and knowledge. If midwives perceived there to be difficulties between them, this was not apparent to the mothers, who commented on the high quality of care provided by MMU midwives. The teams might have functioned more effectively early on, however, if some of the these difficult issues had been thought through and addressed in advance of the MMU opening.

Of particular importance when setting up the MMU had been liaison with the host unit and although there were a number of early difficulties, most had been resolved. An outstanding problem was the differences in records between the MMU and the host unit but work was ongoing to improve this system and communications generally.

Another problem occurred when the MMU manager left. This left the MMU midwives with no professional lead. In spite of this, and the continuing attention from the media, the MMU appeared to continue functioning satisfactorily. The midwives interviewed felt that they lacked midwifery leadership and a vision for the future during this period although the two team leaders assumed temporary managerial responsibilities. This situation was resolved when Grantham was incorporated into a Single Hospitals Trust for the county.

EDUCATION, TRAINING AND SUPPORT

A particular strength in setting up the MMU in Grantham was that the period between the consultant unit closing and the MMU opening and the quiet periods between births allowed for a comprehensive education programme. The university's link teacher provided a large number of sessions on active birth, suturing, resuscitation and child protection and all the midwives were given the opportunity to attend the ALSO course.

Home births caused some concern for ex-hospital midwives but this was addressed by established community midwives providing support for their colleagues. Not all midwives felt that sufficient preparation had been provided for those without recent experience of working in the community. More attention had been given to training for obstetric emergency scenarios rather than preparing staff to work with women in a non-interventionist community

context. This lack of staff preparation for community work could have been partly responsible for some of the initial friction with GPs. However, by the time of the study GPs and midwives reported that professional relationships and communications were much improved.

CONTINUITY OF CARE AND CAREGIVER

One of the aims of a midwife-led service is to improve continuity of both care and of caregiver for women with low-risk pregnancies. The latter does not appear to have been realised for MMU-booked women as the midwives adopted a team, rather than a caseload approach. Former hospital midwives had not been accustomed to providing continuity of caregiver and therefore when this happened it was considered a bonus. Former community midwives and GPs on the other hand reported a lack of continuity of carer for individual women. A few midwives believed that it should be possible to carry a caseload within the team concept but they recognised that caseloads would need to be shared because of the high ratio of part-time to full-time midwives employed.

Women commented that they had met most members of their team during their pregnancy and that it did not matter to them which one assisted them at the birth as the midwives were well known in the town, and were all pleasant and good at their job. The *Changing Childbirth* report (Department of Health 1993) has perhaps caused this problem of loss of continuity of midwife antenatally and postnatally by suggesting that the majority of women should know the person who cares for them during their baby's birth. There is increasing evidence in the literature that though this might be desirable it is not an essential target and that others, such as one-to-one care in labour, are more important (Fraser 1999).

THE ROLES AND RESPONSIBILITIES OF MIDWIVES

A year after the MMU opened it was clear that the midwives' range of opportunities to provide intrapartum care was variable. This was of concern not only to midwives themselves but also to managers, GPs and consultant obstetricians. A number of midwives worked 'on the bank' at their nearest consultant unit but this was very much up to the individual midwife. Two midwives who used to work on the Special Care Baby Unit had taken it upon themselves to keep updated in neonatal resuscitation and provide in-service training. Although this has proved a satisfactory arrangement in the short term, unless the paediatricians from the host unit offer support and advice to MMU midwives in the future it is questionable whether these skills can be maintained. The consultant obstetricians were prepared to offer advice to the MMU midwives when necessary. This included giving a second opinion on fetal heart rate tracings when midwives had concerns about progress in labour or fetal well-being. There was no evidence of a systematic training needs analysis, however, and it is unclear whether service needs, as well as the perceived needs of individuals, are met.

One area where a service needs review could be useful is the 24-hour examination of the newborn. It seems sensible, especially in light of the Government consultation paper, 'A Health Service of all the talents' (Department of Health 2000), to use staff according to who is the most appropriate in a particular situation. GPs and midwives in Grantham might benefit from deciding who should take on the 24-hour examination of the newborn, and indeed the postnatal examination at 6 weeks, as suggested in the Department of Health's 1999 report, 'Making a Difference'. There was no evidence that quiet times on the MMU had been used proactively to look at the scope of practice for midwives or to identify ways in which additional roles might enhance the service provided.

A problem arose in relation to records and record-keeping for MMU births, home births and for women transferred in labour. A significant number of records had incomplete data or were missing complete sections. Although the teams had lacked midwifery leadership for a few months prior to the evaluation, the teams did include supervisors of midwives. It could be that the supervisors were aware of the location of the missing sections of notes but this was not made known to the research team. The development of systems for completing and collating hand-held records appeared to have been neglected. Although the inadequacy of record-keeping could be attributed in part to problems with the management of the MMU facility and the lack of clinical leadership, it was disappointing that individual midwives, and supervisors of midwives in particular, needed this evaluation study to highlight the problem.

A SAFE PLACE TO BE BORN?

Much political, media, public and professional debate concentrates on the safety of births centres in terms of physical morbidity and mortality. More recently there has been much more attention paid to the psychological and emotional sequelae of the birth experience (Marmion 2000). It has been assumed that, provided no physical trauma (outside normal parameters) is sustained, then the providers of the maternity services have been successful in achieving a satisfactory standard of provision. Stories from women tell a different picture (Kirkham 2000). Health professionals have also found that the belief women have in their own body affects outcomes. Recent years have seen increasing strength of opinion both in favour of and opposed to intervention. The National Institute for Clinical Excellence 2001 guidelines on the use of cardiotocograph monitoring in normal labour have gone some way in swinging the pendulum back to normality. In contrast, arguments continue as to whether women should be allowed to choose an elective caesarean section when there is no medical or obstetric indication (Kaufman & Liu 2001).

Evidence from this study suggests that an isolated birth centre is a safe place to be born provided sensible booking criteria are in place and the midwives responsible for the service and the women who access the unit believe that labour and birth should proceed with minimal intervention (Standing Nursing and Midwifery Advisory Committee 1998). Inevitably there will be times when a labour becomes complicated or a normal birth is followed by problems with the third stage of labour. The management of these potential complications does not require midwives who view childbirth as 'normal in retrospect' but midwives who are well educated, who base practice on an expectation of normality, best evidence and good research, and who are accomplished in the 'fire drill' elements of obstetric practice.

Because women's choice and control is so important to their childbirth experience, it is no longer ethical to use randomised controlled trials to research safety issues surrounding choices about where to give birth. From the evidence from small evaluation studies of birth centre outcomes it would seem that birth centres are no less safe than consultant-led obstetric units for low-risk labours. Indeed it could be argued that in the longer term they are safer. Women have less analgesia and they know that epidural analgesia (with its potential complications) is not an option–yet they appear to cope well without it (Bick et al 2002). There also seems to be a lower incidence of perineal trauma but comparisons between similar groups are difficult and our incomplete data set makes it unsound to draw general conclusions in this area. (This could also be a temporary phenomenon as more hospital-based midwives become more skilled in determining whether an episiotomy is really necessary.)

Women who experienced giving birth in the MMU were positive about their birth experience, commenting on the reduction in anxiety resulting from knowing that they would not have far to travel and their confidence in a known team of midwives. Proximity to home was a major factor for the majority of women and this may be an important aspect when decisions are taken about opening birth centres. A few of the consultant obstetricians in this study argued in favour of a midwife-led service adjacent to a consultant-led service, believing this to encompass all the advantages and none of the risks. However, when comparing the transfer outcomes of isolated versus same-site birth centres, Saunders et al (2000) commented that of the 441 women

going to the Edgware Birth Centre in labour:

... 54 (12%) transferred during labour to a hospital for delivery. In comparison ... a randomised controlled trial in Aberdeen of a midwifery-led unit on the same site as a consultant unit produced a 34% antenatal transfer and 16% intrapartum transfer rate using very similar selection criteria to the Birth Centre (Hundley et al 1994).

The differences in practice over time between these two studies could have accounted for this 4% difference in transfer rate. If similar differences were to be found in future studies, however, this would add to the evidence for the safety of isolated birth centres, given that transfer may sometimes be associated with unnecessary intervention.

While it is clear that women who successfully birth in their place of choice are generally satisfied and very positive about their experience, it can be useful to focus on those who are transferred. It might be assumed that these women would not recommend a birth centre to their friends and relatives and indeed could be likely to request intervention in subsequent pregnancies and labour. The majority of these women had apparently 'safe' outcomes but five out of the ten stated on the questionnaire that they would not recommend the MMU as a birth option. Their fear and anxiety about death, of themselves or their baby, were compelling reasons for these recommendations.

CONCLUSIONS

Balancing risks and benefits is difficult in the maternity services and a model in one area is not necessarily appropriate elsewhere. The best option for one woman might be the least preferred for another. What was evident from this study was that the MMU in Grantham is providing an excellent service for a minority of women. However, the data showed that the MMU facility is not cost-effective (but could be argued to be cost-beneficial) as managed at the time of the evaluation. The ratio of midwives to the number of childbearing women is high but compares favourably with other isolated midwife-led units in rural areas. In terms of affordability for the

Grantham Hospital budget, the new model for the maternity services in Grantham is superior, although it could be argued that costs have merely been shifted to other individuals or groups.

Small towns in rural communities have particular problems with the allocation of resources and the recruitment and retention of staff. They cannot make economies of scale and therefore need to be positively weighted when distributing resources. Grantham had no shortage of midwives committed to the success of the MMU and, if they had not been employed in Grantham, they might have been lost to the profession because of family commitments and restrictions in travelling.

Whether the birth centre will be retained and the criteria for admission expanded was uncertain at the time of this study. If the opinions of childbearing women, midwives and GPs provide any such influence on the outcome, however, then this birth centre is here to stay.

REFERENCES

Bick D et al 2002 Postnatal care evidence and guidelines for management. Churchill Livingstone, Edinburgh

Clothier C, MacDonald CA, Shaw DA 1994 The Allitt Inquiry. The Stationery Office Books, London

Department of Health 1993 Changing Childbirth: Report of the Expert Maternity Group. The Stationery Office Books, London

Department of Health 1999 Making a Difference. Strengthening the nursing, midwifery and health visiting contribution to healthcare. The Stationery Office Books, London

Department of Health 2000 A Health Service of all the talents: developing the NHS workforce. The Stationery Office Books, London

Fraser DM 1999 Women's perceptions of midwifery care: a longitudinal study to shape curriculum development. Birth 26(2): 99–107

Hundley V et al 1994 Midwife-managed delivery unit: a randomised controlled comparison with consultant-led care. British Medical Journal 309: 1400–1404

Kaufman T, Liu D 2001 Should caesareans be performed only on the basis of medical need? Nursing Times 97(38) September: 17

Kirkham M 2000 The midwife-mother relationship. Macmillan, London

Marmion S 2000 Reflections on emotional disturbances after childbirth. British Journal of Midwifery 8 (9): 539–543

National Institute for Clinical Excellence 2001 The use of fetal monitoring. Inherited Clinical Guideline C. May. NICE, London

Royal College of Obstetricians and Gynaecologists and Royal College of Midwives 1999 Towards Safer Childbirth: Minimum standards for the organisation of labour wards. Report of the Joint Working Party. RCOG and RCM, London

Saunders D et al 2000 Evaluation of the Edgware Birth Centre. Barnet Health Authority, London.

Stake RE 1995 The art of case study research. Sage, London

Standing Nursing and Midwifery Advisory Committee 1998 Midwifery: delivering our future. SNMAC, London

Yin RK 1994 Case study research: design and methods, 2nd edn. Sage, London

5

The Crowborough birthing centre story

Richard Hallett

INTRODUCTION

This is the story of how a small under-used (but highly valued) GP maternity unit that refused to be closed became a thriving midwife-led unit. In the process (though this was never the aim) the unit has become nationally known, receiving visits and requests for information from all over the UK. In 2000 the birthing centre won the Tesco/Royal College of Midwives Millennium award. A number of midwife-led regional study days have also been held and the birthing centre is now used for student training by Brighton University.

High Weald Primary Care Group area has a population of around 90 000. The largest town in the area is Crowborough, which is the largest inland conurbation in East Sussex, with a population of 24 000 and a high proportion of young families. Uckfield with a population of around 20 000 is some 8 miles south. Crowborough War Memorial Hospital is a community hospital with a local history that dates back to 1911. Eastbourne and County Healthcare Trust operate it, and for many years one wing of the hospital has operated as a six-bedded maternity unit. In recent years this has been 'rented out' to Eastbourne Hospitals Trust who staff and manage the unit.

Only Crowborough provides the option of a small low-tech maternity unit within the area shown in Figure 5.1. These are usually called 'isolated' units but to the women who use them they are local and community-based.

Crowborough's location in East Sussex

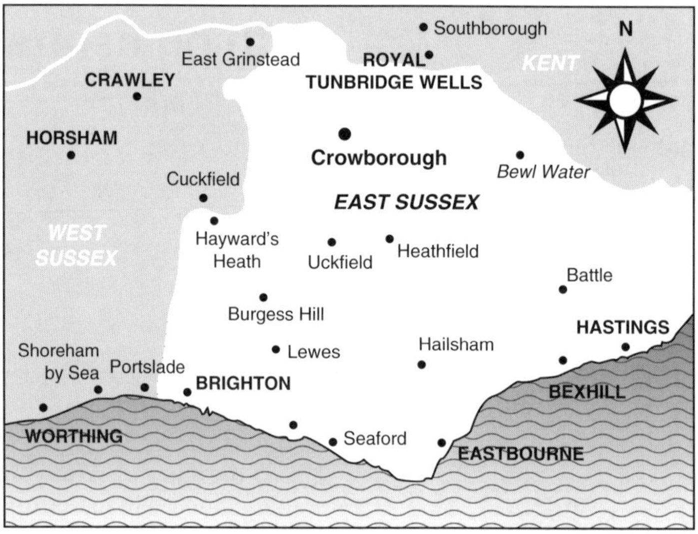

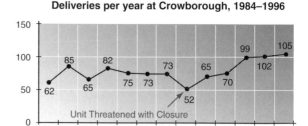

Figure 5.1   Crowborough's location in East Sussex.

Consultant-led maternity care is available at Pembury (12 miles across the county border in Kent), at Princess Royal in Haywards Heath (19 miles across the western county border in West Sussex), or 'within area' at Eastbourne District General Hospital (26 miles away on the south coast).

Over the years the unit struggled on with threats of closure in 1984 and 1990. In 1989 it was recorded in a written answer in Hansard that in the decade 1979–1989 the *only* isolated maternity unit reprieved by Ministers was at Crowborough Hospital. This was the result of a determined campaign, strongly supported by the local MP who took an appeal to the Under-Secretary of State for Health.

One of the lessons of the Crowborough story is that continued threats of closure, especially those that involve 'shock and horror' headlines, will always affect women's confidence in a unit. This was especially noticeable in 1991, following the 1990 closure threat due to the alleged 'undue risk' of the unit (see Fig. 5.2). Continued threats of closure, even if never pushed through, can bring about the same effect simply by creating a climate of fear and uncertainty. These threats of closure affect not only women's confidence in

Deliveries per year at Crowborough, 1984–1996

Figure 5.2   Deliveries per year at Crowborough.

the unit, but also the confidence and morale of the midwives who staff them.

THE CAMPAIGN OF 1996

In April 1996, for legal reasons, local GPs felt unable to continue providing medical cover during labour. This prompted the Health Authority to announce a 'review' of the unit's future. The initial consultation document of August 1996 did not even include the continuance of the existing six-bed inpatient maternity unit as one of the options and allowed for only 6 weeks of consultation (East Sussex, Brighton and Hove Health Authority, 1996a). After a rather stormy and packed public meeting a second consultation document in October (1996b) and a lengthened consultation period were provided. This prompted debate on four main options:

1. That GPs reinstate medical cover during labour.
2. That the unit should be replaced by midwife-led home deliveries and delivery within a consultant-led unit.
3. A midwife-led inpatient maternity unit.
4. A Domino unit.

The first option was known to be impossible as the local GPs had made it quite clear they could not continue to provide medical cover. The second option, though it did not use the word 'closure', was actually just that!

The Health Authority's recommendation (the fourth option) was for a Domino (**Dom**iciliary **in** and **o**ut) unit. This would have consisted of a few rooms set aside within the hospital which would have been unstaffed and unused except when a community midwife opened it up with a woman already in labour. There would be no inpatient postnatal facilities so that women would return home soon after delivery. In comparison with the six-bedded unit already in existence this would have been tantamount to closure and was indeed seen locally as the 'closure by stealth' option. The real fight, therefore, was over 'Option 3'–to change the GP maternity unit into a midwife-led birth centre.

COST ISSUES

There is an almost universal assumption that small units are expensive. Direct comparison was made with Pembury Hospital, the nearest district general hospital, where the cost per birth was £1540. The Consultation Document of August 1996 stated:

Option 3…seeks to develop an isolated midwife-led inpatient maternity unit….average cost per delivery

would increase to between £2500 and £3000, being over £1000 greater than the cost of deliveries elsewhere. It would require substantial cuts in other services to finance it. (East Sussex, Brighton and Hove Health Authority 1996a)

The claim made in the last sentence of this statement became almost vitriolic, with the Health Authority listing a number of possible cuts, such as 2000+ district nurse visits, 200 day-case hernia repairs, 19 hip replacements or 10 coronary artery bypass grafts. The consultation document even went on to say: 'Individuals are also invited to indicate which services could be cut to pay for maternity provision in Crowborough.'

The definitive statement that costs per delivery would rise to £2500–£3000 per delivery (over £1000 more than elsewhere!) was linked to an assumption on women's choices–the argument appeared to be that if there were no doctors and no consultants, then women would not choose Crowborough! The campaign therefore depended on challenging the assumption that women would not choose midwife-led care. The available evidence, though not plentiful, actually showed the opposite to be true. Local surveys among North Weald women strongly indicated that substantial numbers would choose midwife-led care. Some supporting evidence was available from the small maternity unit in Darley (South Derbyshire). The number of GP-led births there had been steadily dropping over the previous three years. It was the introduction of midwife-led care, advertised as 'home-from-home', that reversed this trend and enabled the unit to continue as a viable option.

Information was also available from Wiltshire and Somerset, where there are seven stand-alone units with a consultant unit at Bath, just across the county border in Avon. Some of these units were not dissimilar to Crowborough. In Wiltshire this model of small stand-alone units is a significant provider of maternity care, with 1310 births in 1995. The consultant obstetrician in charge of these units supported the local campaign and spoke at the Crowborough Maternity Unit Forum they organised in November 1996. This forum was chaired by the local MP and gained the attention of the Health Authority, the Community Health Council, senior managers within the provider Trusts, and the local community. One of the most telling statistics used in the campaign was that the 1310 births in Wiltshire represented about 50% of all births within the areas served by these small units. This underpinned the prediction that numbers at Crowborough would not only be maintained, but could be expected to increase to around 200 births per year.

In addition to this, most local surveys demonstrated that what women wanted most was shared care, with their GP providing care from 'cradle to grave' and midwives providing care from 'pregnancy to cradle'. Analysis of the 1995 Crowborough statistics showed that, in practice, GP's were the 'lead professional' in only 3% of deliveries and were only present (even as the 'second professional') for 43% of deliveries. It demonstrated that the answer to the question, 'Who delivered?' was already usually 'A midwife'.

A COST-EFFECTIVE MIDWIFE-LED UNIT

The Health Authority eventually agreed to a 2-year trial period of running the service as a midwife-led unit (though not without some financial assistance from the Hospital Friends) and this began on April 1st 1997. A monitoring group was set up to report back to the Health Authority on the progress made during the trial period. The results were dramatic (see Fig. 5.3). After years of struggling along at around 70 births per year, numbers rose in 1997/98 to 179 births, and to 185 births in 1998/99. This confirmed the campaign's contention that women *do* choose midwife-led care!

By April 1999 the results during the trial period were sufficiently good for the future funding of the unit to be confirmed. A good quality publicity leaflet was then produced and distributed. This, combined with an increase in women's confidence following confirmation of the unit's future, produced a further dramatic increase in activity levels. With regard to the

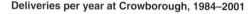
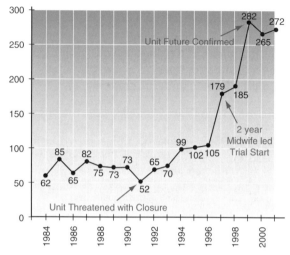

Deliveries per year at Crowborough, 1984–2001

Figure 5.3 Deliveries per year at Crowborough.

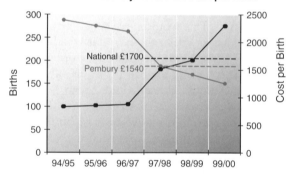

The effect of Activity Levels on Cost per Birth

Figure 5.4 The effect of activity levels on cost per birth at Crowborough 1994–2000.

evidence being gathered by the campaign, a significant statistic was that the 282 births in 1999/2000 did represent about 50% of 'available births' in North Wealden (though the unit has also begun to attract women from some way 'out-of-area').

As the number of births at Crowborough rose so the costs per birth fell sharply, even allowing for some additional staffing (Fig. 5.4). From around £2400 per birth in the previous 3 years the cost per birth dropped to around £1250 for 1999/2000. The Health Authority prediction in 1996 had been that the costs would rise to over

Table 5.1 Comparison of midwife staffing costs per birth in Eastbourne and Crowborough

	Eastbourne	Crowborough
1997/1998	£1120	£1156
1998/1999	£1097	£1100
1999/2000	£1136	£1042

£1000 more than the cost elsewhere. In fact the cost per birth *fell* by over £1000 and dropped below that at Pembury, which had been used as a benchmark, and the national average.

In order to eliminate differences in overhead costs a comparison was made of midwife staffing costs at Eastbourne District General Hospital and the stand-alone unit at Crowborough. Table 5.1 shows that, with appropriate activity levels, small units can be just as cost-effective. This is perhaps not surprising. In maternity units generally some 83% of all controllable costs are staffing costs (N Edwards, presentation for the conference 'Changes in Maternity Services', Royal College of Obstetricians and Gynaecologists, unpublished, July 19th 1999). Provided that staffing and workload are kept in balance then Crowborough can remain as cost-effective as larger hospital units. The latest nationally published data (*Sunday Times* July 15th 2001) shows Crowborough to have a midwife to birth ratio of 1:32, which is close to the national average.

In addition to this, the 'cost per birth' figure is misleading. It was adopted as a benchmark measure because the Health Authority had used it in the consultation document as the yardstick of cost-effectiveness. As a 'real measure, however, it understates the full range of antenatal care, locally held consultant clinics (if appropriate), intrapartum care and good quality residential postnatal care. The centre also acts as a local '24/7 drop-in maternity help centre', with over 2000 attendees per year.

A key benefit gained from residential postnatal care was the improved establishment of breastfeeding, with an 85% rate on discharge compared with 65% for local district general hospital units. This has a general economic benefit in terms of reduced incidence of infant gastroenteritis, although this is difficult to quantify.

An average 3 days of residential postnatal care was also found to *reduce* midwifery staffing costs locally. This paradoxical finding was explained when it was realised that residential postnatal care can be provided with no additional resources because the birth centre midwife is already available 24 hours a day. If women go home immediately postpartum additional community midwife home visits are required for those 3 days. In 1995 the cost saving through provision of residential postnatal care was estimated to be the equivalent of nearly one community midwife.

These overall results on cost-effectiveness at Crowborough are supported by conclusions reached elsewhere. The cost of deliveries at the Edgware Birth Centre was significantly cheaper (by up to 30%) than that for similar women who delivered in local hospitals. Although these somewhat rudimentary conclusions are based on limited evidence from geographically diverse units, they do suggest that, contrary to the universal assumption that small units are expensive, small midwife-led maternity units can be cost-effective.

DEVELOPING A MIDWIFE-LED BIRTH CENTRE

The first crucial decision was to find and appoint a Senior Midwife who had the ability to lead a local team. Secondly it was vital to have a proactive approach to the supervision of midwives, and it was helpful that the primary care manager responsible for transition of the unit to 'midwife-led' was a recognised Supervisor. As well as supervision, teamwork was critical to success as the midwives would have to become a self-managed team. The unit could not be well managed from a distance and both management and morale improved when the team devised their own work and cover rotas and made joint decisions about the unit.

This system led to real job satisfaction for the midwives in the unit, with significant growth evident in confidence and in professional development. Confidence was a real issue for many of the midwives in the unit as many had lost sight of their role as autonomous professionals. A great deal of confidence was gained from working together to develop evidence-based guidelines appropriate for running a small midwife-led unit, working through various difficult issues in a setting in which the midwives could be open about their fears and mistakes.

Midwife recruitment and retention is a fast developing crisis, with job stress and dissatisfaction a significant problem, but there is a waiting list for midwife positions at Crowborough! This Crowborough midwife's view is not unique among small stand-alone units:

I trained and worked at some superb hi-tech units, and I thought intervention was the norm. It wasn't until I came to Crowborough that I began to realise what real midwifery was all about. It has made the job much more satisfying and uses my midwifery skills to the full. (Midwife Debbie Gowers, 1999)

Small units not only have something to offer the women who use them, but also something to offer the midwives who staff them. There is a very real (but often hidden) benefit of high morale in terms of lower absenteeism cover and recruitment costs.

The statistics in Table 5.2 tell only part of the story of the transition to a midwife-led unit. Behind these statistics there lies a story of a group of midwives gaining in confidence, developing an ethos and dealing with new challenges, some of them unique to a small midwife-led unit, such as:

- resisting the temptation not to transfer women who should be transferred when numbers of births were critical to a successful two year review.

- accepting and caring for primigravida women (never before admitted to the unit)
- developing vital new working relationships with local GPs and the nearby consultant units
- providing an integrated service in the community and the unit to cover antenatal, intrapartum and postnatal care.

The antenatal transfer rate was monitored closely and on some measures it could be considered high. In fact it demonstrates both sensitivity to deviation from the norm, resulting in appropriate referrals to consultant care, and the wish of some women to use their local birth centre as an access route to maternity care, regardless of their ultimate choice of type of care.

PROFESSIONAL DEVELOPMENT

Over the 2-year trial period a comprehensive set of evidence-based guidelines were developed and implemented that were in line with the ethos of the unit. Input was invited from local GPs and the associated consultant. These guidelines now form a substantial document that is constantly being updated (Crowborough Birthing Centre 2002). Eastbourne Hospitals Trust midwifery management has introduced the same set of guidelines at the consultant unit in Eastbourne in order to provide consistency of ethos, quality and care. This innovative approach ensures that both ends of the pathways between low-tech and high-tech provision work with the same vision and philosophy of quality and care. Improved continuity of care is now provided for women as they move between consultant and midwife-supported care.

Table 5.2 Crowborough Birthing Centre statistics

	GP Unit (1996/1997)	1997/1998	1998/1999	1999/2000
Percentage primigravida births	—	26%	33%	38%
Percentage multigravida births	100%	74%	67%	62%
Antenatal transfer rate	26%	33%	32%	34%
Intrapartum transfer rate	13%	9%	12%	13%

Some of the issues facing stand-alone midwife-led units are not well documented in the professional literature. The midwife team has therefore set up its own audit system. In particular audits have focussed on intrapartum transfers, water births, second-degree tears, and the physiological third stage. Additionally, in circumstances in which guidelines have not seemed to be appropriate, where mistakes have been made, or where there have been critical incidents, a review is organised with the team, not just with one individual. This has been important in creating a supportive environment for midwives to practise their profession.

The Crowborough Birthing Centre now has an empowered team of midwives who in turn empower women to have positive birth experiences. Use is now made of Crowborough for professional development, for midwife placements and as a refresher in 'normal birth' for acute hospital unit midwives. The midwifery manager uses Crowborough as a confidence-building placement for midwives who need particular help. This is a two-way process, with placements at Eastbourne being used to help Crowborough midwives maintain their technological skills.

The ethos of the Crowborough unit is not only to be 'woman centred', but also 'midwife centred', enhancing the role that the midwife can play as a health professional. *Towards Safer Childbirth* (RCOG and RCM 1999) concludes:

There is agreement that the midwife plays a central role in the care of women in labour... It is the unanimous view that one midwife to one woman should be the standard. There is clear evidence that the provision of continuous skilled support not only enhances maternal satisfaction with labour, but also reduces the need for a wide range of medical interventions.

This one-to-one focus on the woman in labour and the motivation to provide personal support and care is where small units excel and can be a model of excellence without requiring disproportionate resources. Their ability to provide improved quality of care in a cost-effective way is at least partly due to their small size. They provide an environment in which it is easier for midwives to function more effectively in their supportive role.

USERS' VIEWS AND EXPERIENCES

Happy midwives make happy women! Small units where midwifes have high job satisfaction and where their role is enhanced by their environment, are generally highly rated by service users. The supportive care received is usually long remembered and has positive effects on confidence and self-esteem. It is often the local 'community value' that has ensured these units' survival. User perspectives on the Crowborough Birthing Centre are perhaps best expressed in their own words:

I couldn't have asked for anything better, both during the birth and afterwards. First class. Every midwife that I met was incredibly kind, patient and helpful and made my stay here comfortable and even fun! Crowborough midwives have really helped one new mum in her initial journey into motherhood and I now feel confident and happy to get on with the job.
(Jenny, first-time mum)

My water birth was a wonderful experience and my care has been truly special. It has been good to spend quality time with Thomas as he is my number three.
(Jessica)

The midwives here are special, giving support when needed and staying clear when not.
(Maeve)

What a super team. The postnatal care has been first class.
(Dad)

The birth of my daughter was the most wonderful experience and this was very much due to the caring and relaxed approach that you all have within your friendly team.
(Alison)

BIRTH CENTRES IN THE FUTURE

There are those who regard small maternity units like Crowborough as '*quaint relics from a glorious past*'. The conclusion reached from the experience of the development of Crowborough Birthing Centre since 1997 is rather different:

For the majority of women with low-risk normal pregnancies, small midwife-led maternity units can provide cost-effective high-quality care that delights both midwives and users alike. The significant benefits that small units can provide, along with their local availability to users, means that they are well suited to become a popular mainstream choice within enlightened maternity care provision. (R Hallett, 'The Crowborough Story', Friends of Crowborough Hospital, unpublished, 2000)

There are some 90 small maternity units in the UK. Crowborough has a limited population catchment area. In more densely populated areas, particularly urban areas, the potential for this type of unit is enormous. Not only could they provide a significant additional choice for women generally, but their size allows them to focus on the specific needs and cultural requirements of local population groups. They would also go some way towards attracting and retaining midwives in areas where staffing shortages are a significant issue.

The Crowborough Birthing Centre operates as one 'satellite unit' in an outlying area, providing its own supportive quality of care and a 'community gateway' to consultant care where appropriate. The annual birth statistics for Eastbourne Hospital Trust show that some 20% of births now take place away from the consultant unit. The midwifery manager for the two units identifies real benefits from this joint working both for the small midwife-led unit and for the larger consultant unit. One of the wider lessons learned from the Crowborough story is that if small units were to be developed as community satellite units around consultant units it would mean that those consultant units could be smaller and therefore more focussed on the women who need medical intervention and technology. Because these consultant units could be physically smaller and would be handling fewer women they would actually provide improved and more personalised care to the women who really need them.

ACKNOWLEDGEMENTS

The author would like to acknowledge the input and assistance from Helen O'Dell (Head of Midwifery, Eastbourne Hospitals Trust) and Russell Wakefield (Vice-President of the Friends of Crowborough Hospital) in the preparation of this chapter.

REFERENCES

Crowborough Birthing Centre 2002 Evidence-based Care Guidelines. Available from Crowborough Birthing Centre, South View Road, Crowborough, East Sussex, TN6 1HB

East Sussex, Brighton and Hove Health Authority (1996a) Consultation Document–Maternity Services at Crowborough War Memorial Hospital. August 6th: 3

East Sussex, Brighton and Hove Health Authority (1996b) Additional Consultation Paper–Maternity Services at Crowborough War Memorial Hospital. October 4th: 5

Hansard 1989 Written answer from Roger Freeman (Secretary of State for Health) to Michael Latham MP (Rutland and Melton), February 23rd

Royal College of Obstetricians and Gynaecologists and Royal College of Midwives 1999 Towards Safer Childbirth. Report of a Joint Working Party. RCOG & RCM, Section 5.1.3: 12

The Edgware bir

6

Users in the driving seat

Elizabeth Manero
Linda Turner

THE DIRECTION OF TRAVEL

1994 was a year of turmoil and change for the NHS, both nationally and locally, in Barnet and Edgware. In 1992 Sir Bernard Tomlinson had presented his *Report of the Inquiry into London's Health Service, Medical Education and Research* to the Secretaries of State for Health and Education. The summary concluded:

There is likely to be a significant fall in the requirement for inpatient beds...the continuing trend in the efficiency with which inpatient beds are used, which will enable services to be provided within a smaller estate...could mean that between 2000 and 7000 beds could become surplus...closures and mergers will be necessary.

By 1994 this policy had started to filter down to local level in Barnet. There were two district general hospitals in the borough, Barnet General Hospital in the east and Edgware General Hospital in the west. There was much talk and subsequent disquiet about what the future held for Edgware General Hospital once the planned rebuilding of Barnet General hospital had been completed, 5 miles away and within the same Health Authority boundaries. At this stage inpatient obstetric and maternity services were being provided exclusively at Edgware (after the closure of a maternity hospital in Barnet a few years before) but 'state of the art' facilities were being built at Barnet and expected to open in 1997.

Policy on maternity services at this time seemed to be taking a different route from other acute services. Although in some areas birth was still seen as just another acute 'episode of care', elsewhere it was becoming recognised as an important and life-changing event with implications for both individuals and society as a whole. Instead of rationalisation and the need for efficient use of resources, the talk was of 'women-centred services'. Women were starting to assert themselves in maternity services, the beginning of 'patient empowerment'. A by-product of the internal market, this reform sought to turn patients into consumers, although women having babies are really the only users who truly fit this definition because they are not disempowered by illness and have 9 months in which to think about what sort of care they want.

The 'Winterton Report' of the all-party Parliamentary Select Committee on Health had been published in March 1992. The report had challenged the guidance given to Health Authorities by the Maternity Services Advisory Committee in *Maternity Care in Action* in 1984 that 'as unforeseen complications can occur in any birth, every mother should be encouraged to have her baby in a maternity unit where emergency facilities are available'. Winterton's conclusion was rather different: 'On the basis of what we have heard, this committee must draw the conclusion that the policy of encouraging all women to give birth in hospitals cannot be justified on grounds of safety.'

In response, the Government soon established the Expert Maternity Group (EMG), chaired by Baroness Cumberlege, to draw up recommendations about the future of maternity services. Eileen Hutton, President of the National Childbirth Trust (NCT) served as a member, putting user involvement right at the heart of formulating Government policy. In August 1993 *Changing Childbirth* (Department of Health 1993) was produced, which made wide-ranging recommendations to be implemented within 5 years. The publication of this document marked a sharp change of direction in the development of maternity services and laid the foundation for the 'patient-centred NHS' which has become the mantra of the NHS today.

A CHANGE OF DIRECTION

The NCT's excellent 1994 document, *The Challenge of Change* describes the changed policy:

'[After a public consultation]…in January 1994 an NHS Management Executive Letter was issued endorsing all the recommendations, making them Government policy…The Executive Letter defined a 'Changing Childbirth' service as one where:

- purchasers and providers are asking women what they want and testing levels of satisfaction;
- the service has the support of local women; and
- the service provides good clinical outcomes.'

It is hard in retrospect to overstate the effect on users of *Changing Childbirth*. Everywhere one went it was being studied and discussed. At conferences, Community Health Council or Maternity Service Liaison Committee meetings the report and its implementation were almost the sole topics of conversation. The effect of empowerment on lay people and users of the service was profound. The three central tenets of choice, continuity and control for women now gave them the tools and the credibility to start really getting somewhere in discussions about local services, whether with clinicians, managers or the health authorities which purchased the services. Instead of being limited to a rather reactive role of commenting on local maternity services, users and lay people now felt able to take a much more proactive role in suggesting and pushing for changes in the way local services were delivered. Further help and support for women came in the NHS publication *The Patient's Charter: Maternity Services* and the Commission for Racial Equality's *Race Relations Code of Practice in Maternity Services*, both published in 1994. These documents set out the rights that women already had and the ways in which maternity care should improve during the next 5 years in response to *Changing Childbirth*.

One of the effects of the raised profile of maternity services was the sharing of good practice and a greater awareness of different models of care. The home-from-home unit at

Leicester Royal Infirmary, the Darley Unit in Derbyshire, and the midwife-led unit in Bournemouth were all talked of as examples of maternity services which met most of the *Changing Childbirth* criteria and demonstrated that such services could be delivered in different ways. Discussion of alternative and acceptable maternity services was stimulated perhaps most of all by the services that were provided by a number of satellite stand-alone units scattered throughout Wiltshire, centred on the consultant unit at Bath. Lay people began to ask whether some of these models of care could be successfully reproduced in urban or inner-city settings.

USERS GETTING ON BOARD

A different emphasis in policy for maternity services was the first of the two key movements that began to gain momentum around 1994. The second, and perhaps ultimately more powerful and long-lasting, was the recognition of the need for public involvement in planning, delivering and monitoring all aspects of health care. The world of maternity services led the way in this. By this time women having babies, the only NHS users who were not actually ill (and perhaps better informed than their mothers had been), had already begun to question many aspects of the care they received during pregnancy and childbirth.

The introduction of Maternity Services Liaison Committees (MSLCs) had given local women a real opportunity to contribute. As *The Challenge of Change* (National Childbirth Trust 1994) noted:

MSLCs began as one of the recommendations of the Maternity Services Advisory Committee in the early eighties. Their main recommendations on MSLCs were as follows:

• Every district health authority (DHA) should establish and maintain an MSLC to help implement, in the light of local circumstances, the Committee's advice on good practice and plan for action.
• An MSLC should act as a multidisciplinary forum, reaching agreement between the different professions and drawing on the experiences of consumers.

• Each Committee should represent all the professions, to ensure integration between the hospital and community services and between the different professions. It should be led by a person of standing who has the enthusiasm and time to make it work effectively.

The position of MSLCs was further strengthened by the publication of both the 'Winterton Report' (Parliamentary Select Committee on Health 1992) and *Changing Childbirth* (Department of Health 1993). It became common for lay people, including National Childbirth Trust members, to be asked to chair their local MSLC and many MSLCs adopted the model terms of reference written by Helen Lewison for the NCT (1994). These terms of reference stated that MSLCs were to 'advise the purchasing authority and the provider(s) unit on all aspects of maternity services, particularly on policy matters'. Lay people rose swiftly to the challenge, reiterating time and time again that woman-centred maternity care was Government policy and that health professionals were required to ask their views. The Greater London Association of Community Health Councils (GLACHC) document *Listening to people: user involvement in the NHS* had come out in 1992. These publications gave enormous support to lay people who were trying to get the recommendations of *Changing Childbirth* taken seriously at local level.

Public involvement had also been institutionalised for some years in the form of Community Health Councils (CHCs). Established in 1974, they took different approaches to their role. By 1994 they were well established and had recognised powers to refer proposals of major changes in the provision of local services to the Minister for Health. They also had to be consulted on major changes of use or on closures of local facilities. The expectation of a visit to provider premises by a group of CHC members still stirred hospital managers into action and the publication of a critical or damning report following on from such a visit was something that Trust Boards wished to avoid.

Barnet CHC was fortunate in having quite a few members and a chief officer who were interested in maternity services. Two of these members (one of them the CHC's Chair) chaired the MSLC between them for a number of years. MSLC meetings had started in Barnet around 1986 and for the first year comprised a meeting over a cup of tea between the Deputy Head of Midwifery and the first two lay representatives! However, a more recognisable MSLC was quickly formed as membership expanded.

Between them the two lay representatives were able to ensure other broad user representation, which included women from the local NCT branch, the La Leche League and the Postnatal Depression Association, and a member from one of the minority ethnic groups. Barnet MSLC was perhaps also fortunate in having the interest of the Health Authority. Fortuitously, it was a midwife working in public health who serviced the committee and the Director of Public Health and Assistant Director of Commissioning often attended. The MSLC worked hard and tackled many thorny issues such as ultrasound screening and the frequency of antenatal visits. A 'where to have your baby' information leaflet for women was produced entitled 'It's Your Choice'.

The public consultation document on the closure of Edgware as an acute hospital (Barnet and Brent and Harrow Health Agencies 1994) included a somewhat reluctant reference to the possibility of a stand-alone midwife-led unit, which had been suggested by local users:

'During the process of producing the consultation the Agencies canvassed opinion on the viability of a GP or midwife-led unit on site. The balance of opinion was against such a unit. The Agencies would welcome the view of the local Maternity Services Liaison Group on this question.'

A STORMY POLITICAL CLIMATE

It is important to recognise the part that party politics played in the establishment of the Edgware Birth Centre. The closure of accident and emergency services at Edgware was one of the most controversial 'reconfigurations' going on at the time. The local population across the borough had put up with seemingly endless promises of service improvements and changes that invariably seemed to lead to contraction of services. The constituency of the former Prime Minister, which was within Barnet and adjacent to the constituency in which Edgware was located, was served by Barnet General Hospital, where a new hospital had been promised for over 20 years. The relentless bureaucracy of securing funding for a new building in the NHS, punctuated by changes in government and government policy, meant that it still had not been delivered and patients were still being cared for in temporary huts which had been erected in wartime to look after the war wounded. Because of the high profile of one of the former local MPs, every development or proposed development was a sensitive issue.

Meanwhile, to the west of the borough in Edgware, a community in which some of the most deprived people in the country were living, the local hospital was becoming increasingly run down, with no promise of new local services. The 1991 Jarman Deprivation scores for Burnt Oak, West Hendon and Colindale were between 37 and 21 while those around the Barnet Hospital site ranged from 21 to −2 (higher scores indicating higher levels of deprivation).

Other significant factors contributing to local people's frustration were the serious mistakes made by the local NHS management and their reluctance to bring them out into the open. When the internal market reforms began in the early 1990s the Wellhouse Trust was established to run Edgware and Barnet hospitals. Due to errors during this process a predicted overspend of £500 000 actually materialised as a deficit of £2.98 million when the accounts were audited. The Wellhouse Trust began its life with a large deficit, necessitating cuts in services and hours of management time spent in 'balancing the books'. The worsening financial position was disclosed in a report by auditors Touche Ross revealing 'an inability to advise both individual budget holders and the corporate boards of the probable financial position within an acceptable level of accuracy'.

Against this background, a proposal was made to close the Accident and Emergency Department at Barnet, closely followed by another proposal to close the Accident and Emergency Department at Edgware instead, with all its associated acute and maternity services. This was the last straw and a group of community activists formed the 'Hands off our Hospital Campaign' and set out to stop the closure. This most contentious of issues, the closure of a hospital, took off in one of the most sensitive locations, next to a former Prime Minister's constituency, at a time when the Conservative Government had a majority of only two.

This was the political context in which the proposal to establish a stand-alone midwife-led unit at Edgware when the hospital was changed to a community hospital was first put on the table. Politically, the Health Authority needed to be seen to be giving something to a community which was reacting vociferously against a loss. The two local Conservative MPs threatened to withdraw the whip unless the Edgware Accident and Emergency Department remained open, which would effectively have defeated the Government.

Barnet CHC, the local statutory watchdog on the NHS, had for some years been quite high profile. When the CHC considered the consultation on the Edgware closure the outrage in the community was extreme and the political rhetoric intense. The CHC, which is required to operate with political impartiality, had the unenviable task of trying to represent the public interest in this politically charged situation. It referred the proposal to close Edgware as an acute hospital to the then Secretary of State under its statutory powers. This took the closure decision away from the local Health Authority and gave it to the Secretary of State. The closure was approved. The CHC worked with the 'Hands off our Hospital Campaign' to try and turn the loss into a gain for the community by developing new ideas for what could be provided in a community hospital. A low-risk birth unit, or 'birth centre' continued to be one of these ideas.

EVIDENCE–THE REAL DRIVER

It was at this point in 1996 that the new Chair of Barnet MSLC was also elected as Chair of Barnet CHC. The local population in Edgware had had access to maternity services locally for many years. Although the service attracted the usual amount of criticism local women were not happy with the prospect of travelling to Barnet, Northwick Park Hospital in Harrow or to the Royal Free Hospital in Hampstead instead. Women believed that a hospital was the only place in which they could give birth. There was no general expectation that birth in any other setting was possible.

The culture in the local NHS at the time seemed to be 'manager knows best'. The idea that patients or the general public could have ideas worth listening to on service models was not an attractive one. However, the political heat meant that there had to be a dialogue. Barnet was fortunate in having a Director of Public Health with a more open mind than some. It seemed clear that, too often, decisions were made with no real evaluation of the evidence. Prejudice served as a quick way to make decisions and, on maternity services in particular, it was very hard to shift.

There was great resistance to the idea of the birth centre locally: 'Don't set yourself up to fail' was the advice given to the MSLC Chair by the Director of Public Health in the car park after the MSLC meeting. An irresistible challenge! The midwife manager from the Darley Unit was invited to come and present to the MSLC about her home-from-home stand-alone unit in Derbyshire. The Edgware Birth Centre owes her a great debt. Watching the MSLC's reaction to her measured, comprehensive description of how her unit worked was like watching a light being switched on in a dark room. Free from local political sensitivities, she showed that a stand-alone unit was possible, did work and, above all, that doing things in a new way need not be so threatening. One of the GPs on the Committee lent the MSLC Chair his copy of *Where to be Born* (Campbell & Macfarlane 1993), an analysis of the evidence on place of birth. Reading this review of the evidence, it became clear just how weak the evidence base was for the claimed lack of safety of the stand-alone model: '...there is no evidence to support the claim that the safest policy is for all women to give birth in hospital'. A stand-alone unit became feasible.

The decision-making process was bureaucratic, involving a full Health Authority meeting. The MSLC needed to put forward its formal response, agreed by the entire committee. This would not be easy. The best tactic seemed to be to take up the objections one by one and test them against the facts.

STOP–GO

'GPs will not refer to such a unit'.

This was tested with a survey of GPs. Only 23 GPs responded out of 116 surveyed (a 19% response rate). Four opposed the plan, nine supported it and ten said they would refer to it but required reassurance about obstetric and paediatric backup.

'Local women do not want it'.

This was tested by a survey which was approved by the national 'Changing Childbirth Team'. Local students, who had no connection with the discussions, were recruited to undertake face-to-face interviews with 164 women in 16 local antenatal clinics. The survey specifically stated: 'The unit will be run by midwives; there will be no doctors in the unit.' When asked if they would deliver in such a unit 61.6% answered 'yes'.

'The sort of women delivering in Edgware are not suitable for midwife-led care'.

This was tested by analysis of the case notes of women who had delivered at Edgware the previous year by the Health Authority to see how many had had midwife deliveries. Seventy-five

percent (1751 out of 2331) of women who had delivered had been attended only by a midwife. This certainly did not mean that 75% of women would be suitable to deliver in a stand-alone unit, or would wish to do so, but it provided a starting point for discussion.

'The Royal Colleges will not support it'.

This was tested by inviting representatives from the Royal Colleges of Obstetricians, Midwives and GPs to join a local expert panel and deliberate the matter. The majority view was that a midwife-led unit on the Edgware site was supportable.

'Midwives cannot cope if there is an unexpected emergency'.

This was tested by analysing the skills needed in a stand-alone unit, including those a consultant might have which might be transferable, and seeing if they could be transferred to midwives through training. It was agreed that neonatal resuscitation, intravenous cannulation and other skills needed to stabilise mother and baby in an emergency (see Ch. 8) would be included in an appropriate training package.

'The ambulance service will never wear it'.

This was tested by discussions with the London Ambulance Service. They expressed their concern that the removal of maternity services from the area would result in a higher number of births in transit. They were happy to support the proposal, subject to agreement of protocols governing transfer arrangements for women needing intrapartum transfer from the unit to hospital.

'Childbirth is so unexpected–you never know when something might go wrong.'

This was tested by multidisciplinary discussion on selection criteria, based on those developed at the Darley Unit. This discussion involved midwives, consultants, the Director of Public Health, a GP and user representatives. We were fortunate in having at least one highly support-ive obstetrician.* An Independent Evaluation was commissioned by the Health Authority with funding from the Department of Health to test safety, user-satisfaction and cost-effectiveness (see Ch. 12).

*['It is not cost-effective to run a unit like this for a small number of women.']

As central money was obtained for the unit from the Department of Health, a unique opportunity presented itself to test the financial viability of such a service, insulated from the endless pres-sures of local deficits and cost cutting. The Independent Evaluation would evaluate whether or not it was financially viable without such protection (see Ch. 13).

The approach taken by the MSLC was that evidence must be the universal language of deci-sion-making and that the user perspective is a critical part of that evidence. Even if there is no clinical evidence available, assertions and opin-ions should not be accepted instead. In drafting its response to the Health Authority consulta-tion, the MSLC needed to try and put this princi-ple into practice. The draft response submitted to the committee included a blank space for the response of the obstetricians–this space was never filled.

THE DESTINATION

In the late summer of 1996 the Health Authority finally made a decision to proceed with the Birth Centre pilot, with funding for 2 years from the Secretary of State. All three local Trusts had decided that they wished to collaborate in pro-viding the service. The old Ophthalmology Unit at Edgware was refurbished as a home-from-home unit, comprising five single rooms with ensuite bathrooms. It was a bit of a struggle for the user representatives on the MSLC to get their ideas on 'home-from-home' accepted by the local NHS: the plan to paint all the rooms different colours and furnish them with different

soft furnishings was strongly resisted at first but eventually it was even agreed to use ordinary bedroom furniture and carpeting on the floors. At the insistence of the users, even the ceilings of the rooms were designed to look like ordinary bedroom ceilings for women lying on a bed in labour.

The Independent Evaluation reported in April 2000 with positive results (see Ch. 12). This marked the start of a broader national campaign to get birth centres accepted as a viable model of care. The policy of stand-alone midwife-led units had been put into practice in a number of areas. This policy was given a kick-start by the political situation at Edgware, giving us both an opportunity and a responsibility–an opportunity to test out an important model of care, and a responsibility to try and make the most of that opportunity for the sake of the wider community.

When a primiparous woman walks into a delivery room to give birth, she is 'just' a preg-nant woman–when she comes out she is part of a family and has acquired responsibilities which are likely to remain with her for the rest of her life. The way this transformation happens is surely important. An interventionist approach to childbirth can save lives when needed–but can also cause real harm. Enkin et al summarised this in their *Guide to effective care in pregnancy and childbirth* (1995): '. . . such harm can result from unwarranted intrusions into women's private lives, from superfluous interventions and treat-ments, from creating unnecessary stress and anxiety and from allocating scarce resources to areas where they are not needed'. The possibility that the birth centre model of care may prevent unnecessary interventions, limiting this 'harm' and releasing resources for patients, must be thoroughly explored.

A social model of care in its fullest sense must be one that society recognises as consistent with both its values and its diversity, including diver-sity of choice. This means that we must avoid replacing one dogma, that 'all births must take place in hospital', with another–that 'all low-risk women should give birth in a birth centre'. Birth centres should be only one part of the spectrum of care models on offer to women. The users of services need to be closely involved in designing *all* services and in monitoring them, to make sure that they remain the sort of services they want them to be. In the case of maternity services this should lead to childbirth being seen as something women do–not something which is done to them.

REFERENCES

Barnet and Brent and Harrow Health Agencies 1994 Changes in service provision in the Edgware Area

Campbell R, Macfarlane A 1993 Where to be Born–the debate and evidence. National Perinatal Epidemiology Unit, Oxford

Commission for Racial Equality 1994 Race Relations Code of Conduct in Maternity Services

Department of Health 1993 Changing Childbirth. Report of the Expert Maternity Group. The Stationery Office Books, London

Enkin et al 1995 A Guide to effective care in pregnancy and childbirth

Greater London Association of Community Health Councils 1992 Listening to people: user involvement in the NHS. GLACHC, London

Lewison H 1994 Maternity Service Liaison Committees: a forum for change. National Childbirth Trust/Greater London Association of Community Health Councils (GLACHC), London

Maternity Care in Action. Report of the Maternity Services Advisory Committee published in three parts 1982–1985

National Childbirth Trust 1994 The Challenge of Change, National Childbirth Trust,

National Health Service Executive 1994 The Patients Charter: Maternity Services

Parliamentary Select Committee on Health 1992 Second Report on the Maternity Services. The Stationery office Books, London

Tomlinson B 1992 Report of the Inquiry into London's Health Service, Medical Education and Research. The Stationery Office Books, London

7

A public health perspective

Stephen Farrow

THE BACKGROUND

During the creation of the Edgware Birth Centre professional opinion was mostly antipathetic, and at times hostile. From the point of view of those who were promoting the project, the situation was difficult but not impossible. There were, after all, champions amongst the midwives and on the Maternity Services Liaison Committee (MSLC), and the Public Health Department of the Health Authority was relatively neutral and prepared to facilitate the debate. Perhaps the most important factor was the requirement to compensate for the loss of a large district general hospital and provide services for local people so that they would not have to travel to the new hospital in Barnet. Although only 5 miles away as the crow flies, this would have meant a difficult journey by public transport and, with increasing traffic density, a long one, even by private transport. Those living around Edgware were also less likely to have their own transport and were more likely to be disadvantaged generally. The placing of several innovative services on the Edgware site was strongly promoted by local MPs and by the Government.

Although obstetricians and paediatricians were opposed to the birth centre their opposition was publicly argued on the basis of safety. Both professional groups had worked at Edgware when it had its own obstetric unit and they continued to work there after April 1st 1997 in its outpatient departments. Their opposition appeared to be rational rather than based on conviction. The general practitioners' views were mixed. A number were eloquent in their vocal opposition, most were opposed or neutral and some were mildly supportive. Many had only limited personal involvement in maternity care although that did not in itself limit their enthusiastic involvement in the debate.

The midwives also held varied opinions. They ranged however, from the enthusiastic to the doubtful. Some of these doubts related to the overall needs of the midwifery service and to workforce and staffing issues. Those at a senior level were worried that they would not be able to sustain the new obstetric unit, a developing team-based approach in the community and a new birth centre. They were concerned that even if the birth centre secured special funding this was likely to be time-limited and that after the honeymoon period was over there would be increased pressure on the maternity budget.

THE STRATEGY FOR CHANGE

The strategy depended on the formation of an alliance between the various groups and individuals who were supportive of the idea. The principal alliance was that of the Chair of the MLSC and key midwives who had worked at the Edgware Midwifery Unit. They were driven by the idea of a more focussed service that put the needs of women first. They were strongly supported by the publication of *Changing Childbirth* (Department of Health 1993) that argued the case that the woman's choice should be paramount. That document set out three key principles of choice, continuity and control for women using maternity services:

[The Select Committee's view is that]... the medical model of care should no longer drive the service and that women should be given an opportunity for choice in the type of maternity care they receive, including the option, previously largely denied to them, of having their babies at home or in small maternity units.

[Purchasers should] as part of their strategic plan, review the current choices available to women regarding the place of birth. Following consultation, these should be developed as appropriate for their locality.

[Providers should] review their current organisation and practices to ensure that real choice about place of birth is available.

At the same time Informed Choice leaflets (MIDIRS 1997) were being distributed at a national level. These leaflets had been commissioned by the National Centre for Research Reviews and Dissemination and sponsored by MIDIRS, the midwife organisation that provided an information service to practitioners on effective practice. These leaflets covered many issues relevant to antenatal care, care in labour and postnatal care. One of these leaflets dealt with place of birth.

The initial momentum for change came from the MSLC who produced a detailed response to the Health Authority's consultation document on the future of Edgware Community Hospital.

THE MSLC RESPONSE TO THE EDGWARE COMMUNITY HOSPITAL CONSULTATION DOCUMENT

The response was dated March 1996. Although the Community Health Council (CHC) had submitted a separate and detailed response to all aspects of the consultation document it was the response from the MSLC, with its entire focus on the proposed birth centre, that had the most impact. They quoted *Changing Childbirth* at length. They also tackled head-on the issue of risk. They recommended that the birth centre should be established and that midwives be given additional training. They made reference to a letter from the Royal College of Midwives to the Barnet MSLC, dated January 1966, that confirmed that it was RCM policy to support women's choice as described in *Changing Childbirth*. They stated that midwives were fully trained and competent to provide care in midwife-led maternity units and to refer women on to high-risk units or to general practitioners should this become necessary.

The MSLC made reference to the responses from the Wellhouse Trust midwives and from the Women's and Children's Directorate. This suggested a staged approach to allow protocols and skills to be developed.

The MSLC were concerned with another set of issues–emergency transport, paramedic and obstetric back-up. What was envisaged was that ambulances would be called in the same way as in a home delivery and that women would transfer from birth centre to obstetric unit as an emergency transfer, accompanied by a midwife. It would not involve calling out an obstetric flying squad.

The MSLC response emphasised the need to finalise selection criteria for booking in the birth centre, and for protocols for antenatal, intra-partum and postnatal transfer. They were concerned about continuity of care and the need for birth centre midwives to be involved in care if the woman needed to be transferred for any reason to the obstetric unit.

One issue of great importance was the size of the demand for this service. The MSLC had organised a number of surveys to assess the issue of demand as well as the attitude of GPs and midwives to the proposed birth centre service. They also referred to an earlier document from the Wellhouse Trust (January 1995) that made two key points. The first was the importance of proximity of the chosen place of birth to home. The second was the prediction that the demand for home births would rise.

THE GPs' VIEW

A survey was sent to 116 GPs who practised within a 5-mile radius of Edgware General Hospital. There were only 23 responses. Of those who replied:

- ten stated that they would refer to the centre if there was adequate obstetric and paediatric back-up
- nine stated that they would refer to the centre without reservation. Of these, three were enthusiastic

- three stated that they would not refer to the centre
- one stated that referral would only be made if the birth centre were situated alongside a consultant unit.

THE SITUATION ELSEWHERE

The MSLC had arranged for the work of other units to be discussed at its committee meetings. There were midwife- or GP-led units in Aberdeen, Scunthorpe, Eye, Chesterfield (with another due to open in Buxton), Penrith, South Wales and Bournemouth. In the area around Bath there were five stand-alone midwife/GP units, all attached to the main maternity unit. The MSLC also arranged for presentations to be made by managers of these established units. The midwife manager of the Darley Unit presented the experience of her centre, which was 13 miles from the obstetric unit in the district general hospital at Chesterfield: in reference to transfers between birth centre and obstetric unit, in its first year of operation (1994), of the 52 women who had booked to deliver in the centre 10 transferred in labour (19%).

SAFETY

The issue of safety was considered in great detail by the MSLC. Reference was made to the review of evidence carried out for *Changing Childbirth* and to *Where to be Born*, co-authored by Alison Macfarlane of the National Perinatal Epidemiology Unit (Campbell & Macfarlane 1993). Quoting from the latter the MSLC stated, '...there is no evidence to support the claim that the safest policy is for all women to give birth in hospital'. In fact, *Changing Childbirth* went further:

There is no clear statistical evidence that having babies away from general hospital maternity units is less safe for women with uncomplicated pregnancies. It is unlikely that it will ever be possible to know whether there is any difference in mortality: the perinatal mortality rate is now so low, and the number required to achieve a satisfactory sample size to detect a difference within comparable groups in a randomised trial would be prohibitively high.

The MSLC urged the Health Authority to consider the issue of risk in the light of the existing evidence and to focus on outcomes as well as processes. Clearly there would be transfers but these should be seen in the light of the skills of the midwives and the need to develop both selection criteria for initial booking in the centre and transfer protocols.

In conclusion, the MSLC recommended that:

• A survey should be carried out amongst women themselves to see whether they would wish to deliver in the birth centre. This would satisfy the requirement to consult before any change of service.

• Protocols should be developed covering selection criteria for the new centre and transfer to an obstetric unit.

• A staged approach should be adopted while the numbers booking at the centre build up.

• Consideration should be given to the opening of an additional birth centre when the new hospital in north-east Barnet was opened.

THE HEALTH AUTHORITY RESPONSE

The MSLC pursued the questions of selection criteria and transfer protocols through the establishment of a small working group of its own members. The Health Authority welcomed the development of these criteria and was supportive of the proposal to carry out a survey of women's views. Furthermore, they wished to find a way of exploring professional views both locally and nationally to see whether a consensus could be found on the issue of safety. It was decided to convene a special meeting of what amounted to an advisory panel that would include members of the MSLC and invited specialists nominated by four professional groups–the College of Paediatrics and Child Health, the Royal College of Obstetrics and Gynaecology, the Royal College of General Practitioners and the Royal College of Midwives.

All four of the professional bodies agreed to nominate specialists from their own membership and individuals were selected who had no local interest in the politics concerning the survival of the local hospital. The meeting was held in September 1996 and was chaired by the Health Authority's Director of Public Health. The meeting was also attended by local stakeholders–the Consultant Obstetrician and Clinical Director of Women and Children's Services, a second consultant obstetrician, a consultant paediatrician, a general practitioner, the Senior Midwife Community Services, the Senior Midwife of the Local Supervisory Authority, the Nurse/Midwife Adviser to the Health Authority, and the Chair and Past Chair of the MSLC. Written and oral submissions were presented by six of the members of the advisory panel. The conclusions of the meeting were that the Advisory Group:

• noted the extension of choices for women that were proposed in *Changing Childbirth* in relation to alternative methods of managing labour and place of delivery

• accepted the principle of low-risk units run by midwives, separate from consultant-led obstetric units

• considered such units to be best located adjacent to obstetric units

• had considered the conditions that might arise as an unexpected emergency for mother or baby in a low-risk unit and accepted that these risks were similar to those of delivering at home

• concluded that women would need to be informed of the necessary transfer arrangements for emergency obstetric (including caesarean section) and emergency paediatric care

• noted that local clinicians (midwives, obstetricians and paediatricians) would support a unit at Edgware if this was opened, but would strongly recommend siting such a unit at Barnet

• had considered the number of patients who would fall within the admission criteria adopted by the MSLC subgroup. Although the number of eligible women might be high the number who would opt for a low-risk unit might be closer to the number opting for home deliveries. This meant that it was difficult to estimate the likely number who would choose to deliver in the low-risk unit– possibly 100–200 in the first year

- had noted the results of a local survey of women that indicated support for such a unit.

The Advisory Group made the following recommendations:

- The Advisory Group was of the majority view that a low-risk birth unit on the Edgware site was supportable.
- The Advisory Group therefore recommended that the Health Authority pursue this option in terms of cost, accommodation and staffing.
- In view of the reservations of the representatives of the Royal College of Obstetricians and Gynaecology and of the College of Paediatrics and Child Health that such units should only be supported when in close proximity to an obstetric unit, the Advisory Group recommended that the option of a low-risk birth unit on the Barnet site should be given further consideration.

The conclusions of the special Advisory Group meeting give no hint of the argument and debate that went on at the meeting. In recalling the events it is difficult to capture the tone of the arguments–recall is perhaps coloured by a yearning for the dramatic. There was certainly a need to reach consensus among individuals who held strong personal views. Perhaps central to the debate was the contribution from the representative from the Royal College of General Practitioners. While recognising that GPs held diverse views he was an advocate both for community hospitals and for birth centres within them. He admitted that there were few examples of urban community hospitals but argued that the special circumstances of Edgware were in many ways similar to those of rural hospitals in that it was not the geographic distance between Edgware and Barnet that mattered but the perceived distance and the actual travel time.

Another important factor was the opinion of the representative of the Royal College of Midwives who was not a personal advocate of birth centres but, armed with the policy of her College, was willing to support the idea in principle. The views of the other two College representatives were antagonistic but not unreasonably so. Neither was able to produce evidence that addressed the issue of safety and neither was able to state unequivocally that birth centres were inherently unsafe, although that was clearly their opinion.

After consideration of the written and oral submissions the meeting came to an acceptable conclusion, with two College experts on each side of the argument. All four agreed that the Chairman draft a document for the Health Authority that was broadly supportive of the conditional establishment of the Edgware Birth Centre.

The Health Authority accepted the report and so began the next step in making the Edgware Birth Centre a reality.

THE QUESTION OF FUNDING

It was clear from an early stage that capital and revenue funding for the birth centre was unlikely to come from the existing budgets of the acute hospital trust. It was equally clear that the proposal for the birth centre was most likely to succeed if it were linked to the strategic development of Edgware Community Hospital. The Health Authority had agreed at a much earlier date that a new acute hospital would be built on the Barnet General Hospital site in the north-east corner of the Borough. At the time of the birth centre debate the new hospital was nearing completion and the plan was to move acute inpatient services from the Edgware hospital to the new Barnet hospital on April 1st 1997. This was when Edgware General Hospital would be transformed from an acute general to a community hospital.

One of the key issues was the provision of a range of facilities in the community hospital that would give local people a truly local service. There were two other proposals being considered that addressed this: one was the minor injuries unit; the other was the provision of intermediate care beds. These, like the birth centre project, were innovative and it was argued with the Department of Health that all three should have demonstrator pilot site status. Considerable pressure was put on the Department of Health, both at a political level and within the NHS, to support and fund such a proposal. The timing was fortunate in that the then Conservative Government was operating with a single figure majority and the voices of local Conservative MPs were loud and influential. The decision to change the status of Edgware General Hospital had been supported by an earlier Conservative government and the issue was sensitive in that the then Prime Minister was also a constituency MP within Barnet. It was therefore convenient in 1997 for the politicians to be seen to be supporting the development of Edgware Community Hospital because they did not wish the earlier decision to site the acute district hospital elsewhere to be revisited and criticised.

EVALUATION STRATEGY

The evaluation strategy will be only briefly introduced at this point. From early in 1990 Barnet Health Authority had been developing its capacity to evaluate its own services. It had a significant group of researchers in-house, headed by a consultant in public health with a health economics background. It had already developed a system for evaluating new developments and set aside around 10% of the operating budget for this purpose.

When the decision was taken by Ministers to allocate £2 million for the three demonstrator projects at Edgware the same proportion of funding was applied to the evaluation of these projects. Given the high visibility of the projects and the very strong local feeling that the Health Authority might have a conflict of interest if it

carried out the evaluation itself it was agreed that evaluation tenders should be invited from universities for all three projects. In the case of the birth centre the evaluation contract was awarded to Imperial College and this was managed by the Health Authority's Public Health Directorate. This was carried out through the establishment of an Evaluation Project Steering Group chaired by the Director of Public Health.

THE PUBLIC HEALTH PERSPECTIVE

The purpose of this chapter was to describe the public health role in the development of the Edgware Birth Centre. It has so far been mainly a description of events surrounding the origins of the Centre. In attempting to stand back and reflect on roles and responsibilities one runs the risk of overstating the positive aspects and understating the negative.

Public health as a practical discipline has several functions. In relation to health service developments it has to encompass the needs of a defined population within the reality of NHS funding. Within the NHS public health is (or was in 1996/97) based within defined geographical boundaries and in the case of North Central London the population of the London Borough of Barnet was the same population as that which came under Barnet Health Authority. On one side of Barnet were the separate London Boroughs of Brent and Harrow, whose populations came under a single health authority (the Brent and Harrow Health Authority); on the other side of Barnet were the separate London Boroughs of Enfield and Haringey, whose populations came under a single health authority (the Enfield and Haringey Health Authority). Edgware Community Hospital, as it came to be called, was on the border between Barnet and Harrow which meant that the responsibility for the local population, whose families had been using the hospital as its local acute hospital for a hundred years, fell between two local authorities and two health authorities. Although it is quite common for public health departments in health authorities and for environmental health departments in local authorities to work across boundaries this has traditionally been most successful in the management of communicable disease outbreaks. This has not been the experience in health service planning. In relation to the Edgware Birth Centre, joint planning was problematic, not least because budgets were closely aligned to individual organisations and were not pooled. With the emergence of Primary Care Groups and GP fundholding the responsibility for commissioning services was passing from the health authorities to these new bodies.

One of the successes of public health function in Barnet was the existence of a strong Community Health Council and active advisory groups. It would be difficult to cite another health authority district in the UK where the MSLC and CHC functioned at such a high level as champions of the health needs of their public. In many senses they were the second arm of public health and, in the eyes of many, the more vital arm. They had one important advantage over the Health Authority in that they were not constrained by the limited budget. They took the purist view and argued for what was best for women and what was best for the local population. Throughout this period the Public Health Department was involved with both the MSLC and the CHC and sought to facilitate the development of consensus on the issues surrounding the establishment of the birth centre. Given the

initial opposition from significant numbers of health professionals this was no easy task.

Another role for public health was that of advocate for the establishment of services and policies that were effective and safe. In the case of the birth centre this was one of the key issues. There were many practitioners, including public health practitioners, whose interpretation of the literature suggested that home delivery and birth centre delivery were less safe than delivery in hospital. Although there has been a large expansion in the literature of reviews that have considered the evidence of effectiveness it is difficult for the reader to evaluate the quality of these reviews. The argument for the safety of birth centres was strongly supported by the evaluative work that was carried out for and became part of the publication *Changing Childbirth*. Although health authorities themselves may, and in many cases do, carry out their own assessments of the quality of the evidence of effectiveness and safety, these local reviews are often of poor quality. It is unlikely that the Edgware Birth Centre could have been established without expert review of the evidence published in *Changing Childbirth* and in *Where to be Born*.

In conclusion, and with a substantial measure of 'recall bias', the role of public health was central in the establishment of the Edgware Birth Centre. It facilitated, it led (occasionally from the front but usually from behind), it orchestrated, it cajoled and, perhaps most important of all, it remained involved at every step of the way.

REFERENCES

Campbell R, Macfarlane A 1993 Where to be born–the debate and evidence. National Perinatal Epidemiology Unit, Oxford
Department of Health 1993 Changing Childbirth. The Stationery Office Books, London

MIDIRS 1997 Informed Choice leaflets. MIDIRS and The NHS Centre for Reviews and Dissemination, Bristol

8

From concept to reality: developing a working model of a stand-alone birth centre

Olive Jones
Jane Walker

INTRODUCTION

Edgware Birth Centre (EBC) opened in 1997. It is a 'stand-alone' facility sited in a community hospital in an urban area of north-west London. It is unique in that it is a collaborative venture–three different health trusts provide clinical care and a fourth (for the community hospital) provides estate administration. The birth centre is midwife-managed and there is no medical input on site. Clinical and operational guidelines have been developed as part of a risk management strategy. A guiding principle is that no procedure will be undertaken there that cannot safely be provided in a woman's home. If complications arise mothers and babies are transferred by ambulance to one of three consultant maternity units some 4–7 miles distant. For the first 2 years the EBC was a centrally funded Department of Health Demonstrator Project and so the opportunity arose for an independent evaluation of midwifery-led care in the stand-alone setting. It is worth considering how local history influenced the development of this service.

LOCAL HISTORICAL BACKGROUND

Until 1988 there were two maternity units in the Borough of Barnet which worked in partnership. One of these was a stand-alone maternity hospital (the Victoria Maternity Hospital) which had resident obstetric cover but was reliant on paediatric and anaesthetic cover provided by a general hospital half a mile away. There was a tradition of midwife-led care supported by obstetricians in this hospital long before the publication of the 'Winterton' report (Department of Health 1992) and *Changing Childbirth* (Department of Health 1993) and this influenced the subsequent direction of the maternity service. By 1988, however, the provision of paediatric attendance in emergency situations was becoming increasingly difficult and, although babies requiring intensive treatment were transferred to the consultant unit in Edgware, paediatricians deemed it unsafe to provide an obstetric service on a geographically isolated site. This was also a time of difficulty in recruitment and retention of midwives nationally. Taking these two factors into account, a decision was taken to close the Victoria Maternity Hospital and the Chief Executive pledged that the service would be reinstated in the new hospital in Barnet that was to be built in approximately 7 years' time and that two district hospitals would be maintained.

During the period of consultation on the closure of the 'Vic' the notion of a midwifery-only service took root and, although it was dismissed, the vision remained and was to come to the forefront in the mid 1990s. Although a pledge to maintain two district hospitals had been given, Chief Executives come and go, as do governments, and by 1996 it became clear that Edgware General Hospital would close once the new building in Barnet was commissioned.

The notion of a birth centre on the Edgware site was raised again and met with a mixed reception at the many meetings which were held to discuss it. The pivotal point came when a lay member of the local Maternity Services Liaison Committee (MSLC) asked 'Why can't we have a birth centre?'–no one could come up with a valid reason for not having one. From this point the MSLC became a major driving force in taking the development of the birth centre forward (see Ch. 6). Surveys were undertaken of women's views (Manero 1997) and referral intentions of general practitioners (M Meltzer Edgware Birth Centre: survey of GP referral intentions, Barnet Health Authority, unpublished, 1997). The results suggested that approximately two-thirds of women who were classified as 'low risk' would use the centre (although there was an acknowledged bias in that local feelings were running high about the proposed closure of the local hospital). GP opinions ranged from very supportive to total resistance to the concept of birth outside a consultant obstetric unit, and this information alerted us to a critical need for communication.

The Health Authority convened an expert advisory panel and evidence for and against the concept of a birth centre which was geographically separated from a consultant unit was debated (Baird et al 1996, Campbell & Macfarlane 1994, Hundley et al 1994). The outcome of this debate was an agreement that a birth centre would be provided to extend choice for local women and that funding would be sought for this (Fig. 8.1). A project plan and business case were submitted to the Director of Public Health to inform the application for central funding for a demonstration project of 2 years' duration (see Ch. 7). A general election was due in 1997 and the proposed closure of Edgware General Hospital attracted intense media coverage. It is likely in fact that the political agenda assisted us in driving the birth centre initiative forward and in securing financial resources. External funding of the project was critical in order to substantially reduce the financial risk to the participating Trusts, and in particular the host Trust.

THE PLANNING PROCESS

When funding was confirmed, a project leader was appointed to oversee the planning process and to liaise with, and draw together activities undertaken in, the various groups. A steering group was formed to drive the project forward, with midwifery and medical representation from the participating Trusts, GPs, public health representatives, lay members and senior managers. Expert opinions were sought on an ad hoc basis. Two subgroups were established, one to focus on operational issues and the other to develop clinical protocols (Fig. 8.2). Senior midwives from the host Trust took the lead in

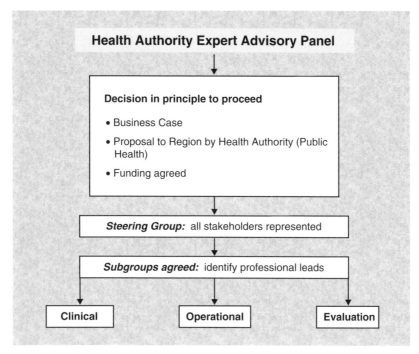

Figure 8.1 Taking change forward.

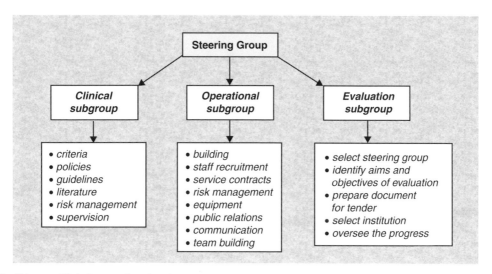

Figure 8.2 Edgware Birth Centre–the planning process.

each of these groups so that there would be 'ownership' of the birth centre as an integral part of the maternity service and to prevent marginalisation of the project. A third subgroup would be formed to initiate the independent evaluation process and this would have its own distinct steering group.

The groups held many meetings, requiring a substantial time commitment by those involved, and it was important that a clear agenda was set and that they were well structured and managed. There is nothing like managing a budget for a project to bring home the expense of meetings! People were generous with their time but sometimes locums had to be employed to free members (e.g. GPs) to attend and this proved expensive.

THE OPERATIONAL SUBGROUP

Extensive structural alterations to the allocated premises were required in order to create a home-from-home environment, with five en suite 'total episode of care' rooms, a sitting room, kitchen, office and storage rooms. A separate project team was responsible for translating our vision into reality and they worked closely with the project leader and operation group to develop a detailed specification. Infection control, health and safety, fire prevention, pharmacy, laundry, cleaning and catering departments all contributed to planning an appropriate care environment. Lay members were closely involved at all stages and chose the decor.

Service specifications were agreed with the ancillary departments that so often 'silently' ensure the smooth running of clinical areas. Specifications had to be made out in minute detail, with decisions having to be reached on items such as how often bins would be emptied, when porters would collect waste for disposal and how often curtains would be washed and carpets cleaned. In practice, we seem to have got it right most of the time. One problem that proved difficult to resolve was the return of duvet covers from the external laundry–eventually a washing machine was purchased and this laundry is now done by midwifery assistants in the birth centre.

Operational policies and procedures were written and approved by the participating Trusts and the Community Trust. The procedure for transfers to consultant obstetric units had to fit with the policy for the community hospital and as it was likely that paramedic assistance would often be required the London Ambulance Service (LAS) worked closely with us in developing a written procedure.

THE CLINICAL SUBGROUP

This group was responsible for developing acceptance and transfer criteria and clinical guidelines. The first task was to decide which women would be accepted for care in the birth centre (see Box 8.1) as the development of client information leaflets depended on this and it was planned that we would start booking women 3 months in advance of opening the centre. Reaching a consensus on acceptance criteria was probably the most difficult aspect of the project, with debate centring mostly on whether or not to accept nulliparous women in view of the high intrapartum transfer rate reported for these women when booked for birth at home or in a birth centre (Chamberlain et al 1997, Hundley et al 1994). To overcome the apparent deadlock it was agreed that only multiparous women (up to their fourth baby) would be accepted in the birth centre and that a review would take place after 6 months. That review resulted in the subsequent acceptance of first-time mothers. Still later, after the evaluation of the service and further consultation, the criteria were extended to include women having their fifth babies.

Much time was saved by securing permission to adopt the guidelines for midwife-led care developed in Leicester (Leicester Royal Infirmary NHS Trust 1997). These were customised for local use and some additional guidelines for managing emergency situations in the birth centre were developed (Jones 2000) and agreed by the three Trusts.

STAFF RECRUITMENT

An initial internal advertisement offering midwives a secondment to the project for a period of 2 years drew a poor response. Reasons cited were uncertainty about the future during a time of great change coupled with a lack of confidence that the substantive posts currently held would still be available if the project failed. The majority of midwives were also more comfortable working alongside obstetricians and expressed fears about the safety of providing

---

Box 8.1   Edgware Birth Centre acceptance criteria

Women should have good general health and an uncomplicated medical and obstetric history. The GP should indicate in the referral letter that there is no medical condition of which they are aware that would indicate the need for a heart and lung examination or require medical supervision of the pregnancy.

Inclusion criteria:

- Full-term singleton pregnancy, 37–42 weeks, with cephalic presentation
- Parity: 1st baby, 2nd, 3rd, 4th or 5th baby without previous complication or where recurrence of a previous complication is not anticipated
- Age: 16–42 years
- Weight: a body mass index of 18–30 before pregnancy.

Women with the following history/conditions should be booked in a consultant unit:

Diabetes	Haemoglobinopathies
Cardiac disease	Factor V Leiden deficiency
Renal disease	Epilepsy
Lung disease	Fractured pelvis
Pulmonary embolism	Congenital abnormality
Deep vein thrombosis	

Asthma: previous hospital admission, systemic medication currently, brittle asthma and where the condition is known to worsen in pregnancy are not suitable for EBC.

Thyroid disease: thyrotoxicosis. (N.B. a patient with correctly treated hypothyroidism may give birth at EBC but care must be shared with a consultant obstetrician and the baby referred to a paediatrician for assessment at age 5 days.)

Any other chronic condition that may affect well-being in the current pregnancy.

Previous caesarean section.

Rhesus antibodies. Other antibodies–seek advice from haematologist/paediatrician.

Significant PPH–consider individually and seek medical advice.

Spontaneous abortion: 3 or more, consecutive and not followed by normal birth.

Severe pre-eclampsia/PIH.

Previous shoulder dystocia.

Previous baby weight of 4500 g or more.

Previous IUGR–seek medical advice.

3° and 4° perineal laceration–seek individual advice.

Major gynaecological surgery including myomectomy and hysterotomy.

Cone biopsy, unless a subsequent vaginal delivery.

Mental health issues should be assessed on an individual basis.

Drug or substance misuse.

Heavy smoker (more than 20 per day).

HIV positive.

Hepatitis B positive.

Previous stillbirth or neonatal death should be assessed on an individual basis.

Last birth before 34 weeks–assess on individual basis.

Other factors at the discretion of GP and midwife in consultation with others involved in care.

---

care for women and babies in a stand-alone facility with no medical staff on site.

A subsequent external advertisement, however, resulted in an overwhelming response from midwives all over the country who were willing to give up their job security for an opportunity to participate in setting up a birth centre, regardless of whether employment contracts were for a fixed period of only 2 years.

Skill requirements for midwives in this stand-alone unit are identified in the job specification/description, which was developed as an integral part of the risk management profile of EBC. At least one year's post-registration experience is required which should if at all possible include out-of-hospital experience and some knowledge of home birth. Perhaps as important, is a willingness to adapt practice and learn new skills,

and to endorse the family-centred philosophy of EBC that engenders what the World Health Organisation terms a 'social model' of midwifery (Wagner 1994). These midwifery skills have been supported by an effective model of peer review and reflective practice through critical analysis of care, developed through the use of an independent Supervisor of Midwives. This innovative model has been described in a recent book on midwifery supervision. (Jones 2000).

The whole-time equivalent of six midwives, appointed from within and outside the Trusts, formed a core team which would provide at least one midwife on duty in the birth centre at all times, supported by a midwifery assistant (see Ch. 11) and community midwives from the three collaborating Acute Trusts (Fig. 8.3). Within 2 months of opening, the core midwives decided

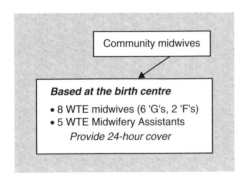

Figure 8.3 Staffing at Edgware Birth Centre.

that 12-hour shifts would be the most practical way of organising the off-duty and so two shifts emerged, 08.00 h to 20.15 h and from 20.00 h to 08.15 h. This was very much easier than trying to balance a three-shift system, especially with the small numbers of staff involved. There are several part-timers among the staff and rotas are managed flexibly, with negotiation and cooperation–again, a much simpler process with a smaller, discrete workforce. No one wears uniforms, but everyone wears a clear name badge which also states the employing Trust and job title. This contributes greatly to the concept of 'home-from-home' informality and to the breaking down of a 'them and us' culture (clients and carers).

Staffing arrangements for the birth centre are organised in such a way as to utilise manpower resources as efficiently as possible. Core midwives working twelve-hour shifts ensures that one midwife is on duty in the birth centre at all times. At weekends and during the night one core midwife and a midwifery assistant staff the birth centre. During weekdays and some evenings, in order to facilitate booking appointments, antenatal care and workshops, two midwives may be on duty. The second midwife is often employed on a part–time contract and the hours required for this additional input suit midwives who can only work during school hours. This provides an opportunity to retain a valuable work force. Core midwives and community midwives may come into the centre in the evening for workshops.

Two full-time community midwifery posts in the host Trust are funded from the birth centre budget, allowing for a community midwife to provide back-up cover for births when a core midwife is the primary carer. The host Trust operates on a 5% vacancy factor to fund bank staff at peak activity times and the birth centre is included in this arrangement. This pattern of working clearly requires great flexibility. It is the view of the authors that continuous team building, the autonomy of self-management and a problem-solving approach are the key motivating factors in the perceived ownership of the birth centre and the willingness of the staff to be flexible in terms of working patterns.

Originally, staffing was based on a prediction of up to 200 births in the first year and of between 200 and 400 births in the second. The number of deliveries taking place in a maternity unit has traditionally been the yardstick for funding and resource allocation. It soon became clear, however, that this measurement is not appropriate for EBC where rates of intrapartum transfers to consultant units are 14–16%. Care of these women in labour is resource-intensive, particularly as a midwife always accompanies the woman to the consultant unit and, when possible, continues to provide care there. The number of women who come to the birth centre *in labour* is now considered the most accurate baseline for activity. The critical volume, given the accommodation available and the requirement to retain a home-from-home ethos, is judged to be 500 women in labour per year and the current staffing is based on this figure.

Although the initial lack of interest from our own midwives was disappointing there was an advantage in the diversity of experience that those appointed brought to the project. It took 3 years for the birth centre to embed as an integral part of the maternity service. Midwives' confidence and interest has increased substantially over time and there is now a waiting list to work there. Several factors appear to have contributed to this turnaround, such as positive clinical outcomes, job satisfaction and, not least, the knowledge that the birth centre is here to stay! This has been reinforced by the Health Authority which has indicated its intention to continue commissioning the service, based on the direct response of users to the service and the outcome of the evaluation. When the centrally funded period ended in July 1999 there followed a period of intense negotiation with the three collaborating Trusts to clarify and agree the funding pathways. Absorption into mainstream funding has followed and permanent contracts issued to all staff.

One midwifery post is allocated to an internal rotation, with midwives from all three Trusts taking it in turn to work in the birth centre for 6 months. This arrangement has contributed greatly to a shared understanding of the nature of care in the different workplaces and has done much to resolve the 'them and us' culture that existed in the early days.

THE CARE PATHWAY

Women can access EBC via their hospital or community midwife, their GP, an obstetrician or by direct self-referral (Fig. 8.4). An information leaflet is available in GP surgeries, antenatal clinics and some local chemist shops and at least 25% of women self-refer. They can be accepted for care at any time in their pregnancy if they meet the agreed criteria, but they cannot be accepted for care once in labour, unless a formal booking has been confirmed. Women have been known to find out about the unit at 39 or 40 weeks of pregnancy, visit, book and return in labour all within 24 hours. According to the statistics most women are booking at around 28 weeks, perhaps when they feel reasonably confident that their pregnancy is progressing normally.

Once a woman has made initial contact with EBC she is informed of the criteria for acceptance before any other steps are taken. In most cases this avoids the woman coming to visit, wanting to book and then being disappointed. If all appears well she will be invited for an informal visit and she will be encouraged to bring along her partner or members of her immediate family. This is so that the nature of the care available can be discussed, i.e. midwifery-led care, no doctors or emergency facilities, and transfer in labour to an acute hospital if there are complications. The tenth 'Informed Choice' leaflet is used to facilitate this discussion (MIDIRS 1997).

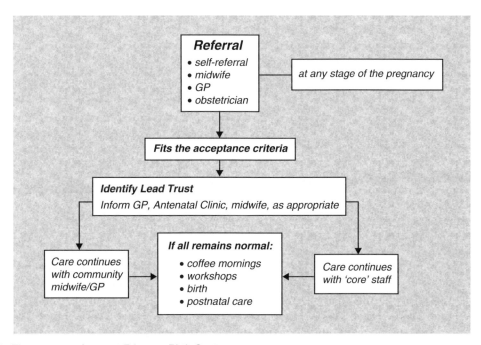

Figure 8.4 The process of care at Edgware Birth Centre.

It was initially envisaged that the focus would be on continuous care from one or two community midwives throughout pregnancy, birth and the puerperium, supported by the core team midwives, who would have a very small caseload of women who came from out of the district. As time went on it became clear that, for a variety of reasons, a large number of women were requesting to be booked with the core team. Sometimes it was because of a perceived resistance to the birth centre on the part of a GP or midwife; sometimes it was because there was no community midwife attached to the GP practice; and it was sometimes because it suited women to be able to come to the birth centre for antenatal care in the evening or at weekends, even though this would result in care being shared by a greater number of midwives. As a result, focus has shifted from continuity of carer to a shared philosophy of caring, continuity of care and one-to-one care during labour. Consequently two midwives moved to the centre from the community to augment the core team.

What is critical is that there is one-to-one care in labour, with a second midwife available when the birth is imminent. In the first stage of labour, because of the close proximity of the five birth/postnatal rooms in the centre, this one-to-one care may be shared with a midwifery assistant or a student midwife, or the couple may be happy to be together, knowing that there is someone just outside the door. Appropriate observations of maternal and fetal well-being are undertaken, but continuous electronic fetal monitoring is not employed in this home-like environment.

Other midwifery contact with women in the antenatal period will include some follow-up visits (for those women booked under the care of the core midwives); 'preparation for birth' workshops; and opportunities to meet informally with other women who are using the centre at 'drop in' sessions. There are also two workshops that focus on postnatal care: the 'baby basics' session and the 'baby massage' class. The baby massage workshop is held when the baby is approximately 6 weeks old and is not only very popular, but also gives women an opportunity to discuss their births with one another and with the midwives. The informal antenatal 'drop in' sessions also give women the opportunity to create peer support groups and these appear to thrive for some time after birth.

SKILLS ACQUISITION

Midwives were in post for 2 months before the birth centre opened, an orientation period in the consultant unit and an opportunity to gain any skills in managing emergency situations which they considered themselves to be deficient in. The skills which had to be acquired included the management of:

- adult and neonatal resuscitation
- shoulder dystocia
- breech delivery
- postpartum haemorrhage (including intravenous cannulation)
- cord prolapse.

Medical staff, specialist nurses/midwives and the local university collaborated to provide an intensive programme of training workshops.

In addition, midwives had to be competent in the examination of the newborn and in waterbirth. Of course this could not all be achieved within 2 months and some local GPs agreed to come to the birth centre and examine babies until midwives completed the necessary training. One of the midwives had extensive experience of the use of water in labour and birth and she not only facilitated workshops for her colleagues but also offered to come in at any time to assist her colleagues until they gained confidence. Such shared learning and peer support has become the norm and is instrumental in ensuring team cohesion.

COMMUNICATION

It was important not to become insular about the emerging birth centre and to share information and updates on progress with midwives, hospital medical staff, GPs, the public and anyone who expressed interest. We capitalised on media attention and the local newspaper printed articles from time to time and maintained an interest in our progress. Open days were held in the community hospital when the public and professional groups were able to observe progress and ask questions.

A named senior midwife and consultant obstetrician from each Trust, a registrar in public health, two GPs and a supervisor of midwives were identified to act as advisors to the birth centre and take issues back to their peer groups for discussion.

After the birth centre had been open for a few months women who had used the birth centre formed a consumer group. They meet regularly and a representative attends meetings of the management group that replaced the steering group when the project period was concluded. These lay representatives do sterling work on a voluntary basis, expressing consumer views of the service, fundraising, producing a newsletter and making other valuable contributions to the ongoing development of the birth centre.

AUDIT

Audit has become a firmly entrenched tradition in the birth centre. At the outset a detailed audit tool was developed to inform the independent evaluation (see Ch. 12 and Saunders et al 2000). Information on clinical outcomes, including the criteria for transfer to consultant care, continues to be collected and subject to audit. Standards on the following issues were also set and are audited regularly:

- booking in the birth centre
- antenatal screening
- care in pregnancy
- care in labour
- transfer in labour
- neonatal well-being
- maternal well-being
- health outcomes

- seeking women's views
- practice issues
- management of emergencies
- midwifery assistants' skills and role, including stock control and administration.

A final risk assessment took place in the building prior to the admission of the first 'client' and the birth centre opened its doors to business 9 months after the formation of the steering group. This seemed an eminently appropriate gestation period!

CONCLUSION

Although 9 months, from the decision to proceed and to the opening of the doors, is very tight this project was achievable mainly because the concept of a midwifery-led service had been in the minds of many people involved–members of the MSLC and the CHC, and senior members of the maternity services management and of the Health Authority–ever since the closure of the 'Vic'. A precedent for implementing other aspects of the *Changing Childbirth* agenda had already been accepted with the development of community-based midwifery services into teams and group practices: the midwifery leadership was able to build on these strengths.

To others planning a similar service, here are some key points:

- Examine carefully the local demography and evaluate the services already available.
- Seek the views of users of the service. This will establish a potential 'market' for the centre.
- Joint working across disciplines, Primary Care Trusts, Hospital Trusts, professional and 'lay' groups will be essential.
- Don't be afraid to welcome 'users' into the heart of the organisation.
- Meticulous planning is essential.
- Appropriate skills preparation and reflective practice support the risk management process.

The Edgware Birth Centre continues to grow and evolve. The community hospital on which it stands will soon be part of an extensive regeneration programme. The birth centre will then have a purpose-built facility designed within the specifications prepared by users and midwives together. A new phase will begin!

REFERENCES

Baird A G, Jewell D, Walker J J 1996 Management of labour in an isolated rural maternity hospital. British Medical Journal 312: 223–226

Campbell R, Macfarlane A 1994 Where to be Born? The debate and the evidence, 2nd ed. National Perinatal Epidemiology Unit, Oxford

Chamberlain G, Wraight A, Crowly P (eds) 1997 Home Births: the report of the 1994 Confidential Enquiry by the National Birthday Trust Fund. Parthenon Publishing Group, Carnforth

Department of Health 1992 Health Committee Second Report, Session 1991–92. Maternity Services. The Stationery Office Books, London

Department of Health 1993 Changing Childbirth. Report of the Expert Maternity Group. The Stationery Office Books, London

Hundley V A et al 1994 Midwife-managed delivery unit: a randomised controlled comparison with consultant-led care. British Medical Journal 309: 1400–1404

Jones O 2000 Supervision in a midwife-managed birth centre. In: Kirkham M (ed) Developments in the Supervision of Midwives. Books for Midwives Press, Hale

Leicester Royal Infirmary NHS Trust 1997 Evidence-based guidelines: intrapartum midwife-led care for midwives. Leicester Royal Infirmary Trust, Leicester

Manero E 1997 New midwifery unit in North London. 'Changing Childbirth' Update 9 June 1997: 21

MIDIRS 1997 Place of birth. Informed choice for professionals Leaflet 10 P. MIDIRS and the NHS Centre for Reviews and Dissemination, Bristol

MIDIRS 1997 Where will your baby be born–hospital or home? Informed Choice for Women Leaflet 10 W. MIDIRS and the NHS Centre for Reviews and Dissemination, Bristol

Saunders D et al 2000 Evaluation of the Edgware Birth Centre. Barnet Health Authority, London

Wagner M 1994 Pursuing the Birth Machine: the search for appropriate birth technology, Ace Graphics, Australia

9

Trusts in partnership–professional collaboration

Susan Dolman

INTRODUCTION

'Women will die!' The fist smashed down on the table and the room fell uncomfortably silent. This was the reaction of the Clinical Director of Obstetrics and Gynaecology at Northwick Park and St Mark's Hospitals to Barnet Health Authority's consultation paper on the relocation of Edgware General Hospital to Barnet.

It wasn't the relocation of the hospital that he saw as the problem–a small paragraph hidden in the middle of the lengthy document had caught his attention. Amongst the proposals for services to be provided on the Edgware site was the possibility of a midwifery-led birth centre. This had inflamed him and no one was surprised. He was renowned as a leading exponent of active management of childbirth, following the Dublin model and Northwick Park Hospital under his leadership had been well known for its active management of labour policy for 20 years.

Without delay he contacted his network of colleagues and before long both Northwick Park Hospital and Brent and Harrow Health Authority had responded to the consultation paper, indicating that they could not support the concept of a midwifery-only birth centre.

As to the rest of us, because we had had no prior warning of the proposal and could not foresee support or funding becoming available, we awaited Barnet Health Authority's final decision on the relocation of maternity services with no great hope of the courageous decision they would make. Credit must be given to the midwives, managers and supporters of Edgware General Hospital that Barnet Health Authority chose to support this ground-breaking enterprise.

This chapter will attempt to describe how the three local acute maternity units came to work together, how they had to overcome local resistance within their own units and how they were then able to collaborate together to provide support and momentum for the birth centre. It is intended as a practical guide for anyone considering setting up a similar project.

The complexity of the relationships involved was enormous, involving three Hospital Trusts, three Health Authorities, two Local Supervising Authorities (LSAs) and finally a fourth Trust, which was introduced when Barnet Healthcare, a primary health care trust, took over the management of the Edgware site.

The project would not have succeeded without the support and enthusiasm of key local general practitioners and representatives from local women's groups who were often able to contribute practical, objective suggestions and alternatives and were instrumental in maintaining focus. This chapter will highlight aspects of the planning process, the collaboration on preparation of guidelines and training and education programmes, and finally will look to the future and ask how the Edgware Birth Centre may become a model for other maternity care providers around the country.

THE BACKGROUND

The reaction of the Clinical Director will be familiar to many midwives. Consultant obstetricians form their opinions from research and experience of complicated childbirth; most (including our Clinical Director) would happily agree, however, that uncomplicated, normal midwifery is best left in the hands of midwives.

Shortly after this incident, in the spring of 1996 midwifery representatives from Northwick Park and the Royal Free Hospitals were invited to a meeting at the maternity unit at Edgware General Hospital. It was announced at this meeting that Barnet Health Authority was interested in bidding for development funding from the Department of Health to set up a midwifery-only low-risk birth centre on the Edgware site, once the consultant maternity unit had relocated to Barnet.

Due to the geographical situation of the Edgware hospital it was felt that women from the catchment areas of all three of the hospitals represented would be attracted to the unit. It was agreed by everyone at the meeting that the general aim of the unit should be that low-risk women could choose to go there, attended by their own community midwife, who they knew and trusted, no matter which Hospital Trust employed these midwives. This appealed to everyone–GPs, midwives, Community Health Council (CHC) and Health Authority representatives.

There was surprise that Northwick Park Hospital midwives were keen to be involved, given the views that had been widely expressed by that hospital in response to the public consultation. However, the opportunities for both women and midwives appeared overwhelming and midwives from all three Trusts were united in their vision of bringing together all the aspects and recommendations of *Changing Childbirth* (Department of Health 1993), famously summarised in terms of choice, continuity and control.

The timescale of the project was daunting. The Edgware maternity unit was planned to relocate to Barnet in April 1997 and it was hoped that the birth centre could open as soon as possible after that, in little over a year's time. The task of the Director of Public Health at Barnet Health Authority was to secure funding and approval for the project from the Department of Health; the midwives' task was to gain the support of their own Directorates and Trusts, not entirely easy given their views.

Much has been written on organisational behaviour and resistance to change. Robbins (1991) summarised the reasons why individuals may resist change: habit, security, economic factors, fear of the unknown, and selective information processing. All these factors emerged when the project was presented to the individual Trusts and were displayed not least by many of the mid-wives themselves. The midwives, particularly those at Northwick Park Hospital who had worked and been confident with active management of labour for so long, anticipated a complete change in the way they worked, a way which they were essentially very comfortable with.

The first step was to identify individual obstetricians and midwives who would be sympathetic and encouraging towards the project. The Clinical Director at Northwick Park Hospital had changed and the new Director was known to be fully supportive of midwives' taking more responsibility and being accountable for their practice. He was at once enthusiastic and offered to be the obstetrician advisor to the project and to inform the Trust Board about the project. Every opportunity was taken to spread the news of the project–regular midwifery meetings, Directorate meetings, Maternity Services Liaison Committee (MSLC) meetings and Midwifery Education meetings. Meetings were also held with the marketing and finance departments to ensure that they were kept abreast of the anticipated changes.

It became quite clear at a very early stage that not everyone supported the project, but what was particularly disappointing was the number of midwives who were actively discouraging. Kotter and Schlesinger (1979) put forward six suggestions for dealing with resistance to change:

1. Training, education and communication–ensuring that everyone understands the reasons for the change and that they can relate to it and in effect 'buy into' it.
2. Participation–involving people in the planning and decision-making, which makes it more difficult for them to criticise later.
3. Facilitation and support–listening to fears and anxieties and providing for them (e.g. as skills training, provision of expert advice).
4. Negotiation–making clear the advantages of the new way of working, what is gained and what is lost.
5. Manipulation and Co-option–emphasising the attractive features of the project and getting people to take responsibility for planning specific areas of the project.
6. Coercion–making it clear that the project *will* go ahead and that not being involved is not an option.

These processes continued throughout the planning period and the opening of the birth centre and continue today as new staff are introduced who bring with them their own anxieties.

PLANNING

Having started the process of communication, a more formal process of planning was introduced. A steering committee was set up in December 1996, with midwifery representation from the three Trusts, Barnet Health Authority's Director of Public Health, local GPs, the LSA officers, a paediatrician, two obstetricians and lay representatives from Barnet CHC and the National Childbirth Trust. The Department of Health had agreed to fund the birth centre for the first 2 years as a demonstrator project and an independent evaluation on the birth centre would be published in 2000.

The philosophy of the birth centre was quickly agreed–choice would be increased for those local women who would have been suitable for home confinement by providing a small homely unit. Informed choice would be supported and women would be involved in the planning of their care, which would be according to their individual needs and would be evidence-based. Women and their families were to come first. They were to be cared for in such a way that they would feel safe, confident and totally involved in all aspects of their care. The model of care to be adopted was a 'one-to-one' approach (Page 1996). A small core team would be employed to provide 24-hour continuing care and back-up support, while small groups of midwives from the three Trusts would work in pairs, booking a personal caseload of 40 women per year.

A number of subgroups were immediately established within the committee to address:

- clinical protocols
- risk strategy
- manpower planning

- training and education
- supervision of midwifery
- project management.

Midwifery representatives from all three Trusts and lay members were involved with each subgroup and midwifery educationalists, LSA officers and architects were co-opted on to the relevant working subcommittees as required. All three Trusts nominated a number of different midwives as representatives for these subgroups. This not only ensured that no one person took on too much work, but that midwives with particular strengths and interests could become involved and communicate progress back to their own departments.

As time was so short it was imperative that the work was broken down and shared between these groups, who reported back to the steering committee at every meeting. The steering committee initially met fortnightly and it was inevitable that not all members were able to attend every meeting. One of the consultant obstetricians very quickly formed the view that the birth centre was a midwifery project and that decisions should be made by midwives, but added that he would be available to give advice or opinion whenever it was needed. This in itself gave the midwives confidence that they were working in the right way and could achieve their goals.

Barnet Health Authority provided a list of all the GP practices whose referral patterns were likely to change when the Edgware consultant maternity unit moved to the Barnet site. Midwives from Northwick Park Hospital and the Royal Free Hospital visited them individually to introduce themselves, explain the changes and introduce the plans for the birth centre. Most of the practices did indeed change their referral patterns as most women choose to attend their nearest maternity unit, but one or two preferred to continue to refer to the unit they had worked with for years, particularly as the unit at Barnet would be new, modern and purpose-built.

When the Edgware maternity unit finally moved to Barnet a few of their midwives chose to leave and take up posts with either Northwick

Park Hospital or the Royal Free Hospital, partly because of travelling distances from their homes but, more encouragingly, also because in this way they could continue to work with the same GPs and with the women they already knew. This was very good news for these two hospitals as having midwives who already knew the site of the birth centre and the geography of the area helped to integrate the changes. It was not an entirely easy step for these midwives, who had been very happy working at the Edgware hospital, and inevitably they met some resentment amongst their new colleagues who saw them as representing the changes being imposed on them. These midwives were particularly welcome at Northwick Park Hospital as some community midwives immediately volunteered to partner them–they probably wouldn't have had the confidence to volunteer to work in the birth centre without this 'expert' support. The GPs who felt that they were losing 'their' maternity unit also welcomed it, because they were still able to work with midwives they knew and trusted.

The subgroup tasked with drawing up the clinical protocols, after careful research, saved a lot of time by gaining permission to use evidence-based guidelines on intrapartum care developed by another maternity unit (Leicester Royal Infirmary NHS Trust 1997). They were then able to concentrate on developing protocols for emergency situations, breech births, intravenous cannulation, neonatal resuscitation, postpartum haemorrhage and transfer to consultant units.

As these protocols for emergency situations were drawn up they were circulated to all three Trusts to ensure that all the midwives were satisfied and that they were workable. They were circulated amongst paediatricians, anaesthetists, obstetricians and midwives in the three units and returned with suggestions, amendments and improvements incorporated. There was surprisingly little disagreement or conflict because they were evidence-based.

Strict acceptance criteria were agreed by the three Trusts. This reassured the community midwives, as only women with a normal healthy pregnancy and anticipating a normal birth would be accepted for booking at the birth centre.

The London Ambulance Service was exceptionally helpful in drawing up the transfer policy. They appreciated the philosophy of the birth centre and agreed that women should be transferred to the maternity unit of their choice, traffic conditions permitting, rather than to the nearest unit. This usually meant that they went to the Trust unit their community midwife was based at–she accompanied them and very often continued their care. Women occasionally chose one of the other Trusts, but all three trusts agreed that a woman's own midwife should have access to continue to care for her if this was appropriate.

Women were to be asked at booking to the birth centre which hospital they would like to be transferred to in the event of an emergency so that they could give a considered opinion. This also meant that the birth centre could send a list of women's names and their expected dates of confinement to each delivery suite so that should they arrive at the hospital in an emergency there would be some awareness of them. (All women also carry their own records with them.) It was also agreed by all three Trusts that community midwives should be able to refer women directly to consultant care either in the antenatal period or in labour.

The steering group agreed that funding for the core staff should go to the Wellhouse Trust and that a midwife and a midwifery assistant would provide 24-hour continuing care within the birth centre and act as support for the community midwives. Each of the three Trusts would then provide the community midwives to accompany women into the unit. Their funding would depend on their activity.

The subgroup addressing supervision of midwives also considered the risk strategy. Birth statistics and details of adverse incidents were to be kept and reported back to the steering committee and all midwives working in the birth centre were to be invited to attend a weekly peer review meeting. A supervisor of midwives would facilitate these meetings, but midwives would be required to reflect on their practice,

present their own cases, debate outcomes and, if necessary, recommend changes to the guidelines. All community midwives would continue to have a named supervisor of midwives at their own Trust with whom they could discuss care plans and concerns, and they would also have access to a supervisor of midwives on site at the birth centre.

A training needs analysis was conducted and a series of workshops was set up at the Edgware site, attended by midwives from all three Trusts. This allowed midwives to get to know each other, share their concerns and appreciate how daunting the project was for everyone, including these midwives from the host site.

Each of the Trusts found that their midwives needed additional support and training in specific areas. At Northwick Park Hospital, for example, only a few midwives were experienced in caring for women labouring in water as only women who had hired their own pools had had that opportunity. Fortuitously, a new birthing pool was installed at the hospital and so midwives there were able to gain extra training and experience before the birth centre opened.

By this time, enthusiasm and apprehension had led the midwives at Northwick Park Hospital to embark on a complete overhaul of their labour-ward midwifery policies. At that time these reflected the long association there with active management of labour. With the encouragement and support of their link lecturer in midwifery, the midwives decided to use the method of the Leicester guidelines, drawing up their own evidence-based guidelines covering every aspect of midwifery care in labour. These were finally produced in November 1999 and encouraged the midwives to book more clients for midwifery-only care within the maternity unit. This is just one example of how the Edgware project effected change, not only amongst community midwives, but also back in the hospital units.

The steering committee continued to meet, collect and ratify the work completed by the subgroups and started to concentrate on marketing the service in anticipation of the opening. Newsletters were sent out to GPs, women's groups and all local health facilities, articles were printed in local papers and professional journals, and conferences were planned. Everyone on the committee–the representatives of the three hospital Trusts, and the Health Authority, the lay members and the GPs–were committed to spreading the news of the Edgware Birth Centre's opening in August 1997 at every opportunity.

THE FUTURE

The Edgware Birth Centre has been open for some years now and activity increases year on year. The independent evaluation (Saunders et al 2000) provided an almost entirely favourable report and summarised by reporting that it is popular with women, birth centre midwives and midwives from other Trusts, that women experience low intervention rates and few complications, and that it is a less expensive alternative to hospital care for low-risk women.

It would be encouraging if maternity service providers across the country might be stimulated to consider offering a similar service but they would be advised to assess carefully whether it would meet the needs of their own locality.

Coincidentally, a neighbouring health authority, Brent and Harrow Health Authority, set up a public consultation exercise to review their maternity services, producing the report *Changing Childbirth in Brent and Harrow* (1999). This followed the merger of their two NHS hospital trusts (Northwick Park and St Mark's Hospitals Trust and the Central Middlesex Hospital Trust) to form the North West London Hospitals NHS Trust. This consultation was one of the fullest health service public consultations to date. It involved a number of formal and informal public presentations, local media reports, focus groups, independent assessments and conferences over a period of 6 months. The five options for change included the setting up of a midwifery-only birth centre on the Central Middlesex Hospital site, relocating the current consultant unit to the Northwick Park Hospital site. This was the overwhelmingly preferred option at the end of the public consultation period and plans at the North-West London Hospitals NHS Trust are advancing to provide a birth centre based on the model provided by the Edgware Birth Centre.

There is no doubt that the women of Brent and Harrow lived closely enough to Edgware to have read about the unit, to have friends and relatives who had delivered there and to feel that they would also like the choice of a similar facility. However, GPs, obstetricians, paediatricians and midwives were also part of the consultation process. Many of them had taken part in the Edgware project and it is encouraging to find that they want to replicate that experience within their own boundaries.

REFERENCES

Brent and Harrow Health Authority 1999 Changing Childbirth in Brent and Harrow. Brent and Harrow Health Authority, London

Department of Health 1993 Changing Childbirth. Report of the Expert Maternity Group. The Stationery Office Books, London

Kotter JP, Schlesinger LA, 1979 Choosing Strategies for Change. Harvard Business Review March–April: 106–114

Leicester Royal Infirmary NHS Trust 1997 Evidence-based guidelines: intrapartum midwifery-led care for midwives, Leicester Royal Infirmary NHS Trust, Leicester

Page L 1996 Reclaiming Midwifery. Midwives 109 (1304): 248–253

Robbins SP 1991 Organisational behaviour, concepts, controversies and applications. Prentice-Hall International, London, P640–642

Saunders D et al 2000 Evaluation of the Edgware Birth Centre. Barnet Health Authority, London

10

A GP's perspective

Jean Beney

THE INCEPTION

I have been proud to be the GP representative involved with this highly successful unit from its inception. I became involved because for years I had been the GP representative on the Barnet Maternity Services Liaison Committee (MSLC). The Edgware Birth Centre was literally 'born' from discussions held years ago during those committee meetings.

I cannot lay any claim to its vision, other than pointing out initially that I thought a barrier to home delivery locally was the poor and over-crowded living conditions found in the deprived area in which I practise. The birth centre was seen as a compromise, with delivery in a natural, home-like environment. It was also in line with government thinking about increasing the numbers of midwife-only deliveries, while keeping an eye on safety and preserving the rare resource of midwife numbers. Home deliveries are always seen to be labour intensive in terms of midwife-hours per birth. Midwifery assistants are employed at Edgware Birth Centre to help with some of the basic tasks as there are always trained midwives on site 24 hours a day.

The birth centre is midwife-led and is attractive to midwives, enabling them to practise freely and safely in a non-medical setting. A personalised service is offered, more in line with home delivery, but creating a better environment than is found in many homes in the area in which we work. The percentage of the population able to access this kind of service is therefore considerably increased.

The birth centre provides a pleasant, safe environment, pet free, for users and staff alike.

I think my comments about living conditions spurred people on to make the centre environment just like a very attractive, spacious, well-furnished home environment. We have all joked on the committee about 'moving in' ourselves as it is so attractive and homely!

THE FIRST BIRTH CENTRE AT EDGWARE

The rooms are large and attractive, decorated in pastel shades with pretty friezes. The beds are not standard hospital beds but divans with headboards although, of course, due attention has been paid to maintain necessary hygiene. Windows and beds are dressed attractively in a smart domestic rather than clinical fashion. It was decided to install special washable carpet on the bedroom floors to complete the non-clinical feel although this met with some controversy. The en suites are spacious, just like a luxury domestic en suite.

The birth centre is now sited in what was a busy district general hospital with an active obstetric unit, which was closed down after 160 years of successful service, in the centre of the deprived area. This is highly relevant to the story, as it has led to uncertainties and complications in the physical setting up of the birth centre (twice within such a short timespan). It was a shame that the birth centre could not have been set up with a clear run, without so much controversy and political attention. The unit was set up initially in a dark, damp semi-basement of Edgware General Hospital that had originally been part of the eye ward and unit. The conversion into an attractive, functional birth centre was quite extraordinary and I would never have dreamt that a unit of such a high standard could be physically achieved there. Due credit must go to a whole host of people with vision, especially Elizabeth Manero, who pushed the scheme through at several levels under the auspices of the Community Health Council.

There were problems when the birth unit was in its semi-basement, mainly to do with access and security. Some patients found it hard to find. For part of the time it was adjacent to a major building site as the original maternity unit block opposite was gutted and refitted as the regional adolescent psychiatric unit. The noise and dust were a major irritation. At times it was difficult for ambulances to access the unit in an emergency, which was crucial for obstetric unit transfers. Safety was, however, maintained at all times. The ground was on such a slope that it narrowed vertically at one end into an unusable wedge shape, cutting down the available space for the unit.

Some of the midwives felt vulnerable working at night in an isolated unit (with, by definition, low staffing levels) in the middle of this building site. As building work progressed the unit became increasingly separated from areas of the hospital which were occupied at night, such as the wards and the Urgent Treatment Centre. A lot of attention was paid to this, with the installation of heavy locked doors and a video-controlled entrance.

Another problem, however, could not be readily overcome as the birth centre was sited in a 'second-hand' building and the unit upstairs was also a repositioned unit. This unit was the psychiatric outpatients department and the fire escape led straight down from that unit into the birth centre! It certainly did not inspire confidence in the staff, although I think most patients did not realise. The other factor was that if the psychiatric outpatients department was not locked securely at night the birth centre was totally vulnerable.

THE SECOND AND SUBSEQUENT BIRTH CENTRES AT EDGWARE

The move to the second site was necessary because there has been so much controversy and mayhem over the whole of the Edgware site that, relatively late in the day, it was decided to demolish the block that the original birth centre was sited in to make way for a whole new building. In that area of the original hospital site there will be a small, modern purpose-built facility, providing a variety of clinical services as a community hospital.

The second site for the birth centre is far superior–on the ground floor of one of the surgical blocks in one of the old inpatient wards. There is more space available, it is completely above ground, not damp, with higher ceilings and more spacious rooms. The difference in natural light intensity is quite exceptional.

The original design and colour schemes have been copied from the first physical unit, although with some minor 'tweaking', and improvements have been made with the benefit of experience. The midwives feel much happier working in the current unit as they feel safer above ground and the entrance is off the main corridor of the hospital and more secure than the dark, secluded back entrance to the first unit. There is a fire escape at the back of the unit but it does not have any contact with psychiatric patients and the whole unit is currently sited near 24-hour facilities such as inpatient wards and the Urgent Treatment Centre.

A third, and permanent replacement birth centre is planned as part of the new building. As part of the planning process as much attention as possible has been given to privacy. Easy vehicular access to the new unit is planned for patients arriving in labour and for the few that are transferred on by ambulance to a local obstetric unit. The whole idea of the community hospital is still shrouded in controversy although, of course, if the district general hospital had still been up and running there would not have been the space to develop the birth centre and we would still have had the full obstetric unit.

The closure of the hospital was perhaps the biggest mistake in the history of the NHS, of such magnitude that no one will now admit to its authorisation. The main loser in this sorry political 'game' has been the local area, already deprived, and now deprived of its hospital as well. It has also severely squeezed secondary care provision for a vast area of North London and Hertfordshire. The pressures are intolerable, far in excess of those we predicted as we tried to fight the hospital closure.

A BRIGHT NEW FUTURE

The Edgware Birth Centre has been one of a very, very few health developments locally in recent years and has been broadly welcomed as 'something positive happening locally in a sea of such negativity'. It is to the credit of those running the birth centre that it is run so well and in the midst of such adversity, with the hospital reconfiguration, and with yet another physical move planned in the next few years.

The birth centre provides not only a high standard of intrapartum care, but also offers antenatal care and postnatal follow-up. There is an attractive meeting room with large comfortable pink settees which looks much like a large domestic lounge. This room is ideal and is used for meetings and group work. There was a similar room in the original birth centre but the current one is larger and far more suitable for the numbers involved in meetings. There is active follow-up of past patients and social events are arranged, such as picnics. Opportunities for fundraising are also explored.

THE POPULATION SERVED

The local area has an ever-rising population, and is quoted as having the fastest growing population in the country. This is partly due to a high birth rate (the rate in my own surgery is four times the rate of some surgeries only a few miles away) and partly due to settling by poor people, asylum seekers and refugees. The area is characterised by a combination of local authority housing, ranging from a pleasant 1927 'Village Estate' officially designated a conservation area, ugly sixties high-rise blocks of unsound concrete construction, a massive, highly unpopular sixties and seventies concrete jungle of an estate (with most of the problems), a seventies estate of middling quality, some new and attractive (albeit miniscule) housing stock, and some fabulous housing for disabled families.

There is not a lot of self-respect in the area–or respect for others and their property. There is litter, violence, drug use, graffiti, poverty, drunkenness, gambling, poor educational attainment, and general deprivation. The black market is huge, facilitated by shops and individuals that readily exchange goods for money, no questions asked, both purchasing and selling. Cash is often used, and in large quantities, rather than the more traceable cheque and plastic card transactions favoured these days by people with bank accounts. Many of the people who find themselves living there live in fear and stress.

There is a sprinkling of thirties semis near the birth centre and, within a mile or two, some very nice, very expensive houses. Even some of the local authority properties, which have been sold off privately as a result of various past government initiatives, fetch a relatively high price due to their proximity to central London and the general shortage of housing locally.

One of the adverse comments that have been made about the birth centre is that the 'clientele' it attracts does not reflect the socio-economic profile of the local population. This is hard either to confirm or deny as the population, especially once you travel a mile from the birth centre, is very mixed. My own practice has been the highest referrer to the birth centre and certainly most patients live within a reasonable distance. There may be some skewing ethnically, as some patients from ethnic minorities do not meet the (very reasonable) criteria laid down for acceptance for delivery at the birth centre.

THE ACCEPTANCE CRITERIA

A multidisciplinary team, which included the steering group, drew up the acceptance criteria initially but opinions were sought from wider professional groups, including paediatricians. We were very keen from the start to err very much on the side of caution, both for the good of the individual mothers and children and for

the future of the unit as a whole. Any unnecessary morbidity or, perish the thought, mortality would have been completely unacceptable in a new unit working in such a new way. For the sake of brevity and clarity I will mainly discuss the acceptance criteria as they stand now, although they have been reviewed and refined at least four times.

Naturally, as there are no medical staff on site for the unit, women are chosen who are in good general health and who have uncomplicated medical and obstetric histories. GPs are asked to cooperate and not to refer women for booking at the unit who do not meet this basic criterion. It is understood that there is no physical examination carried out of the heart and lungs and any women who require this should be referred to a full obstetric unit for care. Women who require medical supervision of the pregnancy are also to be excluded by the GP and not referred for consideration of delivery at Edgware Birth Centre. I feel there has been good cooperation by GPs locally in this aspect of the patient's care. It avoids unsafe practice and disappointment for the woman and her family who might otherwise be excluded from the unit at a later stage in the pregnancy for complications that could have been anticipated and predicted from the start.

There has been considerable pressure exerted on the unit by women wanting to book but who did not fulfil the criteria. This has generated considerable disappointment and the main reasons for booking refusal have been noted. Periodically, the group has reviewed the criteria. Initially, primiparous mothers were excluded from booking at the birth centre. I supported that view as I was always taught that 'a primiparous pelvis is an untested pelvis'. Primiparous state was such a common reason for refusal that it was reviewed once the unit was up and running.

It was agreed, although I must admit I was a bit hesitant to give primips a trial. It was realised from the start that the rate of transfer to a full obstetric unit would rise once primips were accepted. This was seen as a problem as transfers have always been seen as a 'failure' on the part of the unit. It was felt initially that transfers were a measure of poor selection criteria or poor selection by the staff. This hardly seems fair when there was so much pressure for primips to be accepted. The transfer rate has risen as predicted with the new criteria.

The relation of maternal age and acceptance has also caused a lot of grief for staff. The minimum age was revised down to 16 years, which may seem young. However, there is a large proportion of very young mothers in our local population, when compared to the rest of the country as a whole. This is a reflection of poor socio-economic circumstances, with many young women viewing pregnancy, especially pregnancy early in life, as the only way of securing local authority housing. The girls are also often encouraged by their own families, in a bid to relieve overcrowding in the parental home. Aspirations for educational achievement are also low and provide no bar to pregnancy at a young age, as they might in higher socio-economic communities. The young ones actually do very well as in a more 'natural' society this would be the peak age for reproduction. The younger girls especially welcome the more homely one-to-one care the unit can offer.

Many older women are excluded on a variety of health grounds. There was a request to include multiparous women who do not have any other health complications, up to the age of 45 years. It was concluded by the team that this would be unwise but a compromise has been reached and multips are now accepted up to the age of 42 years.

INCLUSION CRITERIA

1. *Predicted normal pregnancy and labour*:
   a. between 37 and 42 weeks of pregnancy (i.e. term)
   b. singleton pregnancy
   c. cephalic presentation
2. *Parity*–women expecting their first or fifth baby or any baby in-between:
   a. without previous complication
   b. with a previous complication that is not anticipated to recur
3. *Age*: 16 years or over and up to 42 years of age

4. *Weight*: the body mass index pre-pregnancy must lie between 18 and 30. Considerable discussion has been stimulated by this criterion but it was felt that it was important that only those in the healthiest weight range should be included for the pregnancy and delivery. It was also felt that although the ceiling of 30 BMI would exclude some patients this was necessary as the women would be considerably heavier at term. Safety issues were expressed with regard to use of the pool and the physical strength required of the midwives in the event of a woman having to be helped out in an emergency.
5. *Good general health*: obstetric or medical opinion would be obtained in cases of doubt.

EXCLUSION CRITERIA

1. *Medical/Surgical history*: excluded conditions are listed in Box 8.1. Much debate was aroused by the inclusion of asthma as it is such a widely diagnosed condition and specific criteria were laid down to include patients with mild asthma whilst still maintaining stringent exclusions necessary for safety reasons, including:
   a. previous hospital admission for asthma as an adult
   b. women requiring *tablet* medication for asthma
   c. brittle asthmatics
   d. a past history of worsening asthma in pregnancy
2. *Previous obstetric and gynaecological history*: factors are listed in Box 8.1
3. *Mental health issues*:
   a. each case to be considered on its own merit
   b. the effect of medication on the unborn child
   c. the effect of medication on the presumed normal delivery
4. *Paediatric and neonatal considerations*: a number of conditions are not deemed acceptable for delivery at Edgware Birth Centre and a paediatric opinion should be sought (see Box 8.1)

5. *Other exclusion criteria*:
   a. other factors at the discretion of the midwife
   b. other factors at the discretion of the GP
   c. other factors at the discretion of others involved with the woman's care.

The acceptance and exclusion criteria are designed to promote safety and individualised care.

GENERAL PRACTITIONER SUPPORT

Without GP support the unit would not have remained viable. It has not all been plain sailing and I have had to deal with colleagues who are anxious and sometimes frankly hostile. At the same time I have had to consolidate my own beliefs and feelings as senior partner of the adjacent practice. My professional views about the unit are those of a woman and have been influenced by my experience as a house officer working on the obstetric unit 25 years ago at Edgware. More recently I have received feedback from patients and my own excellent attached midwife.

On a personal note, I used the maternity services twice over at Edgware, 23 and 24 years ago, when it was a consultant-led unit. Last year I became a grandmother when my daughter gave birth at the 'local' replacement obstetric unit 7 miles away. I would have liked my daughter to deliver in the birth centre but respected her wishes to deliver in a full obstetric unit. This was my most up-to-date, 'virtually first-hand' experience of modern obstetric care and, quite frankly, I was appalled.

I had rejoiced in the memory of good, sound care from my working in the local unit 25 years ago and my own two children's births. I had no idea that standards had been allowed to fall so unacceptably low in every parameter over the last 22 years. I have no idea of when and how this decline occurred. I thought that the unit where my daughter delivered had a reasonable standard of care or I would have dissuaded her from delivering there. Eight months later, she is still talking about her traumatic experience. Her personal poor experience in what should have been a reasonable obstetric unit has further influenced my determination to foster the birth centre ethos for wider dissemination.

WHAT IS DIFFERENT ABOUT A BIRTH CENTRE?

There is more to birth centres than normal deliveries and no doctors! I feel we should be using the high standards of maternal and family birth experience enjoyed at Edgware Birth Centre as the gold standard for full obstetric units to aspire to.

Historically, even good units paid little attention to maternal or family wishes about such things as maternal position of delivery. In certain high-risk cases, unfortunately, personal requests do have to be overridden because of the necessarily interventionist nature of the delivery. However, even women having completely straightforward, normal, quick deliveries without the slightest complication would not have been given any choice of birth position. The standard 'on your back' position must be the most unnatural and least mechanically advantageous position for giving birth naturally that could possibly have been conceived (pardon the pun!). I was never taught such an obvious fact as a medical student or obstetric houseman–perhaps my male consultants and registrars did not know either–or just did not care. Any men reading this who are in any doubt just need to imagine 9 months of constipation and decide in what position *they* would finally choose to expel the problem–given the choice. I doubt if flat on their back would be their the first choice.

Edgware Birth Centre facilitates natural childbirth with its holistic approach to care. Staff at all levels demonstrate dedication and commitment. The vision is family-centred and technological intervention is minimised. The centre is feminine in its attention to surroundings and colour schemes. It is deliberately homely and the patients are *valued*. The facility works at the birth experience, allowing the pain threshold to rise naturally, by improving the labour experience. The natural process is demedicalised, putting the woman in control. The midwives concentrate on their supporting and guiding roles. The service focuses around the woman, the couple, the baby, the family, and the wider family. Staff and women in the unit are no longer slaves to the rigid hospital system with its timetables, ward rounds, theatre time, outpatient clinics etc. By definition, any patient needing *medical* intervention is elsewhere.

Edgware concentrates on 'whole concept' birth care. As a GP, the entire concept reminds me of a geriatric unit experiment at the Bollingbrook Hospital which I visited in the mid-eighties, studying aspects of care for the elderly. There, great emphasis was put on surroundings and on maintaining patients' dignity. They were treated as individuals to be valued, with a past to be honoured and revered. At Edgware Birth Centre there is a focus on safety and on celebration of a physiological event, leading to improved outcome and greater satisfaction. The relaxed atmosphere and unhurried environment lead to a better labour, which means less pain, fewer drugs and less intervention. Happier memories have led to better breastfeeding rates and reduced incidence of postnatal depression.

The unit and its ethos are starting families off on the right footing, laying sound ground rules for the future. We have a unit with modern ideas and old-fashioned values. By removing the fear the patient is able to relax, choose her position and improve her performance.

This aspect of care, along with alternative methods of pain relief, is emphasised at Edgware because it is recognised that for the mother, father, siblings and wider family giving birth is a significant life event for that family which should be a positive and unifying experience. It should not be a painful, distressing, miserable catastrophe that everyone around tries to blot out of his or her memory. I firmly believe that women and their families in the unit are able to feel great confidence around the time of the birth. Many patients, having experienced the birth process at the Edgware Birth Centre, have expressed those thoughts to me as their GP.

The vast majority of mothers unfortunately experience pain at the time of delivery. Without using major interventionist methods it can only be eased, not eliminated. This is usually the one aspect that the mother-to-be and her family dread the most. Edgware, by definition, does not support epidurals and caesarean sections. However, much attention has been given to all basic and 'natural' methods of pain relief. The birth pools are a delight. Much attention is also given to TENS, although 'gas and air' is employed as necessary and of course midwives, as practitioners in their own right, can prescribe and administer pethidine as necessary. I firmly believe that the ethos of birth facilitation also has a positive effect on the degree of discomfort experienced.

The information GPs give to patients can be quite influential on a woman's choice of birth venue. I have offered the birth centre as an option for delivery to all women in my practice who have booked for maternity care and who I felt would meet the criteria. My attached midwife, who has been heavily involved in the birth centre from its inception, has also given out information to patients. Sometimes, talking to a second enthusiastic professional has facilitated patients' consideration of the birth centre as an option. Any patient who has delivered at the birth centre has enthused about the standard of care and the whole birth experience.

THE QUESTION OF SAFETY

From the start safety has been the paramount issue in my mind. I do feel that with good selection and rapid and comprehensive back-up from a full obstetric unit the necessary criteria have been met, a view shared by many local GPs. Some of my GP colleagues, however, have not shared my confidence. Views have ranged from indifference (women could apply but it was 'on their own heads'), to vociferous non-participation, to frankly hostile.

I think that this wide range of local GP feeling mainly boils down to two personal factors.

Firstly, virtually all GPs locally will feel their practical skills in this area to be rusty. Some will never have participated in intrapartum obstetrics as a postgraduate and the rest of us participated so long ago that our skills must be considered null and void. Everybody realises that *medical* intervention would only be required if a complication arose that was beyond the bounds of the very highly trained and competent midwives. GPs are right to feel that their intervention in such circumstances would be inappropriate or even unsafe. Although I have personally tried to explain to many of my colleagues that they would *not* be called upon in cases of complications, when the patient is transferred to a full obstetric unit, I do not feel that I am always believed. In other words, their personal professional role with regard to birth centres is not fully understood by some GPs.

Secondly, GPs' personal experiences colour their opinions–as mine do. One GP said he did not support birth centres because his wife had had twins. Obviously, multiple births are completely outside the remit of birth centres but that experience was enough to make him feel that they were completely unacceptable for *any* of his patients, even though, statistically, the vast majority must be singleton pregnancies. I can accept that some people's obstetric work in the past makes them wary–they may have witnessed seemingly completely normal cases deteriorate into complicated cases, for example. I can understand their views, and the full obstetric unit back-up is crucial from the safety angle. On the other side of the coin, how many 'normal' cases become 'abnormal' through fear and lack of good hands-on support by competent midwives who are not allowed to practise in the manner as laid down in the birth centre? We might never know the answer to that.

COMMISSIONING OF THE BIRTH CENTRE

Primary Care Groups locally have not taken a great interest in the service as yet–they have their own difficulties and it forms only a tiny proportion of an overwhelming agenda and workload. Perhaps the greatest interest initially was shown by a neighbouring Primary Care Group which repeatedly declared that if our PCG had a birth centre, they wanted one too! Though frustrated at not having our birth facility in *their* area, they were awash with their own facilities (to our local detriment) in other areas. The local PCG agenda has now moved on and any work achieved in terms of the birth centre has been swept away and lost.

Responsibility for primary care in the area has now been taken over by one large Primary Care Trust (PCT), the biggest in the country, and the Health Authority has merged with two other health authorities. These huge new organisations seem to focus their time and energy on trying to cope with their own revised internal infrastructure, rather than on dealing with anything as mundane and localised as a birth centre. People are only human and when faced with the threat of redundancy every few months, due to the relentless and unremitting reorganisations, they are bound to be distracted from the work they should be responsible for and undertaking. There does not seem to be much input into anything outside their own internal affairs as the Primary Care Trust is gearing up to merge with Social Services.

The Health Authority faces merger with yet two more health authorities and the grand plan seems to be for health authorities to reach such a massive size that they become totally unworkable and then have to be disbanded.

I would like to think that once the PCT is able to sort itself out locally, it can move on to look at essential services, such as the birth centre. At present that feels a very vain hope.

YET MORE PROBLEMS

The birth centre is also vulnerable in that some people view it as an 'add-on luxury'. I think the only element of luxury is the rooms, which are comfortable compared to those in other local units, whose interiors could only be described as 'uncomfortable'. This is not a luxury service but a way forward for the future, a pioneer unit. The funding for the birth centre is seen by some as a possible 'pot of extra money' that could be acquired for 'their' unit. Sometimes this attitude has come from obstetric units and sometimes from other, completely unrelated units that are finding it difficult to make their books balance.

The new, enlarged Health Authority has even disbanded the Barnet MSLC, which saw through the 'birth' of the Edgware Birth Centre. Once the full obstetric unit at Edgware was closed it became difficult to keep track of maternity provision for Barnet women, as they had to go far and wide for maternity care. Most women went to Barnet General Hospital, Northwick Park Hospital or the Royal Free Hospital and so attention was focused on those three hospitals.

Trying to cover three separate units meant that it was difficult to fit everything on the agenda and meetings sometimes became unwieldy. They often had different protocols, working methods, problems and positive features. The MSLC was still relevant to the Edgware Birth Centre in the format in which it had been running for the last 5 years, however, as these three hospitals share the back-up obstetric responsibility for the birth centre.

Members of the old committee view the 'new' MSLC proposed by the new enlarged Health Authority with dismay. I have resigned as the GP on the committee. One of the hospitals where local women go has been left off the hospital list and has been replaced by a large number of distant hospitals that certainly have no relevance either to me as a GP or to my patients. A replacement GP will presumably be found although it seems hard to believe that any GP will have contact with all those hospitals over such a wide area. Or will the wishes and interests of Primary Care be ignored?

The Committee as proposed could never be run with any relevance to any *one* of those hospitals. Presumably, it will be like the huge, unwieldy Local Medical Committee that has just been formed to mirror the huge Health Authority, with a massive agenda with little individual relevance. There is little relevance for even reasonably sized groups of individuals or institutions. I doubt whether parts of the merged Health Authority have even heard of Edgware General Hospital, apart from the scandal of its closure, which at the time was constantly in the national news. I also very much doubt whether much is known about (or whether there is much interest in) Edgware Birth Centre.

I do feel strongly that the Edgware Birth Centre has been made more vulnerable by the removal of the MSLC to help overview it and champion its cause.

The birth centre has also had to withstand a lot of negative impact from what should have been the supporting surrounding obstetric units. Most of the units have viewed the birth centre budget as something to be rifled and one unit even 'top-sliced' the budget! From the start staff could never be employed at the level which was initially intended due to an artificially reduced budget, which lowered morale generally.

There was supposed to be a lot of infrastructure support put in by the main obstetric unit, though this was often difficult to identify in practice. Managers from the obstetric unit repeatedly did not turn up for management meetings. A senior member of the birth centre staff, who was excellent, did not have her contract renewed by the obstetric unit, presumably as a cost-saving exercise.

The birth centre was also viewed by local obstetric units as a kind of 'repository' for midwives, that could be raided at will when there was a shortage of midwives in the obstetric unit. A shortage of midwives was part of the problem in the unit where my daughter delivered and danger point had well and truly been passed there in my opinion. Another local unit is reckoned to have the worst ratio of midwives to mothers in the country. And yet there is no incentive for midwives to remain in post–the situation will only worsen in that unit as midwives leave. Our own attached midwife comes from that unit and she has just resigned after 16 highly successful years with us.

My midwife has complained for years about having to cope with the most basic of equipment continually in short supply and with dire staffing levels. She was expected to do endless extra duties for no extra pay and yet money was found to pay agency midwives. I thought it was only doctors who were forced to put in excessive hours for free. In this sea of local adversity there is bound to be a knock-on effect on the birth centre, which will most likely not be allowed to flourish to its full potential.

EVERYBODY ELSE ON THE BANDWAGON?

Other areas too are looking at opening birth centres, not as an enhanced facility for maternity care in a family-friendly environment, but as a cost-saving exercise and to ease the closure of yet more full obstetric units. Another birth centre is planned a few miles from Edgware, following the planned closure of a busy full obstetric unit, part of which will transfer to another obstetric unit a few miles away. The birth centre planned for that hospital would be the only maternity facility on that site. Unlike Edgware, there is a very high local Afro-Caribbean population in that area: the criteria for booking at Edgware exclude patients with haemoglobinopathies for safety reasons and it is debatable whether they will have a big enough client base for a birth centre at that hospital. At the moment, birth centres are free to draw up their own acceptance criteria, but presumably they would take into account the complications that haemoglobinopathies can bring to the situation.

I do not feel it is fair to view birth centres as a cheap downmarket option. They are providing a very special service, in harmony with a very special life event, for the whole family. I feel the ethos of birth centres is forward-looking and that they should not simply be viewed by budget-minded managers as a downmarket, cost-saving facility.

A BRIGHT NEW FUTURE FOR ALL?

Edgware Birth Centre has attracted a lot of interest from other birth centres and from around the world. Senior figures from the birth centre have lectured abroad and the centre has been inundated with requests for information and conducted tours from organisations around the world. Many of these requests have been honoured and the staff feel very proud of what they have achieved to gain such international interest and recognition. At one stage, the centre was receiving so many requests for tours from interested bodies that it was felt some requests would have to be turned down–the birth centre is a busy working unit and it was felt the number of tours was becoming too disruptive and taking up too much staff time! Sometimes success does have its own cost.

I will do my utmost to foster this futuristic, family-friendly facility. I sincerely hope it will also influence the ethos in consultant units nationwide, perhaps worldwide. After all, childbirth is a natural physiological event. The pregnant state is the natural state for the sexually mature premenopausal female, not the non-pregnant. Once we have filtered off the unfortunate patients who suffer complications, we should be focusing on normality, not abnormality, in childbirth. Let's try to make this normal event, which should be a happy event for the whole family, as memorable as possible for all the right reasons. This major life event should be celebrated. Where nature has allowed it to progress without problem or complication, it should not be left to the medical, nursing and managerial professions to try to ruin it.

11

Midwifery assistants: a place for non-midwives in a midwifery service

Jane Walker

INTRODUCTION

As part of the Edgware Birth Centre (EBC) project, midwives have had the opportunity to explore new roles and relationships and have taken a lead on developing a role for midwifery assistants. These midwifery assistants (MAs) are mostly mature women with no previous experience of NHS work. They work directly under the supervision of the midwives at EBC. The experience at Edgware has led the midwives to feel very positive about the potential for establishing this new role within the maternity services in the UK, both in acute and primary care settings, and they have approached local universities to see if they will consider developing tailored educational programmes.

BACKGROUND TO THE INITIATIVE

In common with others (Francomb 1997, Spiby & Crowther 1999), the original project leader for the EBC, following a visit to the Netherlands in 1992 to observe the role of the Dutch 'maternity aides', had developed an interest in the transferability of this role to the UK maternity services. She was impressed by their level of knowl–edge and by the obviously invaluable help they were to the midwives and women with whom they worked (Van Teijlingen 1990). In the Netherlands it is the custom for midwives to work in group practices, much as GPs do in this country, and to give women full ante-, intra- and postpartum care. The midwives carry caseloads of over 120 women per year (B Smulders, personal communication, 2000) so the maternity aides are an integral and essential part of the workforce. Although their counterparts working in the EBC would not be subjected to the intensive 3-year educational programme followed by the Dutch maternity aide, clear interest was voiced about the development of a similar role.

When the business plan for EBC was being prepared and staffing issues were considered, it was decided that the 24-hour cover should be made up of one midwife and one health care assistant (HCA), to be known as a 'midwifery assistant' (MA). One of the reasons for choosing another name for this person was the desire to break the mould of the traditional 'auxiliary' or HCA and to be free to construct a different kind of job, based more on the Dutch maternity aide model.

THE FIRST APPOINTMENTS

As recruitment of staff for EBC began in the middle of 1997 a personal specification and a job description were prepared for the proposed

midwifery assistants (see Fig. 11.1 and Box 11.1). These posts were offered first to existing HCAs in the maternity service. It was explained that these posts were to be considered as secondments from their current posts, with a view to their returning to their normal employment after the initial 2-year contract if they so wished. No one applied for the posts in the birth centre. External advertising then followed. Advertisements were put in local papers, with a brief description of the service that was being proposed and the information that these posts would be 2-year, short-term contracts (A grade). It was made clear that applicants did not need to have previous experience within the NHS and that training for the role would be given 'on the job'. It was made explicit, however, that applicants would need to demonstrate an understanding of the needs of women in childbirth; be flexible in their working hours, in order to cover a 24-hour service; and be willing to undertake a whole range of duties designed to support the smooth running of the service and the midwives working there.

The advertisements attracted 60 applicants for five whole-time-equivalent posts. Many of these applicants appeared very suitable for the proposed posts and short-listing was difficult. Each subsequent recruitment process has generated a

Personal specification

- No previous experience required
- Pleasant personality
- Communication skills, both written and verbal
- Able to work in a team
- Aware of issues around birth for women
- Willingness to learn a range of new skills
- Comfortable with the non-interventionist philosophy of the unit
- Flexibility

Role and Function

- Administration
- Clinical support to the midwife
- Housekeeping duties
- Act as labour/birth support person
- Computer work/data collection

Always under the supervision of the midwife

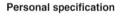

Figure 11.1 Personal specification and role description for midwifery assistants.

Box 11.1 Job description for Edgware Birth Centre midwifery assistants

The Edgware Birth Centre (EBC) is a 'home from home' unit run by midwives that seeks to extend the boundaries of choice around place of birth for local childbearing women. Here birth is viewed as a normal human process and the emphasis is on giving personalised care to women and their families; recognising what an important event birth is in the life of a family and working to facilitate a good outcome, physically and emotionally. There are no doctors on site and the nearest obstetric department is 7 miles away. The midwives and midwifery assistants therefore work closely together on all aspects of care and in the general running of the Centre. If problems arise in pregnancy or labour the woman's care will be transferred to an obstetrician.

The midwifery assistant:

- will at all times work under the auspices of the midwife present in the unit
- will be accountable to the midwife she is working with and also to the midwife manager of the unit
- will be required to work on a rotational basis, i.e. on day and night duty and with a flexible attitude to working arrangements.

ROLES AND DUTIES
Assisting the midwife

1. Preparing the rooms for women attending for antenatal, labour or postnatal care.
2. Help the midwife preparing for and carrying out antenatal/postnatal support groups. This includes: preparing the room, helping with refreshments, equipment and generally being available to help.
3. Assist the midwife with general (non-midwifery) care in labour.
4. Work closely with the midwife giving antenatal and postnatal care and assisting where appropriate.
5. Once appropriate training has been given, carry out simple observations of temperature, pulse and blood pressure, if required and under the instructions of the midwife, always reporting your findings to the midwife.
6. Make phone calls calling for assistance for the midwife if the midwife is unable to leave the client and according to agreed protocols. This will sometimes be an emergency situation and it will be the ambulance service that you are calling.

Assisting the mother

1. Welcome the mother and her partner/birth supporter to the birth centre, escort them to their birthing room and help them to settle in.
2. Attend to her non-midwifery needs while in labour, acting as a 'doula', encouraging and supporting her and her partner/family.

3. Help with the filling and the emptying of the birthing pool if required.
4. Help with the non-midwifery care of mother and baby, e.g. bathing and showering and helping to clear up after the birth.
5. Assist the mother with the care of her baby, demonstrating nappy changing and baby bathing where appropriate.
6. Support women with infant feeding, under the guidance of the midwife and according to agreed guidelines.
7. Accompany mother and baby to an arranged transfer Trust and support them in this (non-emergency transfer only).

General duties

1. Welcome clients, their families and other visitors to the birth centre. Introduce them to the facilities and the kind of service provided at the centre.
2. Help and sometimes host the coffee morning/drop-in sessions.
3. Answer the telephone in a friendly and helpful manner; take messages and refer to the midwife if midwifery advice is required; arrange appointments and informal visits with reference to the work diary.
4. Undertake general clerical duties that may be associated with the smooth running of the birth centre. This may include computer data entry for which instruction would be given.
5. Liaise with other departments in the Community Hospital regarding day-to-day administrative needs.
6. Undertake simple errands if required.
7. Check stock levels of supplies, stationery and other non-medical equipment and prepare order forms for the midwife.

Housekeeping Duties

1. Make beds and tidy the rooms during and following the care of a woman and her family.
2. Arrange for the cleaning of rooms and facilities as agreed, ensuring that this has been satisfactorily undertaken.
3. Assist with the provision of drinks and light snacks for those using/visiting the birth centre and clear up afterwards.
4. Audit the condition of crockery, cutlery and other non-medical equipment.
5. Monitor the supplies of linen and CSSD, reporting to the midwife any problems with availability.
6. Liaise with the catering department for the supply of pre-packed meals and other catering needs, as required.
7. Use the washer/dryer for the cleaning of the special birth centre linen (duvet covers and pillow cases). Some ironing of this linen may be required.

Box 11.1 *(Continued)*   Job description for Edgware Birth Centre midwifery assistants

OTHER CONSIDERATIONS

- The midwifery assistant will be required to have a caring approach to women and their families; to have good communication skills; and to be comfortable working in an informal care environment.
- Pregnancy and childbirth is a very important time for women and their families. At the birth centre we

seek to respect the concerns and needs of each individual, recognising social, economic, cultural and religious diversity.

- All staff are required to be flexible and adaptable as the work covers a wide range of care and activity.

Reviewed November 2001

---

long list of applicants, demonstrating the size of the potential workforce that is available within local communities (Department of Health 1999). Many of the women (they were all women) were holding responsible jobs in other organisations but were very keen to move into an area of work they felt to be interesting and important to other women. Only one or two were already working in the NHS. One or two actually took a drop in salary to take up the posts. Part-time work was readily offered and accepted as many of the women had family responsibilities. An essential requirement, however, was the ability to work flexibly, so that the 24-hour periods would be covered. One of the successful applicants later wrote:

I first learnt about the Edgware Birth Centre through an article in the local press. I was glad that this kind of service was being offered to women, even though it had come too late for me. My two experiences of childbirth had been in hospital where active management was very much favoured. So, when I saw the job description for midwifery assistants I applied, and once I had looked round the centre on the day of my interview I knew that it was the job for me. I felt that I could help women get the care and the positive birth experience that I never had.

At the time of the initial interviews it was felt that there were going to be some distinct advantages in recruiting women who had not worked in the NHS and, in particular, in acute hospital maternity departments before. The midwives were keen to introduce and develop a new approach to the care of pregnant women and their families and employees who were already socialised into the hierarchical, task-orientated

working patterns so common in maternity departments might have found it difficult to adjust to a more cooperative and flexible way of working. The informal atmosphere of the birth centre is important–no one wears uniform.

It transpired that these first appointments were to set the standard by which later appointments would be judged. One woman in particular demonstrated natural leadership skills which she was encouraged to exercise and which were to prove critical to the successful organisation of the birth centre.

THE FIRST MONTHS

The first MAs took up their posts in October 1997. Most of them had been chosen because of the personal qualities that they would bring to the job and because they appeared able to work as members of a team, excited by the prospect of being part of the development of a new facility with a new role. Many of them had not worked in the health service before or had not been involved in clinical care. This presented EBC with the challenge of developing a learning programme that would not only help them to develop the skills that would be required of them, but would also help them to integrate into the midwifery working environment. An initial orientation programme was developed by one of the EBC midwives who was also a midwifery lecturer (see Boxes 11.2 and 11.3) and a named midwife mentor was allocated to support them in the first months. Advantage was taken of an existing HCA

Box 11.2 Edgware Birth Centre midwifery assistants: planning the introductory programme

The development of the Edgware Birth Centre (EBC) is an exciting initiative that has attracted significant local and national interest. Underpinned by the concepts expressed in the *Changing Childbirth* agenda, the EBC midwives seek to establish new patterns of working and the integration of midwifery assistants into the staffing of the centre is one of those initiatives.

The women recruited as midwifery assistants are chosen because of the personal qualities that they may bring to the job and also because they appeared able to work as a member of a team, and excited by the prospect of being part of the development of a new facility and a new role. Many of them have not worked in the health service before, or have not been involved in clinical care. This presented the challenge of developing a programme of learning/orientation that will not only help them prepare for the skills that will be required of them, but that will also help them to integrate into the midwifery working environment.

PHILOSOPHICAL APPROACH

As adult women they will bring a wide variety of life experience and a maturity that usually contributes to a well-motivated learner. Education is a dynamic and lifelong process in which personal development and change are part of the learning process. These women will be encouraged to consider the ways in which their personal experiences will help them to develop their supporting role within their new work environment. Their varied experiences will be valued and they will be encouraged to learn from and support each other.

THE PROGRAMME

The women will participate in an introductory programme of 7 days which will be extended or developed further in response to the women identifying for themselves further educational and practice issues.

AIMS OF THE PROGRAMME

1. To provide an initial opportunity to explore the role and function of the midwifery assistant (MA) in the context of a 'home-from-home' birth centre.
2. To introduce the MA to the structure and function of the Health Service and the significant current influences upon it.
3. To introduce the MA to the physical and emotional experience of childbirth and the ways in which they can support women and their families at this time.
4. To help the MA consider the role of the midwife in the continuum of childbirth and the ways in which the MA can support the midwife in the context of the birth centre.

OBJECTIVES OF THE PROGRAMME

On completion of the initial orientation programme the MAs will be able to:

- understand the function and purpose of a 'stand-alone' midwifery-led unit
- describe the advantages and disadvantages of such care
- organize their day-to-day working patterns
- identify their role and function within the EBC
- assist the midwife in a rudimentary way with the care of women antenatally, in labour and postnatally
- start a reflective portfolio of experience.

TEACHING AND LEARNING STRATEGIES

1. Lectures/discussion
2. Interactive participation
3. Role play and practice simulation
4. Skills sessions
5. Journal and reflective portfolio.

---

programme being run by the 'host' Trust and the MAs were able to participate in some specific sessions within that programme.

As a new facility, the work at EBC naturally took time to build up. October 1997 was quiet enough to enable the midwives and midwifery assistants to have some very useful time to spend together–getting to know each other, developing procedural guidelines for referrals, learning administration and computer skills, experiencing clinical situations (and using these to reflect on their roles and responsibilities) and team building.

These first months of activity were very skilfully guided by the initial project leader as she helped midwives and midwifery assistants to function in a non-threatening environment where everyone's opinions were valued and heard. This was not as easy as it may sound. The main tool for personal and group development was the weekly reflective meeting. At first, midwives were uncertain about discussing clinical situations that had arisen with MAs at the meeting. This was possibly because, as midwives working in other clinical environments, they had not before had the opportunity to discuss care in

---

Box 11.3   Introductory/orientation programme for midwifery assistants at Edgware Birth Centre

Day 1   09.00–16.30
1. Meeting new people–welcome and introductions
2. Introduction to the Health Service
3. Introduction to the Maternity Services
4. Introduction to the Trust and the background to EBC
5. *Meet the midwives over lunch*
6. Human Resources and occupational health all afternoon.

Day 2   09.00–16.30
1. Health and Safety at work–Part One
2. 'Drop in' coffee morning for mothers and babies using EBC
3. *Lunch*
4. What is a midwife? Part One: roles and responsibilities; brief historical overview; 'with woman'–what does this mean?
5. The role of the midwifery assistant in the birth centre: brainstorming/discussion with EBC midwives; examination of job description; off-duties and working arrangements.

Day 3   09.00–16.30
1. Health and Safety at work–Part Two: manual handling
2. Communication–Part One: listening and talking; messages and emergencies; non-verbal communication
3. *Lunch*
4. Overview of care in pregnancy.

Day 4   09.00–16.00
1. Health and Safety at work–Part Three: control of infection+practical session

2. Communication–Part Two: record keeping; preparing client records; introduction to PAS
3. *Lunch*
4. Overview of care in labour.

Day 5   09.00–16.30
1. Helping women in labour: meeting with women who have recently given birth–listening to their experiences
2. Helping women in labour, practical session: the birthing pool; preparing for delivery; positions in labour
3. *Lunch*
4. Introduction to portfolio work and reflective writing.

Day 6   09.00–16.30
1. Overview of postnatal care
2. Introduction to infant feeding issues and breastfeeding
3. *Lunch*
4. Learning from women: meeting and talking to women about breastfeeding
5. Introduction to baby massage.

Day 7   09.00–16.00
1. Fire lecture
2. Specific aspects of the role of the midwifery assistant
3. *Lunch*
4. Role play and other experiential learning
5. Planning follow-up days, which would include: introduction to NVQs, specific clinical skills, reflective workshops.

---

a 'blame-free' culture and open enquiry initially made them feel vulnerable, even when discussing births with positive outcomes, as was usually the case. It was not long, however, before it became clear that these meetings provided excellent learning opportunities for everyone. Critical incident analysis also helped everyone to develop an awareness of the need for partnership and collaboration. The first emergency situations that were dealt with were a rich source of later role play and role clarification.

As part of their personal and clinical skills development each MA was encouraged to keep a portfolio of her experiences. This included reflective writing about births they had been involved with. Midwives were encouraged to ensure, particularly early on, that they set aside time to 'debrief' the MAs and answer questions

about care and about why certain clinical decisions were made. The MA portfolios became very impressive documents. Very quickly, it seemed, midwives and midwifery assistants became a well functioning team.

ORGANISING THE WORK
Non-clinical work

It is important to remember that EBC is a 'stand-alone' unit, which means that, although midwives and midwifery assistants based at the centre are employed by the 'host' Acute Trust, they are physically set apart from that Trust by being on the community hospital site. EBC is therefore administratively self-contained–there are no clerks or secretaries. It would therefore usually be a midwifery assistant who would answer the telephone and deal with initial client enquiries or take messages for the midwives from GPs, other Trusts or from other midwives. Their customer care skills are important as they will often be the first point of contact for potential and booked clients. They are also responsible for inviting women to visit the centre prior to formal 'booking' for care and for explaining the nature of the care provided. The clients seem to value this aspect of the care and the midwives find that the women and their families form strong relationships with the MAs.

It became apparent early on that in order to encourage the MAs to become a cohesive workforce they needed an opportunity to spend time together as a distinct group, as well as spending time with the midwives. Initially facilitated by one of the midwives, these group meetings quickly became self-organising. The MAs would arrange a meeting and chair it themselves. The meetings would be used for very practical reasons, such as problem-solving or the planning of administrative duties. They would also raise concerns at these meetings which would then be brought to the attention of a senior midwife or brought to the weekly reflective meeting for discussion or decision by the whole team.

As the months passed it was clear that the MAs were making a significant contribution to the ethos and the smooth running of the birth centre. A decision was made to enhance their sense of group identity and responsibility by facilitating the development of group autonomy. Among the MAs a form of democratic leadership emerged. They began to identify particular areas of responsibility amongst themselves: one took responsibility for maintaining the stock levels and ordering; one became responsible for the laundry and linen; one became a skilled 'computer person' and helped with collecting monthly statistics; one emerged as a natural administrator, organising the filing cabinets and the paperwork and reminding midwives when they 'forgot' to complete all the necessary booking forms! They organised their own off-duty, annual leave and even sickness cover when possible–always referring to the senior midwife

for checking or confirming arrangements. One midwifery assistant described her job like this:

It is very difficult to describe exactly what the job involves as there are so many aspects to it. It can be about cleaning rooms and making beds, answering phones and general office duties and helping with the everyday running of the centre, but I think one of the most important things we do is to build up a relationship with the women and their families. This happens from the time we show them round and then at the antenatal coffee mornings and then in the workshops before and after the birth.

After one year, the MAs worked with the midwives and the project leader to rewrite the job description.

Direct client care

The job description (Box 11.1) details some of the aspects of direct client care which the MAs are involved with. There are two aspects of this direct clinical care that are important. Firstly, they always work under the supervision of the midwife. Secondly, clinical decisions about care are made by midwives, in full discussion with the clients.

Some of the MAs have developed particular areas of interest, for example breastfeeding or baby massage, and the midwives have helped them to develop the knowledge and skills required. All the MAs help the midwives to run the preparation for birth workshops and so become quite knowledgeable about certain aspects of care. They also coordinate workshops, inviting families who have recently given birth at the centre to come and share their experiences with the women attending. After about 18 months the MAs decided that, in response to requests from the women, they would develop a 'postnatal' workshop on care of the new baby–baby bathing and other practical aspects. This was planned with the support of the midwives, who helped them with group-work techniques and sat in with them until they gained confidence. This workshop is known as 'Baby Basics' and is very popular.

Another very important aspect of care that the MAs provide can be likened to the role of a 'doula' (Kirkham & Walters 1997). Their involvement in this particular aspect of care is more significant at night and at weekends when there are fewer 'extra' people around, such as student midwives, to take the role of birth supporter.

Because the birth centre is physically small (five en suite birth/postnatal rooms) the staff caring for a woman in labour are within close contact. If a midwife is undertaking an antenatal follow-up check, for example, and there is a client in labour, the MA will 'keep an eye' on the labouring woman, talking to her and walking round with her. She will often be directly involved in preparing the pool for use in labour (there are three pools at Edgware, all in frequent use). A common scenario starts with the client telephoning the birth centre, thinking that she may be in labour. The MA passes her to a midwife and the midwife invites her to come in. The passing comment to the MA is: 'Get the pool ready–she's on her way!' Welcoming the woman into the centre, the MA shows the woman and her labour supporter into the prepared room where the pool is filling. The midwife undertakes the initial assessment of well-being and progress and the MA helps the woman to settle in. Once she is in the pool the midwife or the MA will stay with her. The midwife will alert a second midwife to the fact that a birth is imminent or contact the on-call community-based midwifery team planning to look after this client. All the time the MA is around to help, making cups of tea, looking in on a postnatal client in another room, talking with the labouring couple and encouraging them, particularly when the birth is imminent and the midwife is concentrating on preparing for the birth. Walters and Kirkham (1997) discuss in depth the important function of a doula: 'The doula explains what is happening as labour progresses, helping to ease the anxiety that comes with unfamiliarity ... .'

If an emergency situation develops it is often the MA who is asked to make the 999 call to the ambulance service and alert the Acute Trust to the impending transfer while the midwife concentrates on dealing with the situation.

ROLE CONFLICT AND CONFUSION?

One of the questions most frequently asked when the subject of 'midwifery support workers' is raised (Francomb 1997, Kaufmann 1999) is one about the potential for role conflict and confusion. The RCM Position Paper 5a on support workers in the maternity services states that: '...it is important that their role does not undermine, conflict with or obstruct the role of the midwife' (Royal College of Midwives 1999).

While acknowledging the controversies surrounding this issue and about which there must be much more debate, we believe that the strengths of the Edgware model of midwifery assistants lie in the fact that they were recruited from the locality of the birth centre and that a role developed that encompasses organisational, clerical and clinical elements. This role has been fostered as a partnership and the ethos is one of mutual respect. There has generally been no role confusion but there is a real valuing of everyone's contribution to the whole.

It has been interesting to note the reaction of some visiting midwives and student midwives to the presence of non-midwives involved in care. EBC midwives and MAs have sometimes observed a tendency either to disregard the presence of the MAs, or to decline to involve them in client care, other than in a subordinate role. (They may instruct the MA to go and clean up after the birth in a rather traditional hierarchical way, for example.) After discussing this phenomenon at an EBC meeting it was decided that a file would be prepared for visiting staff that gave them all kinds of basic information about the birth centre and its philosophy and guidelines for care. The midwifery assistants' job description was included near the beginning of the file.

It has been interesting to consider why it is that the potential for role confusion has not been apparent at EBC. One suggestion that has been made is that in EBC the MAs are able to observe midwives taking a more autonomous professional role than they might in large acute units, where midwives may be perceived as deferring to medical opinion on many aspects of care in pregnancy and birth. A well-developed ability to make appropriate, autonomous decisions is a critical requirement in the context of risk management and safety for birth in a stand-alone unit. MAs have also witnessed emergency situations in which skilled care is pivotal to a satisfactory outcome for both mother and baby and they have not demonstrated any desire to interfere with or contest professional boundaries.

CONCLUSION

I feel as midwifery assistants we play a key role in the running and the success of the birth centre.

The midwifery assistant who made this accurate observation has recently begun her preregistration midwifery course. There is a strong consensus of opinion among the midwives at EBC that one of the strengths of the midwifery assistant role is its potential for widening the gateway into midwifery practice. What better preparation for midwifery education could there be than working with women experiencing normal pregnancy and birth and with midwives who are confident in their skills and knowledge both in normal childbirth and in those situations when referral for obstetric opinion or emergency care is required.

It is the EBC experience that many of the extremely capable local women recruited into the service as MAs are representative of many women in our communities, who may not possess the standard entry requirements for midwifery education but who are highly motivated and interested in assisting women and midwives during childbirth. Suitable educational and career pathways are required for midwifery assistants. A national vocational qualification (NVQ) designed specifically to develop the knowledge and skills to support women and midwives in the birth centre setting may offer a solution.

REFERENCES

Department of Health 1999 Making a difference– strengthening the nursing, midwifery and health visiting contribution to health and healthcare. The Stationery Office Books, London

Francomb H 1997 Do we need support workers in the maternity services? British Journal of Midwifery 5 (11) November: 672–676

Kaufmann T 1999 Working with healthcare assistants: threat or promise? RCM Midwives Journal 2 (10) October: 316–317

Kirkham M, Walters D 1997 Support and control in labour: doulas and midwives. In: Kirkham M,

Perkins E R (eds) Reflections on Midwifery. Baillière Tindall, London

Royal College of Midwives 1999 Support workers in the maternity services: RCM Position Paper 5a. RCM Midwives Journal 2(10) October: 317–318

Spiby H, Crowther S 1999 Dutch maternity aides: a transferable model? RCM Midwives Journal 2 (1) January: 20–21

Van Teijlingen E R 1990 The profession of maternity home care assistant and its significance for the Dutch midwifery profession International Journal of Nursing Studies 27 (4): 355–366

12

Evaluating a new service: clinical outcomes and women's assessments of the Edgware Birth Centre

Mary Boulton   Jean Chapple
Dawn Saunders

INTRODUCTION

It cannot be assumed that all new services are better than (or, indeed, as good as) the ones they replace or augment, even if they have full support from professionals and client groups. *Changing Childbirth* (Department of Health 1993) stated: 'New patterns of service should be designed to allow evaluation of both their effectiveness and their acceptability to women using the service.' In an evidence-based health service systematic evaluation of all aspects of a new service by independent researchers is essential, especially if service providers and clients hope that their service will act as a template for future services elsewhere. An evaluation must also include an assessment of the likely transferability of results to other parts of the country.

Our aims in undertaking an evaluation of the Edgware Birth Centre were:

1. To describe the extent to which it is able to deliver a safe, woman-centred alternative to hospital care and the comparative cost of doing so.
2. To describe the preferences, expectations and degree of satisfaction of women who choose the birth centre as their place of delivery.
3. To describe the operation of the unit and its acceptability to the unit midwives and to the wider community of professionals in maternity care.

A full account of the evaluation is provided in the final report (Saunders et al 2000). In this chapter, we will consider the experience of the women who booked to deliver at the Edgware Birth Centre (EBC) in terms of their clinical outcomes and their assessment of their birth experience.

WHOM DID THE BIRTH CENTRE SERVE?

The lifestyles and social background of women have an important effect on the outcome of pregnancy (Office for National Statistics 1998). It is therefore important to know something about the social circumstances of women who live in Barnet and those who booked at the birth centre before deciding whether this model of care is suitable for other areas.

Barnet is a geographically small health authority (about 12 km north to south and 12 km west to east) on the outskirts of London, covering one local authority. North–south transport links are quite good, with the Northern tube line traversing the district and with many bus routes. The borough and its immediate surroundings are relatively affluent areas. Using a scoring system based on unemployment, overcrowding, non-ownership of a car and low social class (Carstairs 1989), Barnet is in the top ten of the least deprived London boroughs and ranks 130th out of 354 local authorities for district-level deprivation throughout England (although this masks some pockets of severe deprivation). In 1996 22% of Barnet residents were from ethnic groups other than 'white'. The largest minority ethnic group was 'Indian' (8%), with 4% classifying themselves as 'other Asian' (Barnet Health Authority 1998). About 4000 women living in Barnet have babies each year.

CLINICAL OUTCOMES FOR WOMEN WHO BOOKED TO DELIVER AT THE EBC

The rarity of perinatal mortality and of life-threatening morbidity in mother or baby meant that we could not use these outcomes alone to assess the relative safety of the Edgware Birth Centre (Field et al 1988). Recent studies focus on proxy measures of serious morbidity, such as low Apgar scores and resuscitation rates in neonates; of non-life-threatening morbidity, such as tearing or episiotomy in women; and of intervention rates and process measures such as transfer rates. Antenatal, intrapartum and post-delivery transfers were also studied as outcomes of care, as transfers cause anxiety for both mother and carers and add to the cost of services in free-standing maternity units.

METHODS

Outcomes were analysed by intended place of delivery (birth centre or hospital) and compared for three groups:

1. *Group A*: Women booked to deliver at EBC (589 women). Data were obtained for 589 out of 602 (98%) women who delivered during the evaluation period and who had booked to deliver at the birth centre. Some women were lost to follow-up because they transferred to other more distant units antenatally.

2. *Comparison Group B*: Women delivering over the evaluation period at home or in hospitals in North West Thames Region who fulfilled EBC's clinical criteria (19 529 women). Data were obtained for 19 529 women who fulfilled the birth centre criteria, selected from the regional St Mary's Maternity Information System (SMMIS) database. SMMIS is made up of routinely collected, pooled data from 14 hospital trusts in the North West Thames Region and between 1997 and 1998 included 73 223 singleton deliveries (75 607 deliveries in all). This database includes home deliveries conducted by trust midwives. The selection criteria restrict EBC deliveries to women aged between 18 and 40 years with a parity of between one and four and without a poor obstetric history. The age range for primigravidae is 18 to 36 years. The SMMIS comparison group, which fulfilled the eligibility criteria for booking at EBC, represented 27% of the total SMMIS population.

3. *Comparison Group C*: Women in Group B who had a normal vaginal delivery (14 125 women, 72% of Group B).

The inclusion criteria used to select the comparison groups are shown in Box 12.1. The variables from the SMMIS database (used to derive the comparison group) were complete, with missing values of no more than 1%, with three exceptions: antenatal hypertension had 17.5% of values missing; maternal height had 26.4% missing; and body mass index had 32.7% of values missing. The last two reflect that some units no longer routinely measure height or weight of mothers. Body mass index is an important factor in outcome of pregnancy, especially for mode of delivery, so we hope that midwives everywhere will record height and weight at least once in each pregnancy.

Pregnancy outcomes were analysed on where the women *intended* to deliver rather than where they actually did deliver. This is based on the intention-to-treat principle (Newell 1992). This means that all women who booked at EBC, intending to give birth there, have been included in the analysis, regardless of their actual place of delivery. The analysis therefore includes women who transferred their care at any stage during pregnancy or labour. The group intending to deliver at the birth centre differs from the general obstetric population as they are self-selected by choice and by standardised selection criteria.

Data on women intending to deliver at the birth centre were obtained from all relevant sources, including the birth centre's own records, local computerised maternity information systems, and birth registers at the birth centre and at other local units (such as Northwick Park, Barnet General and the Royal Free hospitals) for women who transferred. During the 2 years of the evaluation period to September 1st 1999 a total of 602 women who had booked at the birth centre gave birth.

PERINATAL AND MATERNAL DEATHS

There were no deaths of mother or baby in the evaluation period.

ANTENATAL TRANSFERS

Of the 602 births in the evaluation period, 64.8% of women delivered at the birth centre, 33.5% delivered in hospital and 1.7% gave birth at home.

There were 144 antenatal transfers to hospital. The majority of the transfers (115, 80%) were for clinical reasons, including two miscarriages (2%) and three premature labour (3%); 29 (20%) transferred care for non-clinical reasons. The majority of the medical transfers in the antenatal period were for postmaturity and induction of labour (40 transfers, 35%). Prolonged pre-labour rupture of membranes, with or without meconium, accounted for 12 transfers (10%) and pregnancy-induced hypertension for nine cases (8%). The remaining 49 transfers were for a variety of other reasons, including 26 (23%) not specified.

TRANSFERS IN LABOUR

Of the 602 women who gave birth, 441 (73%) went to the birth centre in labour, intending to deliver there, and 387 of these 441 women (88%) delivered at the birth centre.

Box 12.1   Eligibility criteria for evaluation study groups

Group A–women booked to deliver at EBC (589)
Maternal age between 18 and 40 years
Maternal height greater than 149 cm
Parous but less than four
No previous history of diabetes
No previous history of epilepsy
No previous history of hypertension
No antenatal renal disease
No antenatal cardiac disease
No antenatal proteinuria
No antenatal hypertension
Smoking less than 20/day
No previous caesarean section
Less than three previous miscarriages
Weight of previous baby less than 4500 g
Singleton birth
Body mass index (BMI) between 20 and 25

Group B–women delivering in hospital in North West Thames Region (19 529)
As above

Group C–women in Group B who had a normal vaginal delivery (14 125)
As above, but had a normal vaginal delivery

First stage of labour

Forty-four women transferred to hospital during the first stage of labour (10% of those intending to deliver at the birth centre). Of these women, 28 (64%) were primigravidae. The main reasons for the transfers, as described by the midwives, included 11 for delay in the first stage of labour (25%), seven for meconium in the liquor (16%), four for fetal distress (9%), four in response to a request for stronger pain relief (9%), two for pregnancy-induced hypertension (5%) and 16 for a range of other reasons (36%).

Second stage of labour

Ten women (2%) were transferred to hospital during the second stage of labour. The reasons for the transfer were: seven for delay in second stage of labour, one for abnormal fetal heart and failure to progress, one for maternal exhaustion and one for having no urge to push and wanting an epidural. All the transfers took place by ambulance. From the time of the ambulance being called by the birth centre to the time of its arrival there was an average wait of 11 minutes, with a range of 5 to 27 minutes. For the three transfers for which we have information, ambulances took 13, 18 and 31 minutes to arrive at the hospital. The longest journey started at 13.34 h and the shortest at 22.00 h.

Three of the women transferred in the second stage had epidural anaesthesia and two had spinal anaesthetics in hospital. Two women used Entonox only for analgesia. For three women we have no information on analgesia used. Two of the women had emergency caesarean sections, two had a Ventouse delivery and two a forceps delivery. One woman had a normal delivery and the mode of delivery was not known for three women.

POST-DELIVERY TRANSFERS

A total of 32 (7%) women transferred to hospital following delivery at the birth centre. Sixteen women transferred for maternal complications, including seven for postpartum haemorrhage (PPH) or symptoms of PPH, five for retained placenta, two for suturing of an extended episiotomy and two for other reasons. A further 16 women transferred because their baby needed care not available at the birth centre. Reasons for transfer associated with the baby included increased respirations (tachypnoea) (five), jaundice (two), low Apgar score (two) and a variety of other reasons (seven).

COMPARISON OF OUTCOMES

GROUP A AND COMPARISON GROUP B

The women who intended to deliver at EBC (Group A) were compared with the women of SMMIS Comparison Group B. Outcomes of pregnancy for these groups are shown in Tables 12.1, 12.2 and 12.3. There were significantly higher rates of normal vaginal delivery in the group intending to deliver at the birth centre, although one-third actually delivered in hospital. There were significantly lower rates ($P < 0.001$) of induction of labour, Ventouse delivery, elective caesarean section, episiotomy, and postnatal stays of more than 3 days among those women who intended to deliver at the birth centre. There was no significant difference in emergency section or forceps delivery rates. Use of clinical analgesia such as pethidine and epidural anaesthesia was also lower in the group intending to deliver at the birth centre (Table 12.4).

It was not possible to compare the use of water, massage, aromatherapy or change of positions as these are not currently entered into computerised maternity data. However, there was much less use of clinical analgesia among the women intending to deliver at the birth centre than in the SMMIS Comparison Group B.

DELIVERIES AT EBC AND SMMIS COMPARISON GROUP C

Deliveries at the birth centre were compared with deliveries in other hospitals. Secondary analysis was done on actual rather than intended

Table 12.1   Delivery methods for Group A and SMMIS Comparison Group B women

	SMMIS Comparison Group B (n=19 529[1]) %	Booked and intended to deliver at EBC (n=589[2]) %	Difference (95% CI) % CI	P value
Normal delivery	72.3	85.6	13.3 (CI, 10.2 to 16.2)	<0.001
Emergency caesarean	9.3	5.8	3.5 (CI, 1.5 to 5.5)	0.004
Forceps delivery	5.1	2.0	3.1 (CI, 1.8 to 4.3)	0.001
Ventouse delivery	9.5	1.9	7.6 (CI, 6.3 to 8.6)	<0.001
Elective caesarean	3.3	0.3	3.0 (CI, 2.3 to 3.6)	<0.001

[1]100 missing any values.
[2]26 missing any values.
NB: Proportions have been worked out using the number (n) for each column, but results are slightly lower due to the missing values in each row.

Table 12.2   Perineal morbidity and postpartum haemorrhage in Group A and SMMIS Comparison Group B women

	SMMIS Comparison Group B (n=19 529[1]) %	Booked and intended to deliver at EBC (n=589[2]) %	Difference (95% CI) % CI	P value
Intact perineum	43.3	46.7	3.4 (CI, −0.8 to 7.5)	0.114
First-degree tear	14.6	19.4	4.8 (CI, 1.4 to 8.1)	0.002
Second-degree tear	22.6	22.6	0.0 (CI, −3.5 to 3.4)	0.98
Third-degree tear	1.0	0.2	0.8 (CI, 0.4 to 1.2)	0.08
Episiotomy	18.9	5.1	13.8 (CI, 11.9 to 15.8)	<0.001
Postpartum haemorrhage (PPH) >500 ml	7.1	6.8	0.3 (CI, −2.4 to 1.9)	0.86

[1]100 missing any values.
[2]26 missing any values.
NB: Proportions include all missing values.

place of delivery. Table 12.5 shows the outcomes for the 386 women who laboured and delivered at the birth centre and the 10 who delivered at home compared to the 14 125 women in SMMIS Comparison Group C who fulfilled the birth centre criteria and had normal deliveries in hospital.

Perineum

There were significantly fewer episiotomies among the women who delivered at the birth centre: only six were carried out over the 2-year period. There was no difference in the proportion of perineal tears between the groups.

Blood loss after delivery

There was a significantly higher rate of postpartum haemorrhages of more than 500 ml in the

birth centre group. Of those who delivered at the birth centre, data on management of the third stage of labour is available on 375 women. Sixty percent of women (221/375) had a physiological third stage of labour (no oxytoxic drugs given and the placenta delivered by maternal effort only). Of these, 3% (6/221) had a postpartum haemorrhage of 500 ml or more. It is not possible to compare the management of the third stage of labour in the EBC deliveries with the Comparison Group C subset as this data is not recorded on the computerised maternity information systems.

Use of analgesia

Table 12.6 shows the use of Entonox and pethidine were significantly lower in the birth centre group, while the use of TENS was significantly

Table 12.3 Other outcomes in Group A and SMMIS Comparison Group B women

	SMMIS Comparison Group B (n=19529[1]) %	Booked and intended to deliver at EBC (n=589[2]) %	Difference (95% CI) % CI	P value
Meconium-stained liquor	17.4	15.6	1.8 (CI, −1.3 to 4.9)	0.281
Induction of labour	16.8	7.3	9.4 (CI, 7.2 to 11.4)	<0.001
Postnatal stay >3 days	14.9	2.9	12.0 (CI, 10.5 to 13.6)	<0.001
Transfers to Special Care	5.6	3.7	1.8 (CI, −0.1 to 3.4)	0.07
Antenatal stay >3 nights	4.0	1.5	2.5 (CI, 1.4 to 3.6)	0.003
Stillbirths	0.4	0.2	0.2	—

[1]100 missing any values.
[2]13 missing any values.
NB: Proportions include all missing values.

Table 12.4 Use of analgesia in Group A and SMMIS Comparison Group B women

	SMMIS Comparison Group (n=19529[1]) %	Booked and intended to deliver at EBC (n=589[2]) %	Difference (95% CI) % CI	P value
Entonox	67.4	53.1	14.3 (CI, 10.1 to 18.5)	<0.001
Epidural	30.7	11.4	19.3 (CI, 16.5 to 22.0)	<0.001
Pethidine	25.5	7.8	17.7 (CI, 15.4 to 20.0)	<0.001
Combined spinal/epidural (CSE)	5.0	1.7	3.3 (CI, 2.2 to 4.5)	<0.001
Spinal	4.6	2.4	2.3 (CI, 0.9 to 3.6)	0.0128
TENS	3.7	6.6	2.9 (CI, 0.8 to 5.0)	<0.001
General anaesthetic	2.8	1.0	1.8 (CI, 0.8 to 2.7)	0.02
Massage	—	16.0		
Aromatherapy	—	9.5		
Change of position	—	50.9		
Water	—	45.2		

[1]100 missing any values.
[2]13 missing any values.
NB: Proportions include all missing values.

higher. Entonox, TENS and pethidine are the only analgesics available at the birth centre which can be recorded on the SMMIS system so comparisons could not be made for other analgesics.

Births in water

Of all the women giving birth at the birth centre, 184 (50.5%) gave birth in one of the two birthing pools. Of those babies delivered in water, seven (3.8% of all babies) were transferred to the acute unit for special care facilities. Four of these babies had tachypnoea, and three had non-respiratory problems (jaundice in two and failure to pass urine in one). Seven babies not born in water were also transferred, three because of tachypnoea, one with a congenitally dislocated hip, and three with problems at delivery (shoulder dystocia, low Apgar score and meconium at delivery). Place of delivery (i.e. in or out of water) was not recorded for the two other babies transferred to the acute unit.

It is not possible to make comparisons between the groups as place of delivery is not recorded on SMMIS. However, national data shows that this is an exceptionally high proportion of births in water. From April 1994 to April 1996 only about 2000 births (approximately 0.6%) in England and Wales took place in water each year (Gilbert & Tookey 1999).

Table 12.5   Comparison of outcome by actual place of delivery (Groups A and SMMIS Comparison Group C)

Outcome	SMMIS Comparison Group C (normal deliveries only) ($n=14\,125^1$) %	Delivered in EBC/home ($n=396^2$) %	Difference (95% CI) % CI	P value
Normal delivery	100	100	—	—
Intact perineum	41.4	47.0	5.6 (CI, 0.4 to 10.6)	0.0317
First-degree tear	19.0	23.2	4.2 (CI, −0.1 to 8.5)	0.0418
Second-degree tear	28.1	27.5	0.6 (CI, −4.0 to 5.1)	0.8583
Third-degree tear	0.8	0	0.8 (—)	—
Episiotomy	11.0	1.5	9.5 (CI, 8.1 to 10.9)	<0.001
PPH >500 ml	3.1	5.6	2.5 (CI, 0.08 to 4.8)	0.0081
Induction of labour	15.0	0	15.0	—
Meconium-stained liquor	14.7	12.6	2.1 (CI, −1.4 to 5.5)	0.2862
Transfers to Special Care	3.8	1.5	2.3 (CI, 0.9 to 3.6)	0.0257
Stillbirths	0.3	0	0.3	—
Antenatal stay >3 nights	3.2	0.3	2.9 (CI, 2.2 to 3.6)	0.0014
Postnatal stay >3 days	5.1	0.3	4.8 (CI, 4.1 to 5.6)	<0.001

[1]Missing values, max 7.
[2]Missing values, max 3.
NB: Proportions have been worked out using the number (n) for each column, but results are slightly lower due to the missing values in each row.

Table 12.6   Use of analgesia in women delivering at EBC (Group A) and in Comparison Group C

	SMMIS Comparison Group C (normal deliveries) ($n=14\,125^1$) %	Delivered in EBC/home ($n=396^2$) %	Difference (95% CI) % CI	P value
Entonox	74.9	52.3	22.6 (CI, 17.5 to 27.7)	<0.001
TENS	4.0	7.8	3.8 (CI, 1.0 to 6.6)	0.0003
Pethidine	26.5	3.0	23.5 (CI, 21.5 to 25.4)	<0.001
Epidural	19.9	0	19.9	—
Spinal	1.3	0	1.3	—
Combined spinal/epidural	2.0	0	2.0	—
General anaesthetic	0.6	0	0.6	—

[1]Missing values, max 7.
[2]Missing values, max 3.
NB: Proportions have been worked out using the number (n) for each column, but results are slightly lower due to the missing values in each row.

WOMEN'S VIEWS

We now look at what the women themselves thought and felt about the care they received at the birth centre. The approach to evaluation taken in this study differs from more traditional approaches, which have largely focused on assessing satisfaction with a set of features which are common to all forms of maternity care. A number of studies have investigated features such as choice over place of birth; continuity of care and carer; control over labour and pain relief; information and communication; and involvement in decision-making (Cartwright 1979, Martin 1990, Spurgeon et al 2001). While all these features are relevant to care at EBC, it was felt that using such broad, generic terms to seek women's views would provide little real insight into the nature of their experience at the birth centre or how well they felt their particular needs had been met. The birth centre was presented as providing a distinctive option for maternity care for 'low-risk' women in North West London and the evaluation, it was argued, should focus on this claim.

The primary aims of this aspect of the evaluation were therefore defined as three-fold:

1. To establish what women themselves saw as the distinctive features of the birth centre, compared with the other options for maternity care available to them.
2. To assess how far women who gave birth at the birth centre felt that these features did, in the event, make a difference to their experience of giving birth.
3. To elicit their views as to whether the birth centre provided the kind of maternity care they wanted.

METHODS

In contrast to the assessment of clinical outcomes, which were based on data routinely collected by health professionals on all births, the assessment of women's views was based on their responses to questionnaires and interviews designed specifically for the birth centre evaluation by the research team. Two sets of questionnaires and interviews were developed.

The first set of questionnaires was designed primarily to explore what women were looking for in booking to deliver at the birth centre, what attracted them to the birth centre and what concerns they had about delivering there. This questionnaire was given out antenatally, at the appointment when women booked to deliver at the birth centre. The initial version of this questionnaire included four open-ended questions about the attractions and drawbacks of a birth at the birth centre, compared with a conventional hospital birth and with a birth at home.

The first 100 antenatal questionnaires returned were analysed to identify the features of the birth centre that the women themselves considered most salient. These included 13 features which were seen as *attractions* of the birth centre (seven compared to a conventional hospital birth and six compared to a home birth) and 11 features which were seen as *drawbacks* of the birth centre (five compared to a conventional hospital birth

and six compared to a home birth). In the second version of the questionnaire the open-ended questions were replaced by statements, written to convey each of these features, and women were asked to indicate on a five-point scale how far they saw each as an *attraction* or a *drawback*.

Questionnaires were distributed to the 596 women who booked to deliver at EBC between February 1st 1998 and August 31st 1999 and were returned by 481 women (81%). Ninety percent were married or living as married and the majority were well educated: half had a degree or equivalent and a fifth had A levels; only 21 (4%) had no formal qualifications. The majority of women were affluent: two-thirds had a household income of over £20 000 and almost a third had a household income of over £40 000. Just under two-thirds owned their own home and four-fifths owned a car. A third of the women described themselves as full-time employed, 9% as self-employed and 17% as part-time employed. Nearly three-quarters (354) described their ethnicity as 'white', 30 (6%) as 'black', 34 (7%) as Indian, 10 (2%) as Pakistani or Bangladeshi and 35 (7%) as 'other'. This is a similar distribution to the population of Barnet as a whole. Nearly one-fifth of women indicated that they did not speak English as a first language but 92% regarded themselves as speaking English very well or fairly well.

The evaluation report (Saunders et al 2000) gives full details of the response to these questionnaires. In this chapter we will focus on the findings of a second set of questionnaires, which were sent postnatally to the 481 women who had completed and returned an antenatal questionnaire.

The primary aims of the postnatal questionnaire were to establish how far women's initial expectations had been fulfilled and how far their initial concerns had been addressed in the course of their delivery at the birth centre. The questions developed for the antenatal questionnaire were adapted for the postnatal questionnaire and additional questions on their overall assessment of the birth centre were also included. Because not all women who booked at the birth centre eventually delivered there, four different questionnaires were designed for women who:

1. delivered at the birth centre
2. transferred to hospital before labour
3. transferred to hospital during labour
4. transferred to hospital with the baby following birth.

Questionnaires were sent to 481 women about 3 weeks after they had given birth and were returned by 248 (52%) women, including 173 women who gave birth at the birth centre, 44 women who transferred antenatally and 31 women who transferred during labour. Eight women had transferred with the baby following delivery. A total of 204 women who returned the questionnaire had laboured at the birth centre.

ATTRACTIONS OF THE BIRTH CENTRE

Compared with a conventional hospital birth

Table 12.7 lists the features of the birth centre which had been identified as its attractions, compared to a conventional hospital. These reflect the high value that women place on an attractive and home-like environment for giving birth and on retaining control over the manner of their labour and delivery. The table shows the proportion of women who felt that each feature had contributed to their birth experience. Three features were almost universally seen as adding greatly to their experience: the relaxed and homely atmosphere; having their own room; and the freedom to do what feels right during labour and delivery. A fourth–not being attached to monitors–was seen as adding greatly to their experience by three-quarters of the women.

Women were also asked to select which two of the features in the list were most important to them. Well over half the women (59%) chose the freedom to do what felt right for them; 54% chose the homely and relaxed atmosphere of the birth centre; and 30% chose having their own room for the whole time they were at the birth centre.

Compared with a home birth

From a clinical perspective, a birth at the birth centre shares many of the features of a home birth.

Table 12.7   Women's assessments of the importance of the attractions of EBC compared with a conventional hospital birth (n=204)

	Added greatly to my experience n (%)	Added a little to my experience n (%)	Made no difference n (%)	Took away a little from my experience n (%)	Took away a great deal from my experience n (%)	Missing data n (%)
The EBC had a homely and relaxed atmosphere	193 (95)	4 (2)	1 —	0 —	0 —	6 (3)
At the EBC I had my own room from the time I arrived until I was ready to leave	189 (93)	6 (3)	2 (1)	0 —	0 —	7 (3)
At the EBC I had more freedom to do what feels right for me during labour and delivery	183 (90)	9 (4)	2 (1)	0 —	0 —	10 (5)
At the EBC I was not attached to any monitors or high-tech equipment	158 (78)	15 (7)	20 (10)	2 (1)	0 —	9 (4)
At the EBC I was looked after by midwives and no doctors were involved	135 (66)	34 (17)	25 (12)	3 (2)	1 —	6 (3)
At the EBC I didn't have to move to another room after I'd had my baby	91 (45)	13 (6)	37 (18)	2 (1)	0 —	61 (30)
At the EBC I could sort out my own food	89 (44)	42 (21)	53 (24)	5 (3)	1 —	14 (7)

Table 12.8 Women's assessments of the importance of the attractions of EBC compared with a home birth (n=204)

	Added greatly to my experience n (%)	Added a little to my experience n (%)	Made no difference n (%)	Took away a little from my experience n (%)	Took away a great deal from my experience n (%)	Missing data n (%)
There were more facilities at the EBC than I could get at home	163 (80)	10 (5)	17 (8)	0 —	0 —	14 (7)
The midwives were always there at the EBC; I didn't have to wait for them to come	161 (79)	15 (7)	13 (6)	0 —	0 —	15 (7)
I did not have to clean up any mess after the baby was born	134 (66)	26 (13)	27 (13)	1 —	0 —	16 (8)
My home and children were not disrupted	104 (51)	22 (11)	62 (30)	0 —	0 —	16 (8)
I got a break from domestic responsibilities	89 (44)	33 (16)	67 (33)	0 —	0 —	15 (7)
I did not have to worry about getting the house clean and tidy before I had the baby	82 (40)	34 (17)	74 (36)	1 —	0 —	13 (6)

Indeed, a remarkably high proportion of women–over a third (74, 36%)–who completed the postnatal questionnaire had considered, at some point in their pregnancy, having a home birth. The women's views on the significance of the features which distinguish a home birth and a birth at the birth centre are therefore particularly interesting.

Table 12.8 lists the features of the birth centre which had been identified as its attractions compared to a home birth. These reflect the high value that women place on having a special, non-medicalised centre in which to have their baby. The table shows, for each feature, the proportion of women who, after they had had their baby, felt that it had contributed to their birth experience. Three features of the birth centre were described as adding greatly to their experience of labour and delivery by the great majority of women: the special birthing facilities at the birth centre (e.g. birthing pool, birthing stool); the fact that the midwives were always there; and the fact that they did not have to clean up any mess after the baby was born.

These views were reinforced in choice of the two attractions that the women selected as most important. The special facilities at the birth centre

were identified by 68% of women and the constant presence of a midwife by 53%. Given what is involved in emptying and cleaning a birthing pool, it is perhaps not surprising that a substantial minority of women (21%) included the fact that they did not have to clean up the mess after the baby was born.

DRAWBACKS OF THE BIRTH CENTRE

Compared with a conventional hospital birth

The features of the birth centre which had been identified as its drawbacks compared to a conventional hospital birth are shown in Table 12.9. These reflect the concerns that women have about the absence of a doctor and the lack of specialist medical facilities. The table shows, for each feature, the proportion of women who, after they had had their baby, felt that it had detracted from their birth experience. What is striking here is that the majority of women found that each of these potential drawbacks did not in practice make any difference to their experience. Only two features–the potential need to transfer to a hospital a few miles away and limited

Table 12.9 Women's assessments of the importance of the drawbacks of EBC compared with a conventional hospital birth (n=204)

	Added greatly to my experience n (%)	Added a little to my experience n (%)	Made no difference n (%)	Took away a little from my experience n (%)	Took away a great deal from my experience n (%)	Missing data n (%)
I would have had to transfer to a hospital a few miles away if I or my baby developed a problem	16 (8)	2 (1)	100 (49)	57 (28)	22 (11)	7 (3)
There was limited specialist equipment at the EBC in case I or my baby had a problem	6 (3)	11 (5)	118 (58)	48 (24)	13 (6)	8 (4)
There was no doctor at the EBC in case of an emergency	12 (6)	12 (6)	135 (66)	33 (16)	7 (3)	5 (3)
Meals were not provided at the EBC	10 (5)	3 (2)	166 (81)	14 (7)	2 (1)	9 (4)
At the EBC I was not able to have an epidural	26 (13)	6 (3)	148 (73)	13 (6)	2 (1)	9 (4)

specialist medical equipment–were identified by what could be considered a substantial minority as detracting from their experience. It is interesting to note that more women found that not having the option of an epidural *added* to their experience than those who thought that this detracted from it.

Again, this picture is supported by the selection women made of the two potential drawbacks of the birth centre which were most important to them. Only one–the possibility of having to transfer to another hospital if a problem developed–was selected as important by the majority of women (59%). Only 47% identified limited specialist medical equipment and only 33%, the absence of a doctor.

Compared with a home birth

The features of the birth centre which had been identified as its drawbacks compared to a home birth are listed in Table 12.10. These reflect the concerns that women have about leaving home and travelling during labour. For each feature, the table shows the proportion of women who, after they had had their baby, felt that that feature had detracted from their birth experience. For all features at least two-thirds of the women

indicated that they made no difference to their experience at all. None of the features of the birth centre were selected as important drawbacks in practice by any more than a handful of women. The feature most commonly selected–having to pack a bag and travel when in labour–was selected, for example, by only 56 (27%) of the women.

WOMEN'S OVERALL ASSESSMENT

In all four versions of the questionnaire women were asked to make a number of global judgements about the relative advantages of a birth at the birth centre. Again, their responses underline how satisfied the women were with the birth centre and provide a very strong endorsement of it.

Comparison with the alternatives and their own hopes and expectations

When asked how far they agreed or disagreed with the following three statements the great majority of the 248 women indicated that they felt that a birth at the birth centre had advantages over a birth elsewhere and that their hopes

Table 12.10   Women's assessments of the importance of the drawbacks of EBC compared with a home birth (*n*=204)

	Added greatly to my experience n (%)	Added a little to my experience n (%)	Made no difference n (%)	Took away a little from my experience n (%)	Took away a great deal from my experience n (%)	Missing data n (%)
I had to pack my bag and travel when I went into labour	4 (2)	7 (3)	146 (72)	29 (14)	2 (1)	16 (8)
I had to arrange my own child care when I went to the EBC to have my baby	4 (2)	2 (1)	145 (71)	19 (9)	1 (1)	33 (16)
I had to bring my food with me to the EBC	6 (3)	7 (4)	153 (75)	15 (7)	4 (2)	19 (9)
I had less privacy at the EBC than I would have had at home	3 (2)	5 (3)	162 (80)	17 (8)	0 —	17 (8)
I did not have all my own familiar things around me at the EBC	4 (2)	3 (2)	166 (82)	16 (8)	0 —	15 (7)
My baby had to get used to a new place when I took him/her home	4 (2)	1 (1)	180 (88)	3 (2)	0 —	16 (8)

and expectations for their birth had been met: 73% strongly agreed and 15% agreed that the birth centre had considerable advantages over a hospital birth; 52% strongly agreed and 29% agreed that it had considerable advantages over a home birth; and 66% strongly agreed and 9% agreed that all their hopes had been met. Inasmuch as a birth at the birth centre most closely resembles a home birth, it is interesting that only 2% of women disagreed that the birth centre had considerable advantages over a home birth, although a further 13% neither agreed nor disagreed. A larger number (9%) disagreed that all their hopes had been met, but these were largely the women who transferred out of the birth centre before or during labour and the great majority had strongly agreed or agreed that they were.

Views on place of birth in the future

Finally, women were asked where, if they were pregnant again, they would like to have their baby and whether they would recommend the birth centre to a friend or relative if they were pregnant. The great majority of women (86%) said that they would have another baby at the birth centre; 7% said they would have a baby in hospital next time; and 4% said they would want a home birth.

An even larger number (96%) indicated that they would recommend it to a friend and only 2% said that they would not do so (in part because they did not believe in recommending anything to others). Four key themes could be identified in what they indicated they would say to others. It is striking that many women who had to transfer to hospital before labour or during labour made comments similar to those made by women who delivered at the birth centre.

The first theme was the relaxed, attractive, home-like environment of the birth centre. Typical comments included:

It's home from home, with a very relaxing and reassuring atmosphere. Everybody is so encouraging, reassuring, approachable and treat you so well. *(Delivered at the birth centre)*

Lovely, homely, comfortable environment. Midwives treat you and baby like you're special and it's a very special moment, no matter how many kids you have. You feel like you're having a baby and not ill or a burden and very confident. (I hope there'll be more like the birth centre and they can have doctors.) *(Transferred out before labour)*

The second theme concerned the confidence that women had in the midwives at the birth centre and in the quality of the maternity care they provided, which meant that they felt safe and secure in giving birth there. Examples of comments include:

The centre was an amazingly warm and relaxed atmosphere. The midwives are wonderful, both in experience and attitude. I *never* felt I was taking a risk being there. *(Delivered at the birth centre)*

Safe, caring, guided by experienced midwives. *Very* good alternative to hospital birth. *(Transferred out after delivery)*

The third theme was the feeling that they counted as individuals at the birth centre and that they received personal care and support, which enabled them to deliver as they chose to:

It is a relaxed, caring, warm and friendly environment where you count as a person and not a number on a conveyor belt. I was totally confident with the midwives who looked after me and I have no hesitation in recommending the birth centre. *(Delivered at the birth centre)*

The birth centre provides an invaluable service to women. The care is truly woman-centred. It seems to be the only place that treats women as intelligent human beings. My experience there is so at odds with what I experienced during hospital care, it is hard to believe it is part of the NHS. *(Transferred out during labour)*

The fourth theme was their sense of control over labour and delivery at the birth centre:

You . . . get woman-centred care in which you are empowered to make your own choices (e.g. birthing positions, use of birthing pool). A non-medicalised birth, birth seen as a natural experience. The birth centre enabled my labour and birth to be an immensely positive and empowering experience. *(Delivered at the birth centre)*

The midwives were excellent and very informative. They allowed me to feel relaxed and be in complete control of my labour. Also, I would emphasise how natural they made my baby's birth seem, not to mention the birthing pool which I couldn't have had a drug-free birth without. *(Delivered at the birth centre)*

As these comments suggest, the four themes are closely linked. Their recognition of the midwives'

skills and concern for them as individuals reassured women and helped them feel 'safe' in delivering at the birth centre, while its home-like environment helped to normalise the birth and gave them the confidence to assert control over their delivery. Together, these contributed to the sense of satisfaction and fulfilment that women found in their birth experience at the birth centre.

DISCUSSION

This chapter has described an evaluation of the Edgware Birth Centre carried out by an independent team of researchers. Health service innovations come with their own, often unexpressed, political agendas, which makes it vitally important that any evaluation is carried out by an independent team. We would like to thank the staff at EBC for their help in collecting data on clinical procedures and outcomes used in the evaluation. However, even with a well-motivated staff and nagging researchers, it proved difficult to get complete data on a number of topics, such as reasons for transfer. Similarly, questionnaires were returned by only just over half the women who gave birth during the study period. These gaps in the data are limitations which must be borne in mind in interpreting the findings reported in this chapter. They also suggest that routine audit may be difficult for service providers to conduct, even in the context of excellent clinical care.

The availability of a regional database of maternity care allowed us to make comparisons of clinical outcomes with similar women delivering at home or in hospital. However, no comparable database on women's assessment of their birth experience in hospital was available and we were unable to assess the preferences and assessments regarding place of birth of women who, despite fulfilling the eligibility criteria, did not choose the birth centre as their place of delivery. The birth centre just reached its targets for deliveries (166 deliveries in the first year of operation and 221 in the second) so it appears that many women were either not told about the birth centre or made a definite choice not to go there. Ideally, we would have assessed the views of these women on features of their place of birth and compared them with those of women who booked to deliver at the birth centre in order to gauge better the strength of support for the birth centre. Although this was not possible, it is clear that the level of satisfaction expressed by women who delivered at the birth centre matches or exceeds that of women reported in other studies who delivered in hospital (Cartwright 1979, Spurgeon 2001).

The two aspects of maternity care addressed in this chapter–clinical outcomes and women's own assessment of their birth experience–provide a positive picture of the birth centre. Several points are worth considering further. Morbidity rates were lower for women who booked to deliver at the birth centre. Birth centre midwives suggested that this was due to the high value they placed on a 'natural' labour and delivery, without medical intervention. As there was no epidural service on site, women did not suffer the complications sometimes associated with this type of anaesthesia (Lieberman 1999). Episiotomy rates were also significantly lower, a finding which is in line with current thinking on routine episiotomy (Lede et al 1996). However, these intervention rates were lower for *all* women who intended to deliver at the birth centre although 33.5% of these women actually delivered in hospital. The group choosing to book at the birth centre were clinically selected and self-selected for non-intervention in pregnancy, so it is likely that the high rates of normal birth in women booking at the birth centre were also due to their own aspirations for natural childbirth (which were supported by the midwives).

Twenty-four hour midwifery cover at the birth centre made it an attractive alternative to a home birth. While for a home birth women have to wait for a midwife to arrive and then see her leave shortly after the birth, the constant presence of a midwife at the birth centre made it feel a safer option. Despite the reassurance of staff on home birth, some women still felt that the birth centre was inherently safer and more accessible to medical back-up than their own home.

More generally, the birth centre was perceived as offering a distinctive option for maternity care, which women who booked to deliver there felt was attractive in principle and, following delivery, described as contributing to a satisfying and fulfilling birth experience. While the 'non-medical' nature of the birth centre was acknowledged as a potential drawback, it was rarely seen to detract from their experience except where transfer to a hospital had been required.

The findings described in this chapter are very encouraging in relation to midwife-led birth centres. However, this positive picture needs to be set in the context of one further consideration: the accessibility of the birth centre to women who would like this type of maternity care. The main factors restricting such women's access to the birth centre were their clinical suitability at the start of pregnancy and the clinical progress of the pregnancy. Requirements for safety at a stand-alone maternity unit led to the implementation of a tight set of criteria for booking at the birth centre. When applied to all the women booking in 1997–1998 at units on the SMMIS database, only 27% would have been eligible to book for care at the birth centre. This 'screening' test of eligibility criteria is not a specific or a sensitive tool. It rules out, from the start, many women who could potentially have a normal delivery (lack of specificity) but also includes many women who later go on to develop complications of pregnancy (lack of sensitivity). This severely limits the number of women who can benefit from the midwife-led care and the non-medicalised birth experience at the birth centre. Further research is needed to refine the eligibility criteria in order to extend further the choices women have in their maternity care.

REFERENCES

Barnet Health Authority 1998 Annual Public Health Report, Barnet Health Authority, London

Carstairs V, Morris R 1989 Deprivation, mortality and resource allocation. Community Medicine 11(4): 364–372

Cartwright A 1979 The dignity of labour. A study of childbearing and induction. Tavistock, London

Department of Health 1993 Changing Childbirth. Report of the Expert Maternity Group, The Stationery Office Books, London

Field D J et al 1988 Is perinatal mortality still a good indicator of perinatal care? Paediatric and Perinatal Epidemiology 2(3): 213–219

Gilbert R, Tookey P 1999 Perinatal mortality and morbidity among babies delivered in water: surveillance study and postal survey. British Medical Journal 319: 483–487

Lede R, Belizan J, Carroli G 1996 Is routine use of episiotomy justified? American Journal of Obstetrics and Gynaecology 174: 1399–1402

Lieberman E 1999 No free lunch on labor day. The risks and benefits of epidural analgesia during labor. Journal of Nursing and Midwifery 44(4): 394–398

Martin C 1990 How do you count maternal satisfaction? A user-commissioned survey of maternity services. In: Roberts H (ed) Women's health counts. Routledge, London

Newell D J 1992 Intention-to-treat analysis: implications for quantitative and qualitative research. International Journal of Epidemiology 21(5): 837–841

Office for National Statistics 1998 ONS Monitor DH3 98/3 August 18 1998. Infant and perinatal mortality–social and biological factors. Office for National Statistics, London

Saunders D et al 2000 Evaluation of the Edgware Birth Centre. Barnet Health Authority, London

Spurgeon P, Hicks C, Barwell F 2001 Antenatal, delivery and postnatal comparisons of maternal satisfaction with two pilot *Changing Childbirth* schemes compared with a traditional model of care. Midwifery 17:123–132

13

The economic implications of the Edgware birth centre

Julie Ratcliffe

INTRODUCTION

This chapter compares the resource use and resource costs associated with the provision of intrapartum care for low-risk women booked to deliver in hospital, at home and in a midwife-managed delivery unit (the Edgware Birth Centre), using 1998 data from the St Mary's Maternity Information System (SMMIS) in the North West Thames Health Authority region. The evidence presented in the earlier chapters suggests that over time, increasing numbers of women are choosing to deliver at the Edgware Birth Centre. From an economic perspective this observation raises the question as to whether the resources used and the costs associated with intrapartum care at the birth centre are lower than those associated with other modes of intrapartum care, in particular with intrapartum care received at a traditional hospital location.

Several previous studies have been undertaken which have compared the costs associated with home and hospital delivery (Anderson and Anderson, 1999, Henderson and Mugford 1997, Stilwell 1979). These studies found that the total costs associated with home deliveries were lower than those for hospital deliveries, although the differences found were not substantial. Two recent studies, undertaken in the United States (Stone & Zwanziger 2000) and Canada (Reinharz & Blais 2000), compared the costs associated with free-standing birth centres and medical models of care. Both studies concluded that there were some differences in the resource use and costs associated with care during the intrapartum period, with birth centre costs being lower, on average, than the care costs associated with the medical model of care. Evidence is currently lacking on the costs associated with the provision of intrapartum care within free-standing birth centres in the UK and on how these costs compare with those of births in traditional hospital or home locations.

METHODS

The vast majority of previous costing studies in the maternity services have taken a 'top-down' approach to the comparison of resource use and resource costs of alternative models of care. However, recent guidelines for costing in economic evaluation studies in the health care sector suggest that a 'bottom-up' approach is more appropriate, whereby all cost estimates are based on actual resource consumption, using local unit costs wherever possible (Drummond et al 1997). This approach has been adopted here. The main items of resource use which data were collected on are listed in Box 13.1. Information on resource use was obtained primarily from SMMIS records, a large and high-quality routine database. Health care resource use and costs were included for care received in the intrapartum period only. Intrapartum care is the most easily definable period of maternity care as there is much more variability between women in the pattern and content of antenatal and postnatal care received. In addition, most women

---

Box 13.1 Items of resource use recorded for cost analysis of intrapartum care

Type of delivery (including duration of labour and delivery, and the staff who delivered the baby)
Frequency and type of investigations carried out
Drug use and interventions for mother and/or baby
Transfers to hospital
Frequency of postnatal admissions
Length of postnatal stay

---

booked to deliver at the birth centre were booked there after 20 weeks gestation and it was difficult to obtain accurate information on their antenatal care resource use prior to transferring to the birth centre.

The total sample size of women to be included in the economic analysis was estimated on the assumption that there are, on average, 3500 deliveries at each acute unit per year. Of these women, it was considered that approximately 25% would be eligible to give birth at the birth centre. A sample of 1 in 25 women, fitting the criteria for giving birth at the birth centre, who were booked to deliver at each acute unit was then taken randomly, resulting in a sample of 33–35 women booked to deliver at each acute unit. A random sample of 1 in 10 women booked to deliver at the birth centre was also used, giving a matching numerical sample of 35 women from EBC.[1]

All data analysis was conducted on the basis of intended place of delivery at booking. Transfers from the intended place of delivery to another location were therefore possible and the resource use and cost data reflected such transfers where these occurred.

The majority of unit cost information was obtained from the Finance Department of Barnet Health Authority for the financial year 1999–2000. Specialised staff time during labour and delivery was costed according to the amount of time spent by identified staff with each woman during the first and second stages of labour. All cost estimates were inclusive of on costs. The type and frequency of investigations, the quantity of consumables and medications used and the cost of each of these were used to estimate the total costs per woman for these items. The cost of deliveries included consumables, equipment and specialised staff time. In the absence of locally available disaggregated information, the unit costs of transfers, general staff time and overheads during labour and delivery and postnatal inpatient admissions were obtained from

---

[1]The total number of women included in the economic analyses was smaller than the research team would have liked ideally but reflected study timescales and the limits of research resources.

a previous study funded by North Thames Research and Development Committee (Lang 1998). The costs of general staff time and overheads were apportioned according to the amount of time spent in labour and delivery at each location for all women in the sample. The costs of inpatient admissions included general staffing costs, all non-staff running costs and overhead costs per 24-hour stay, and were similarly apportioned according to the number of postnatal days for all women in the sample.

Due to the absence of complete information on capital costs at all locations, capital costs are not included in the base case analysis. However the implications of the inclusion of capital costs for the results obtained are considered further in the sensitivity analysis.

STATISTICAL ANALYSIS

Data analysis was conducted on the basis of intended place of delivery, using the Statistical Package for the Social Sciences (SPSSPC) for Microsoft Windows version 9.0. Differences in resource use between alternative locations were reported in the form of frequency distributions and medians and ranges of values where

appropriate. (Due to the small sample sizes and non-normal distribution of the data, it was not appropriate to report means and standard deviations for resource use data).

The mean health service costs and standard deviations for intrapartum care and immediate postnatal stay were calculated for the sample of women booked to deliver at each location. The Kruskal–Wallis one-way analysis of variance was used for comparison of data between the independent samples. All statistical tests are two-tailed and the statistical level of significance was taken where P was <0.05.

RESULTS

Table 13.1 presents a summary of resources used by women booked to deliver at each location for intrapartum care. All of the women booked to deliver in the birth centre sample actually delivered there. The vast majority of these women (94.3%) had a normal vaginal delivery. Of the home birth sample, three women who had been booked to deliver at home (11.5%) were transferred to hospital during labour because of complications. For the two hospital samples,

Table 13.1 Summary of resources used, by location, for intrapartum care

	EBC (n=35) Number (%)	Home (n=26) Number (%)	Barnet (n=33) Number (%)	NPH (n=35) Number (%)
Normal deliveries at home	—	23 (88.0)	—	—
Normal deliveries in hospital	—	3 (11.5)	24 (72.7)	23 (65.7)
Normal deliveries in birth centre	33 (94.3)	—	—	—
Forceps deliveries	2 (5.7)	—	—	2 (5.7)
Vacuum extraction deliveries	—	—	6 (18.2)	4 (11.4)
Elective caesarean deliveries	—	—	1 (3.0)	1 (2.9)
Emergency caesarean deliveries	—	—	2 (6.1)	6 (17.1)
Breech deliveries	—	—	—	—
Transfers during labour	—	3 (12.0)	—	—
Inductions	—	2 (8.0)	18 (54.5)	13 (37.1)
Epidurals	—	—	15 (45.4)	14 (40.0)
Pethidine	—	1 (4.0)	11 (33.3)	8 (22.9)
Entonox	8 (22.9)	10 (40.0)	17 (51.5)	20 (57.1)
Sutures	4 (11.4)	—	15 (45.4)	4 (11.4)
Blood transfusions	—	—	—	2 (5.7)
Baby resuscitation	5 (14.3)	1 (4.0)	2 (6.1)	6 (17.1)

Barnet = Barnet General Hospital.
EBC = Edgware Birth Centre.
NPH = Northwick Park Hospital.

the incidence of assisted deliveries was much higher than for the birth centre sample, with 27.3% of the Barnet General Hospital sample and 34.3% of the Northwick Park Hospital (NPH) sample having an assisted delivery. There was a higher incidence of inductions (i.e. the use of oxytocic drugs to start labour, or during labour to increase contractions) at the hospital centres, Barnet having an incidence of 54.5% and NPH, 37.1%. A high proportion of women also received epidurals (Barnet, 45.4%; NPH, 40.0%) and other forms of pain relief at the hospital centres, relative to the birth centre and home locations. Barnet had a much higher incidence of sutures (45.4%) than NPH (11.4%).

A comparison of postnatal care received, by location, is reported in Table 13.2. The median length of postnatal stay following delivery for all samples was 24 hours, although the range of inpatient days for those admitted at Barnet (1–5 days) was greater than for all other locations.

Table 13.3 presents a detailed comparison, by location, of resources used for intrapartum care. It can be seen that, overall, there was much greater resource use for the two hospital samples, in comparison to the birth centre and home birth samples. A large proportion of women delivered at Barnet (42.4%) and a majority of women delivered at NPH (54.3%) were delivered by a hospital doctor whereas 94.3% of women booked to deliver at the birth centre and 96.0% of women booked to deliver at home were delivered by a midwife or community midwife. A comparison of the time spent in labour and delivery at each location (Table 13.4) reveals that women booked to deliver in hospital spent longer in labour and delivery, on average, than those booked to deliver at the birth centre or at home.

A comparison of the costs to the health service of hospital-booked, home-booked and birth centre booked women is presented in Table 13.5. There were statistically significant differences between locations in the costs associated with monitoring, spontaneous vaginal deliveries, vacuum extraction deliveries, elective caesarean deliveries, inductions, epidurals, and pethidine and Entonox for pain relief. Total mean intrapartum care costs were lowest in the home location (£193.96), followed by the birth centre (£297.01), Barnet General Hospital (£424.35) and NPH (£428.16), and the difference between the mean costs at each location was highly statistically significant ($P < 0.001$). Similarly, the costs associated with postnatal stay in each location differed significantly, with NPH having the highest total mean cost (£296.71). The total mean health service costs were lowest for women booked to deliver at a home location (£217.16), followed by the birth centre (£392.30), Barnet General Hospital (£608.90) and NPH (£635.81), and again the difference between the total mean health service costs at each location was highly statistically significant ($P < 0.001$).

SENSITIVITY ANALYSIS

The Edgware Birth Centre has six whole-time-equivalent (WTE) midwives permanently based at the centre and five WTE midwifery assistants. Within the base case analysis the costs of staff time in attendance was estimated according to the amount of time spent with the woman during

Table 13.2 Comparison of postnatal care received, by location

	Postnatal stay Number (%)	Inpatient days for those receiving postnatal care Median (range)
Edgware Birth Centre (n=35)	19 (54.3)	1 (1–2)
Home (n=26)	2 (8.0)	1 (1–2)
Barnet General Hospital (n=33)	29 (87.9)	1 (1–5)
Northwick Park Hospital (n=35)	19 (54.3)	1 (1–2)

Table 13.3 Detailed comparison of resources used, by location, for intrapartum care

	EBC (n=35) Number (%)	Home (n=26) Number (%)	Barnet (n=33) Number (%)	NPH (n=35) Number (%)
Induction using prostaglandin	—	1 (4.0)	8 (24.2)	5 (14.8)
Induction using oxytocin	2 (5.7)	1 (4.0)	10 (30.3)	8 (22.9)
Artificial rupture of membranes	6 (17.1)	9 (36.0)	17 (51.5)	16 (45.7)
Electronic fetal heart monitor	2 (5.7)	1 (4.0)	28 (84.8)	35 (100)
Fetal blood sampling	2 (5.7)	—	4 (12.1)	6 (17.1)
Inhalational analgesia in labour	7 (20.0)	9 (36.0)	17 (51.5)	20 (57.1)
Pethidine in labour	—	1 (4.0)	11 (33.3)	7 (20.0)
Epidural in labour	—	—	12 (36.4)	12 (34.3)
General anaesthetic in labour	—	—	—	—
Spinal in labour	—	—	1 (3.0)	—
Combined spinal/epidural in labour	—	—	—	—
TENS in labour	—	—	—	—
Inhalational analgesia in delivery	8 (22.9)	1 (4.0)	4 (12.1)	2 (5.7)
Epidural in delivery	—	—	15 (45.5)	14 (40.0)
General anaesthetic in delivery	—	—	—	—
Spinal in delivery	2 (8.0)	—	1 (3.0)	1 (2.9)
Combined spinal/epidural in delivery	—	—	1 (3.0)	3 (8.6)
TENS in delivery	—	—	1 (3.0)	—
Local infiltration in delivery	1 (4.0)	1 (4.0)	1 (3.0)	3 (8.6)
Pudendal block in delivery	—	—	—	—
Spontaneous vaginal delivery	33 (94.3)	26 (100.0)	24 (72.7)	23 (65.7)
Elective caesarean delivery	—	—	1 (3.0)	1 (2.9)
Emergency caesarean delivery	—	—	2 (6.1)	6 (17.1)
Lift-out forceps	2 (5.7)	—	—	2 (5.7)
Rotational forceps	—	—	—	—
Ventouse	—	—	6 (18.2)	4 (11.4)
Assisted breech	—	—	—	—
Breech extraction	—	—	—	—
Delivered by community midwife	11 (31.4)	22 (88.0)	10 (30.3)	2 (5.7)
Delivered by midwife	22 (62.9)	2 (8.0)	9 (27.3)	14 (14.0)
Delivered by hospital doctor	2 (5.7)	—	14 (42.4)	19 (54.3)
Unattended in labour	—	1 (4.0)	—	—
Inhalational analgesia post-delivery	—	—	—	1 (2.9)
Pethidine post-delivery	—	—	—	—
Epidural post-delivery	—	—	4 (12.1)	11 (31.4)
General anaesthetic post-delivery	—	—	—	—
Spinal post-delivery	1 (2.9)	—	—	2 (5.7)
Combined spinal/epidural post-delivery	—	—	—	2 (5.7)
TENS post-delivery	—	—	—	—
Local infiltration post-delivery	—	1 (4.0)	8 (24.2)	7 (20.0)
Pudendal block post-delivery	—	—	—	—
First-degree sutures	2 (5.7)	—	4 (12.1)	1 (2.9)
Second-degree sutures	1 (2.9)	—	11 (33.3)	3 (8.6)
Episiotomy	3 (8.6)	1 (4.0)	4 (12.1)	12 (34.3)
Third-degree sutures	—	—	—	—
Postnatal blood transfusion	—	—	—	2 (5.7)
Resuscitation–mask	4 (11.4)	—	2 (6.1)	3 (8.6)
Resuscitation–intubation	1 (2.9)	—	—	—
Resuscitation–cardiac massage	—	—	—	—
Resuscitation–naloxone	—	1 (4.0)	—	3 (8.6)

Barnet=Barnet General Hospital.
EBC=Edgware Birth Centre.
NPH=Northwick Park Hospital.

Table 13.4 Comparison of time spent in labour and delivery, by location

	Length of first stage (*minutes*) Median (range)	Length of second stage (*minutes*) Median (range)	Total length of labour and delivery (*minutes*) Median (range)
Edgware Birth Centre (*n=35*)	600 (15–2225)	27 (5–600)	648 (25–2337)
Home (*n=26*)	500 (130–1153)	15 (3–134)	528 (135–1201)
Barnet General Hospital (*n=33*)	726 (150–2830)	32 (3–335)	812 (201–2901)
Northwick Park Hospital (*n=35*)	775 (100–1450)	26 (3–347)	783 (110–1620)

Table 13.5 Comparison of costs for hospital-booked, home-booked and birth centre booked women (Figures are in UK £ sterling)

	EBC (*n=35*) Mean (SD)	Home (*n=26*) Mean (SD)	Barnet (*n=33*) Mean (SD)	NPH (*n=35*) Mean (SD)	P value
Intrapartum					
Monitoring	1.29 (5.30)	0.26 (1.30)	2.28 (5.49)	2.29 (6.28)	<0.001[1]
Specialised staff time during labour and delivery	185.88 (116.99)	134.07 (66.27)	214.74 (145.44)	197.77 (100.15)	0.431
General staff time/overheads during labour and delivery	79.87 (50.54)	8.32 (2.26)	89.52 (62.84)	81.28 (43.27)	0.141
Spontaneous vaginal deliveries	18.99 (4.75)	20.15 (4.43)	14.65 (9.11)	13.24 (9.70)	<0.001[1]
Forceps deliveries	2.76 (11.38)	—	—	2.76 (11.38)	0.335
Vacuum extraction deliveries	—	—	8.79 (18.93)	5.52 (15.60)	0.014[1]
Elective caesarean deliveries	—	—	6.37 (36.61)	6.01 (35.55)	0.619
Emergency caesarean deliveries	—	—	12.74 (50.96)	36.06 (80.43)	0.011[1]
Transfers during labour	—	28.43 (4.26)	—	—	0.512
Inductions during labour	—	2 (8.0)	18 (54.5)	13 (37.1)	<0.001[1]
Epidurals	—	—	40.18 (48.93)	45.21 (55.81)	<0.001[1]
Pethidine	—	0.01 (0.15)	0.25 (0.35)	0.17 (0.32)	<0.001[1]
Entonox	0.78 (1.47)	0.72 (1.05)	1.21 (1.41)	1.19 (1.24)	0.114
Sutures	5.19 (10.76)	—	15.41 (13.84)	12.95 (14.43)	<0.001[1]
Blood transfusions	—	—	—	10.22 (42.12)	0.147
Baby resuscitation	2.25 (10.90)	0.004 (0.02)	0.21 (0.86)	0.31 (1.00)	0.284
Manual removal of placenta	—	—	—	0.18 (1.07)	0.448
Total intrapartum care	297.01 (116.11)	193.96 (58.74)	424.35 (175.04)	428.16 (167.10)	<0.001[1]
Postnatal stay					
Inpatient days	95.29 (99.11)	23.20 (68.52)	184.55 (146.23)	296.71 (207.65)	<0.001[1]
Total health service	392.30 (164.29)	217.16 (156.79)	608.90 (253.51)	635.81 (311.96)	<0.001[1]

Barnet=Barnet General Hospital.
EBC=Edgware Birth Centre.
NPH=Northwick Park Hospital.
SD=Standard deviation; *P*=probability.
[1]Statistically significant, *P*<0.05.

the intrapartum period. This is the normal practice for economic evaluation studies in health care and is based on the premise that if the staff were not with the woman, they would be caring for other women at the same or in another location. Due to the relatively low frequency of deliveries over time at the birth centre (less than one delivery per day on average) this may not be the

Table 13.6 Comparison of costs for birth centre booked women according to the proportion of about non-patient-based time spent by core midwives (Figures are in UK £ sterling)

	5%	10%	20%	30%	40%
Proportion of time spent on non-patient-based care					
Total annual cost of time spent on non-patient based care	12 181.00	24 361.00	48 723.00	73 083.00	97 444.00
Mean cost per woman of time spent on non-patient-based care	30.53	61.06	122.11	183.17	244.22
Total intrapartum care cost	327.54	358.07	419.12	480.18	541.23
Total health service cost	422.83	453.36	514.41	575.47	636.52

case for the core midwives based at the birth centre.[2]

In order to reflect fully the costs associated with the core midwives over the time period being studied, several assumptions were made about the amount of time spent per midwife at the birth centre during which direct patient care was not given. The costs associated with this time were then apportioned to the volume of women receiving intrapartum care at the birth centre during the second year of the evaluation, in order to obtain an additional mean cost per woman of non-patient care. This additional mean cost was added to the total cost for each woman included in the birth centre resource use sample and the overall impact on the total mean health service cost for care received at the birth centre was assessed (Table 13.6). It can be seen that when it is assumed that the amount of time spent by the core midwives at the birth centre on non-patient-based care is an average of 30%, the mean total health service costs of care received at the birth centre during the intrapartum and early postnatal period (£575.47) remain lower than the mean total health service costs for care received at Barnet (£608.90) or at NPH (£635.81) during the same period. If it is assumed that 40% of time is spent on non-patient-based care, the mean total health service costs of care received at the birth centre (£636.52) are higher than at either of the hospital locations.

[2]It may also be argued that an allowance for time spent on non-patient-based activities should be incorporated into the costs associated with midwives' time at both of the hospital locations. However, given that the frequency of deliveries is much higher at these locations, it is unlikely that the time allocated to such activities will be as significant.

Table 13.7 Comparison of costs for women booked at Barnet General Hospital and at Edgware Birth Centre, incorporating capital charges

	EBC (n=35)	Barnet (n=33)
Total capital charges per annum	£92 718.00	£750 000.00
Number of deliveries	399	2333
Mean capital charges per woman delivered	£232.38	£321.47
Total intrapartum care	£529.39	£745.82
Total health service	£624.68	£930.37

Barnet = Barnet General Hospital.
EBC = Edgware Birth Centre.

A comparison of costs for women booked at Barnet General Hospital and at the birth centre, incorporating capital charges, is presented in Table 13.7. The capital costs associated with the birth centre are abnormally high as the centre is based at a site that is not being fully utilised at present. Inclusion of the capital charges element (£92 718) to the overall costs of care received at the birth centre, apportioned on the basis of activity during the second year of the evaluation (399 deliveries), results in an increase in the mean total health service costs of care received at the birth centre during the intrapartum and early postnatal period of £232.38 per woman. This estimate represents a 59% increase on the mean total health service costs per woman of care received at the birth centre reported in the base case analysis, which included actual resource use only and excluded capital costs. The mean total health service costs per woman booked to receive care at the birth centre increase to £624.68 when capital charges are included in the cost analysis. Similarly, inclusion of the capital charges element to the overall costs for women booked to receive care at Barnet (£750,000.00), apportioned on the basis of activity during 1997 (2333 deliveries), results in an increase in the mean total health service costs of care received at Barnet during the intrapartum and early postnatal period of £321.47 per woman, an increase of 53% on the mean total health service cost reported in the base case analysis. The mean total health service costs per woman of care received at Barnet increase to £930.37 when capital charges are included in the cost analysis.

DISCUSSION

The results from this study indicate that the total mean health service costs are lowest for women intending to give birth at home, followed by Edgware Birth Centre, Barnet General Hospital and NPH. The low costs for the home birth sample reflect the relatively low resource use by this group, in particular the absence of general staff/overhead costs during labour and delivery and postnatal inpatient admissions for the vast majority of women in this sample. However, the results from this study must be interpreted with caution for three main reasons:

- Firstly, the sample sizes which the resource use and cost exercises have been based on are quite small and hence may be subject to selection bias.
- Secondly, despite the best efforts of the evaluation team during the time-frame of the study, we were unable to obtain locally relevant unit costs for every item of resource use included in the analysis. In particular, the unit cost of transfers, general staff time and overheads during labour and delivery and postnatal inpatient admissions were obtained from a previous costing study carried out in inner London (Lang 1998).[3] It may not be possible to generalise these costs to other centres and it is important

that further work is undertaken to isolate the local unit costs of these items at the locations included within this analysis.

- Thirdly, data on capital costs was not available at all locations and it was therefore not possible to include this information in the base case analysis.

However, the advantage of using an identical set of unit costs throughout (as in the base case analysis) and applying these to resource use data at all locations is that variation in costs between alternative locations can be explained by differences in actual resources used rather than by differences in hospital costing and/or accounting procedures. Ideally, one would undertake two separate analyses: the first analysis including unit costs generated by the finance department at each location; and the second analysis using a common set of unit costs throughout. Unfortunately, we were unable to adopt the first of these approaches due to the unavailability of disaggregated unit cost information at all locations for the majority of resource use items included in this analysis.

Inclusion of the capital charges element inflates the mean total health service costs for women booked to receive care at the birth centre. However, it was found that this increase is not substantially higher than the increase in mean total health service costs incurred at Barnet General Hospital when this element is included. The 'true' extent of time not spent on 'hands-on' delivery care at the birth centre or any other location is very difficult to quantify. Calculations based on assumptions regarding the percentage of time spent on non-patient-based care by the birth centre midwives (5%, 10%, 20% or 30%) show a reduction in the difference between the mean total health service costs per woman at this location relative to a hospital location. When this percentage reaches 40% the cost of care received at the birth centre is higher than at a hospital location. However, in the majority of instances, the results from the sensitivity analysis do not overturn the base case conclusions that the cost to the health service of maternity care for women booked to deliver at

---

[3]The use of these specific cost estimates may partly explain the relatively high cost of care received at NPH despite the observation that their woman-to-midwife ratio is higher than that at Barnet General Hospital.

the birth centre is lower than that for women booked to deliver in hospital but higher than that for women intending to deliver at home.

CONCLUSION

The study results may reflect both the way in which care at the birth centre is managed and the characteristics of women who choose to deliver at the birth centre. It is possible that the higher mean average costs at the hospital locations are a reflection of the relatively high proportion of women receiving epidurals, who then go on to require a higher proportion of assisted deliveries, on average, than women who use other forms of pain relief. In addition, women who require induction are, by definition, always included in the hospital group (some women who transferred from other locations may also have gone on to require induction during labour). The data analysis suggests that women who choose to deliver at the birth centre spend a shorter time, on average, at the birth centre and receive relatively few interventions relative to women who choose to deliver in a hospital location. These differences in actual resources used are reflected in the lower mean health service costs associated with women booked to deliver at Edgware Birth Centre in comparison with Barnet General Hospital and NPH.

REFERENCES

Anderson R E, Anderson D A 1999 The cost-effectiveness of home-births. Journal of nurse-midwifery 44 (1) 30–35.
Drummond M et al 1997 Methods for the economic evaluation of health care programmes 2nd edn. Oxford University Press, Oxford
Henderson J, Mugford M 1997 An economic evaluation of home births. In: Chamberlain G (ed) Home Births. Parthenon, London
Lang H 1998 Options in maternity care. Final report to North Thames Health Authority, North West Thames

Health Authority Research and Development Committee London
Reinharz D, Blais R 2000 Cost-effectiveness of midwifery services versus medical services. Canadian Journal of Public Health 91: 112–115
Stilwell J A 1979 Relative costs of home and hospital confinement. British Medical Journal 2: 259–259
Stone P W, Zwanziger J 2000 Economic analysis of two models of low-risk maternity care. Research in Nursing and Health 23: 279–289

FURTHER READING

Scottish Home and Health Department 1993 Provision of maternity services in Scotland. A policy review. The Stationery Office Books, Edinburgh

Twaddle S, Stuart B 1994 Home and domino births: resource implications. British Journal of Midwifery 2: 530–533

Birth centres
in the wider world

14

The Stockholm birth centre

Ulla Waldenström

INTRODUCTION

The first birth centre in Sweden opened at Södersjukhuset (South Hospital) in Stockholm in October 1989. During the first three and a half years the centre was part of a research project, before being transferred to standard care. This chapter focuses on these first years and the outcome of the evaluation of the birth centre. It also summarises some of the controversies associated with the start of the centre and its transfer from research project to routine care. Finally, I will describe the present status of what has been one of the most controversial maternity services in Sweden over the last 15 years.

In spite of its location (within a hospital) the Stockholm Birth Centre had great similarities with the free-standing birth centres in the US. Antenatal, intrapartum and postpartum care took place in the same homelike premises by a team of midwives. Women were at low medical risk at booking in early pregnancy and the aim was to provide care which would facilitate a natural childbirth. Medical technology, such as electronic fetal heart-rate monitoring, induction, stimulation of labour and pharmacological pain relief, was not available at the centre. If a woman wanted an epidural block or developed some kind of complication she was transferred to standard care. The birth centre was located on the ground floor, just under the ordinary delivery ward, and transfer during labour took only a couple of minutes. The woman was encouraged to take as much responsibility as possible for her own pregnancy and during the antenatal period she kept her own records. In the centre she and her partner had access to the kitchen, which was shared with the midwives. During labour the woman and her partner could lock the door to the birthing room from inside. This was, however, more a symbol of empowerment rather than something practised as routine. Babies were examined by a paediatrician before discharge, which took place within 24 hours after the birth. The midwives visited the new family in their home when needed. Approximately 2 months after the birth the woman came back for a routine postnatal check-up with the midwife.

The centre was staffed by 10 midwives who shared 8.5 full-time equivalent positions. One of them was the charge midwife, with approximately half of her time allocated to administrative work. An obstetrician was responsible for the medical guidelines, and provided antenatal care half a day a week. Intrapartum and postpartum care was provided by the midwives independently, based on the written guidelines. During labour, the midwife decided herself about transfer to the ordinary delivery ward; during pregnancy, transfer to standard antenatal care usually took place in collaboration with the obstetrician providing antenatal care at the birth centre.

A midwife was available 24 hours a day to care for women in labour. If no woman was in the centre she did administrative work, cleaning or other activities related to the maintenance of the centre. She was also able to make home visits during the overlap period between the day and evening/night shifts. At night and over the weekends a second midwife was on call at home. Each midwife provided antenatal care at least one day a week and also ran parental classes. Parental education was given either weekly, as classes with a maximum of six couples, or as lectures once per month to which all expectant parents booked for antenatal care at the centre were welcome. These lectures covered themes like 'how to cope with labour pain', 'how to care for the newborn' and 'breastfeeding'. The centre had a capacity of approximately 400 bookings per year.

HOW IT ALL STARTED

In the mid 1980s Dr Carl-Axel Nilsson visited several birth centres in the US and met with Dr Ruth Watson Lubic who at that time was the director of the Maternity Center Association, the non-profit organisation that opened the first free-standing birth centre in New York. Dr Nilsson, who was the head of the Department of Obstetrics and Gynaecology at Motala Hopital, Sweden, was concerned about the increasing use of medical interventions in obstetrics. He was also in favour of free choice and consequently of the existence of options for care. As a midwife, I shared the same concern about the medicalisation of childbirth. I had recently finished my PhD, which was about early discharge from hospital after normal birth. This work had made me question many of the procedures surrounding labour and birth and the effect of hospitalisation on childbirth. I was also involved in the public debate about natural childbirth which was taking place in the media at the time.

When Carl-Axel and I met we decided we would try to start a birth centre in Sweden. We were both committed to evidence-based care, even though the concept was not in vogue at that time. We wanted to take advantage of the fact that Sweden did not then have any birth centres, which made it possible to conduct a randomised controlled trial: women who opted for birth centre care would have a 50% chance of getting it, instead of no chance at all. Under these circumstances it would be ethical to randomise women into a birth centre group and another group which offered standard antenatal, intrapartum and postpartum care. The experiment would be feasible because it would not be possible for women allotted standard care to go to any other birth centre in the city. We realised that the trial needed to be conducted in Stockholm in order to recruit sufficient numbers of women within a reasonable period of time. The problem was that we did not live or work in Stockholm.

We contacted the Head of the Department of Obstetrics and Gynaecology at Södersjukhuset, the most centrally located of the six maternity hospitals in Stockholm. He supported the idea and we were then able to continue to 'sell' it to the political decision-makers in the Stockholm County Council. We also needed the support of the other five maternity units in the region in order to prevent any of them from opening a similar centre during the project period. This would have impacted in a negative way on the recruitment of women to our research project. We were also keen to encourage a spirit of collaboration with our colleagues practising in the local antenatal clinics, especially the midwives, who could help us by handing out information folders to pregnant women at booking and by telling them about the new alternative in a positive way. This was important as the birth centre concept was completely new for women in Sweden.

To our surprise, we received support from all the heads of the departments of obstetrics and gynaecology in Stockholm at a joint meeting, and a proposal was sent to the Stockholm County Council where the final decision (including an answer to the question of financial support) had to be made. We were surprised because we knew that many of the obstetricians would not be enthusiastic about the birth centre concept. However, they all agreed that the research project could provide important information and that a randomised controlled study would include a control group of women in standard care, which would also produce information about routine care. The fact that the birth centre was to be part of a research project was a prerequisite for the unanimous support.

We went to see the chairmen of the five largest political parties in Stockholm, those in power as well as those in opposition, in order to avoid the introduction of this new model of care becoming a political issue. All parties supported the idea, based mainly on our arguments about the increasing use of medical technology, the need to introduce alternatives to standard care and more freedom of choice, and the possibility of rising costs. In a second round of visits we went to see the chief administrator of the respective political parties. After these months of lobbying it took another year before the final political decision was made, in 1988, which gave financial

support to the new birth centre for a period of 2 years. No money, however, was allocated to the rebuilding of the premises.

An application to the Swedish Medical Research Council for the costs involved in evaluation of the birth centre was approved and I received project money which would cover my own salary for a period of 4 years.

SWEDISH MATERNITY CARE

In order to understand the context in which the birth centre was set up, I would like to say a few words about Swedish maternity care. Sweden has a population of approximately 9 million inhabitants and the number of births per year was slightly more than 100 000 when the birth centre opened. Maternity care is public, except for a few privately run antenatal clinics, and all care (except in home births) is paid via taxes. Antenatal care takes place in local antenatal clinics. During the project period these numbered approximately 600, 70–75 of them located in greater Stockholm, which was the recruitment area for the birth centre. Antenatal care is provided by midwives and in a normal pregnancy women only make one or two routine visits to a doctor. Almost all women give birth in hospital (the home-birth rate is approximately 0.1%) and the length of stay was approximately 4 days at the start of the project. During labour women are assisted by midwives, except during operative deliveries. An obstetrician is often on site on the delivery ward and midwives and obstetricians consequently work in close collaboration, even if the midwives do the major part of all 'hands-on' work.

Swedish midwives have a long tradition of relatively independent practice, but they work within the public system and are employed by the county councils in the same way as the majority of the medical profession. In contrast to many other western countries, however, it is the midwifery, and not the medical, profession which most women associate with normal childbirth. In this context you would think that the birth centre concept would not be a great challenge, but it was.

When the birth centre opened, hospitals and antenatal clinics were still funded via budget.

This was very advantageous because midwives at the antenatal clinics around Stockholm could recommend women at booking to go to the birth centre without any negative financial consequences for their own clinic. However, this changed during the project period when hospitals and outpatient clinics began to be reimbursed according to 'production'.

THE PROBLEMS

Once the political decision was made, the problems began. Without going into details, the Head of the Department of Obstetrics and Gynaecology at Södersjukhuset at the time wanted to take the project over and to exclude Carl-Axel Nilsson and myself. One of the arguments was that we were outsiders who did not work within the Department. However, we came to an agreement and I was accepted as project leader, but without the mandate of such a position. The following months of preparations were extremely difficult and I came to a point where I decided to give up and leave the project. Obviously, this was a necessary step and it resulted in an external audit. This reviewed the process and finally came up with a solution–all our roles were clarified and Carl-Axel and I were able to continue our work according to the approved project plan. Carl-Axel's role was to take responsibility for the medical guidelines and also to be the obstetrician providing antenatal care and participating at the monthly meetings held at the centre. My role as project leader was to take responsibility for the research and to see that the clinical part of the project followed the project plan. After these initial months of conflict the climate changed, a new head of department was employed, the premises had been renovated by money from the hospital, the new midwives came on-board and we were all filled with enthusiasm.

THE MIDWIVES

Altogether, 25 midwives applied for the advertised positions. Experience with intrapartum care was of highest priority as this was the area where the midwives would practise most

independently and also where dramatic events could occur at short notice. Next in priority was experience with antenatal care, followed by personal characteristics and willingness to practise according to the centre's guidelines and philosophy. The 10 midwives employed were, on average, aged 41 years (the range was 35–51 years). They had been practising midwifery for an average of 14 years (range, 7–28 years), within intrapartum and postpartum care for an average of 11 years (range, 4–24 years) and antenatal care for an average of 1.5 years (range, 0.1–7 years). Three of them were also qualified midwifery teachers and seven had children.

During the project period of 3.5 years there was no turnover of staff. The team worked extremely well together and today, after 13 years, we are still very close and meet regularly socially. There are many reasons why the team worked so well. First, it was a selected group of committed people who enjoyed being midwives, who believed that childbirth was a major and positive life event, and whose most important professional goal was to support pregnant women and their families through pregnancy, labour, birth and the first few days with the baby. This had a great influence on their own work and on what happened at the centre. We all met one day a month and all the major decisions were made jointly at that meeting. The day started with 2 hours with the obstetrician, when we discussed medical problems. After this, general issues that needed to be dealt with were raised, followed by 2 hours with a psychologist. During these last 2 hours we discussed psychological problems of individual women in our care as well as problems within the team. Another factor that strengthened and united the team was a certain degree of external pressure.

In 1993 we published a book based on two interviews (in 1990 and 1992) with each of the 10 midwives about their experiences of practising in a birth centre (Waldenström 1993). Their experiences can be summarised in the following quotes from that book:

The major advantage with birth centre care was that antenatal, intrapartum and postpartum care were integrated. This was an advantage for the parents as well as for the midwives. To provide antenatal, intra-partum, and postpartum care and domiciliary visits, as well as having parental education and contraception counselling, made the work varied and stimulating. The midwives learnt to know the parents very well during the extended contact–almost a year from early pregnancy to postnatal check-up. They got involved in 'their' parents, were able to provide individualised care and were better at following up their work than they used to be in other workplaces. The midwives believed that the comprehensive care made the parents feel more secure because they became familiar with the midwives and the premises.

Another advantage with birth centre care was the focus on childbirth as something normal and healthy, and not to use medication and technology unnecessarily. Most of the midwives did not miss pharmacological pain relief, the option of augmenting labour, or electronic fetal monitoring. They were more guided by the woman's own needs than by established routines. The midwives said they had developed their own way of monitoring labour. They felt they were better at interpreting the woman's and her baby's signals, such as movements, sound, facial expression, words and emotional expressions. This was facilitated by the fact that the midwife had the opportunity to be with the woman during her entire labour and she didn't need to spend time on organising medical equipment.

In spite of the fact that all the midwives had extensive professional experience of intrapartum care when commencing at the birth centre, they felt after some time that they had learnt a lot more about pregnancy, labour and birth. They were impressed by the woman's own power, which they hadn't seen so clearly before.

The most important change in the midwives' way of practising after 2 years in a birth centre was an increased attentiveness to the woman's feelings and needs. The midwives felt they were less authoritarian than before. They gave less direction during labour and birth and handed over more responsibility to the woman and her partner than they had done before. They saw the woman's partner more as a participant than as a companion. The small-scale format made the activities within the centre easy to grasp. The midwives felt it was easy to influence both their own work and what happened at the centre as a whole. The work environment was pleasant, physically as well as psychologically.

The midwives believed that the major disadvantage of birth centre care from the parents' perspective was

the transfer to the ordinary labour ward when complications occurred or when the woman needed pharmacological pain relief. This could cause distress and be perceived as a failure.

The midwives listed as the major disadvantage the shortage of stand-ins when someone was sick or otherwise not available. Some of the midwives were concerned about the possibility of losing knowledge about medical complications if they worked in the birth centre over a prolonged period.

THE RESEARCH PROJECT

Information about the birth centre was widely spread. Many of our midwifery colleagues in the local antenatal clinics helped by handing out our information folder. This included a description of the centre and the research project, with its random allocation to birth centre care and standard care. During the 1980s an interest in natural childbirth developed among midwives, expectant parents and journalists. The birth centre was therefore a popular topic in the media. The great interest among journalists, and the fact that many of the pregnant journalists were subjects in the birth centre project themselves, gave us frequent and very good media coverage during the first years.

In my role as project leader I was not involved in the clinical work, but participated at the monthly meetings. The midwives had no part in the research, except for informing women who rang the centre about the research project. They never saw what questions were asked in the questionnaires and they were not informed about any outcomes while the centre was still part of the research project. One factor that we could not disregard was the fact that we were all biased, believing that birth centre care was superior to standard care–that was the reason why we were all there. This was also true for many of the expectant parents. We addressed this problem in many ways. One was to make sure that all the midwives had a thorough understanding of the idea behind a randomised controlled trial. Even if we *believed* that birth centre care was the best of birth options, we did not *know* if this was the case–it might be a good alternative for some parents but not for others, and some aspects might be better than standard care but others might not. There was in fact no evidence available, and that was the reason why we were conducting a trial. We all had to have this in mind and had to be totally objective when we informed parents about the project. Being randomised to the control group was not a negative outcome, but equally important in terms of collecting information about the pros and cons of the two models of care being compared.

The expectant parents were informed in several ways before being randomised: briefly over the phone at the first contact; via the information folder which was mailed to their home address (if they had not received it at a local antenatal clinic); and, finally, at a personal meeting either with me or with a research assistant. They then took a sealed, opaque envelope from a box, which contained a paper strip with either 'Birth centre group' or 'Standard care group' written on it.

The aim of the trial was to study the effect of birth centre care on:

* mothers' and fathers' satisfaction with care
* mothers' and fathers' experience of childbirth
* fathers' involvement in infant care and utilisation of parental leave
* breastfeeding
* medical procedures, such as pharmacological pain relief, induction, augmentation of labour, mode of delivery and transfer rates
* infant and maternal outcomes.

In addition to these aims, we also wanted to study:

* the characteristics of women choosing birth centre care
* midwives' experiences of birth centre care.

Data in the trial were collected by means of three questionnaires: one before randomisation, in early pregnancy; a second by the end of pregnancy; and a third 2 months after the birth. Medical data were retrieved from the hospital records, covering antenatal, intrapartum and postpartum care.

The funding covered only the first 2 years, too short a period to recruit a sufficient number of women to be able to make valid conclusions about infant outcomes such as perinatal mortality and severe morbidity. From October 1989 to February 1992 we recruited 1230 women, 617 randomised to the birth centre group (BCG) and 613 to the standard care group (SCG). Data from these women and their partners enabled us to achieve the first four aims. We then succeeded in getting additional funding and continued the recruitment for another 18 months, ending up with a sample of 1860 women, 928 in BCG and 932 in SCG. The expected dates of delivery of the 1860 women ranged from October 1989 to the end of June 1993. This sample provided the power (confidence interval 95%, power 80%) to detect a reduction in the caesarean section rate from an expected 10% in SCG to 6.3% in BCG, a reduction in the rate of epidural anaesthesia from an expected 16% in SCG to 11.4% in BCG, and an increase in the rate of neonatal transfers from an expected 10% in SCG to 14.4% in BCG. The sample was, however, still too small to detect differences in perinatal mortality.

To achieve the last two aims, a different research design was required. The study on background characteristics required a control group of women who were *not* interested in birth centre care, and the study of the midwives' experiences was an interview study with a qualitative approach. I will present the major findings of the research in reverse order to the list of aims above. The study of midwives' experiences has already been summarised.

CHARACTERISTICS OF WOMEN CHOOSING BIRTH CENTRE CARE

The reason we wanted to conduct a separate study describing the background characteristics of the women who participated in the trial (Waldenström & Nilsson 1993a) was that we suspected that it would be a rather distinctive group of women. If this was the case it would underline the importance of conducting a randomised controlled trial which would prevent us from comparing 'apples with oranges' and, at the same time, increase our knowledge about the population to which the findings could be generalised.

There is always a percentage of the population that is very open to new ideas and willing to test new concepts. Personally, I estimate this group to comprise around 10% of the population and I believe that these individuals are over-represented in certain professions, especially the so-called 'free professions'. My impression when recruiting women into the trial confirmed this view.

The first 1086 women enrolled in the birth centre trial formed an 'alternative group' (their randomisation to BCG and SCG were disregarded for the purposes of this part of the study) and a control group of 630 women was collected from among pregnant women who had chosen not to participate in the trial. This sample was drawn from the registers of the local antenatal clinics in Stockholm and matched with the alternative group regarding choice of antenatal clinic (residential area) and gestational stage when answering the questionnaire, but drawn at random in all other respects. The control group completed the same questionnaire the alternative group had completed prior to being randomised. The response rate was 100% in the alternative group and 70% in the control group. Responders and non-responders in the control group were of similar age, but primiparas were over-represented among the responders.

The study showed that women in the alternative group were older, better educated and had a different professional profile to the women in the control group. Health care workers and 'artists' (actors, singers, writers, journalists etc.) were more common in the alternative group while jobs in business, economics and law and clerical work were more common in the control group. Women in the alternative group had more positive attitudes to and expectations of the approaching birth and a greater interest in not being separated from the newborn and the rest of the family immediately after birth. They were also more interested in being actively involved in their own care. Generally speaking, women in the alternative group were more concerned about the psychological aspects of childbirth. No statistical differences were found in civil status, proportion of native Swedes or parity.

MEDICAL DATA

The major findings relating to medical interventions and infant and maternal outcomes are summarised in the paper 'The Stockholm Birth Centre Trial: maternal and infant outcome' (Waldenström et al 1997). Details about maternal outcomes are summarised elsewhere (Waldenström & Nilsson 1997). The 928 women randomised to BCG were very similar to the 932 women in SCG regarding age (mean, 30 years in both groups), education (mean, 14 years at school in both groups), civil status (93% and 95% respectively were married or cohabiting), proportion of native Swedes (87% in both groups) and gestation at randomisation (20 weeks in both groups). The proportion of first-time mothers was much higher than in the Swedish population but approximately the same in the two trial groups (59% for BCG and 56% for SCG).

In the birth centre group, 80% of the multiparas actually gave birth in the centre but only 51% of the primiparas did so (see Table 14.1). The major reasons for antenatal transfers were breech position (3.3%), high blood pressure or toxaemia (2.2%), post-term birth, >42 weeks (2.2%) and preterm birth, <37 weeks (1.2%). The major reasons for intrapartum transfers were failure to progress in labour (9.9%), fetal distress (5.1%) and need for analgesia (4.4%). Reasons for postnatal transfers were retained placenta (0.6%), sphincter damage (0.6%), haemorrhage (0.4%) and small baby (0.2%).

Data were analysed according to 'intention-to-treat', which means that all participants remain in their allotted group regardless of withdrawals and transfers. The option of transfer from the birth centre to standard care in cases of complications or if a woman needs any pharmacological pain relief is part of the birth centre concept. This explains why some women in BCG have pharmacological pain relief or other interventions (see below) in spite of the fact that these were not available in the centre.

Table 14.1   Maternal outcomes in the birth centre group (Waldenström et al 1997)

	Primiparas (n=544) %	Multiparas (n=384) %	P value	All (n=928) %
Withdrawals	2.0	2.9	0.54	2.4
Miscarriage, abortion	1.5	2.1	0.65	1.7
Antenatal transfer	15.8	9.9	0.01	13.4
Home birth	0.2	0.8	0.39	0.4
Intrapartum transfer	29.4	4.2	<0.001	19.0
Birth centre births	51.1	80.2	<0.001	63.1
Maternal postpartum transfer	2.2	1.3	0.45	1.8

Table 14.2 shows that women in BCG had less pharmacological pain relief than SCG women, but the difference in epidural rates was not statistically significant. There was a lower incidence of induction, augmentation of labour and electronic fetal monitoring in BCG and labour was, on average, 1 hour longer than in SCG. The incidence of surgical procedures, such as operative deliveries and episiotomies, did not differ statistically between the groups. Intervention rates in the group in standard care were generally lower than the national rates, which may be explained by the selection of low-risk women in early pregnancy but also by the selection of rather outspoken women who were able to get what they wanted, even within the standard system of care.

Infant birth weight, Apgar scores and principal newborn diagnoses did not differ statistically between the trial groups. Neither did admissions to neonatal care (11% in BCG and 9% in SCG) but the pattern of transfers differed between primiparous and multiparous women. First-born babies were admitted more often from BCG (15.6%) than from SCG where the rate was 9.5% (p=0.003), while the converse was the case for newborns of multiparous women (4.7% for BCG and 8.4% for SCG, p=0.04). Eight infants had some form of serious morbidity not caused by malformations or preterm birth. Six of these were from the birth centre group and two from the standard care group. In three of the BCG cases possible avoidable factors were identified and described in detail (Waldenström et al 1997). Perinatal mortality, defined as intrauterine death after 22 weeks of gestation and infant death

within 7 days of birth, occurred in eight cases (0.9%) in BCG and in two cases (0.2%) in SCG. Possible avoidable factors were identified in two of the stillbirths in the birth centre group and reported in detail (Waldenström et al 1997).

IS BIRTH CENTRE CARE SAFE?

Even if our study did not show any statistically significant differences in infant outcomes between the trial groups, some of the outcomes for first-born babies caused concern and highlighted the importance of further studies. The analyses of the individual cases of severe morbidity and mortality did not reveal any specific pattern. However, a potential risk factor associated with birth centre care could be the strong focus on normality and the commitment to a common philosophy of natural childbirth among midwives and expectant parents, which may increase the risk of overlooking signs of complications. Not having base electronic fetal heart monitoring on admission and the delay that can arise when a woman in labour is transferred may be other risk factors, and lack of experience with long labours could have been a problem during the first years. At the 30-month interview with the midwives they expressed a greater awareness of the risks of prolonged labour and said that they transferred women earlier than they did at the beginning of the trial.

After the project period ended electronic fetal monitoring was introduced (only as an admission test) and stricter criteria for transfer in cases of meconium-stained amniotic fluid were introduced.

Table 14.2   Medical interventions and outcome of labour (Waldenström et al 1997)

	BCG %	SCG %	P value
Analgesia:			
Epidural	12.1	15.1	0.07
Pethidine	3.7	13.4	<0.001
Nitrous oxide	14.3	46.6	<0.001
Pudendal block	3.4	5.6	0.04
Local analgesia postpartum	25.4	35.4	<0.001
General anaesthesia	6.5	6.1	0.83
Induction	2.7	4.6	0.05
Augmentation of labour:			
Amniotomy	23.3	39.3	<0.001
Oxytocin 1st stage	15.6	24.9	<0.001
Oxytocin 2nd stage	17.9	29.5	<0.001
Monitoring of labour:			
CTG	30.7	84.9	<0.001
Internal monitor	18.4	31.7	<0.001
Fetal scalp blood sampling	2.2	4.1	0.03
Intrauterine pressure catheter	6.1	5.7	0.77
Surgical procedures:			
Caesarean section:	7.1	8.9	0.18
elective	1.9	2.4	0.53
emergency	5.6	6.5	0.29
Vacuum extraction	3.9	4.4	0.74
Forceps	0	0.1	
Episiotomy	7.8	8.3	0.71
Manual removal of placenta	1.4	1.1	0.65
Postpartum haemorrhage:			
>600 ml	12.5	12.7	0.96
Blood transfusion	0.7	0.6	0.98
Length of labour (start of contractions to birth) in hours mean (median)	15.0 (12.1)	14.0 (11.7)	0.05

BCG = Birth centre group.
SCG = Standard care group.

In order to gain additional knowledge about safety, we are now conducting a study of infant outcomes over 10 years, including all 3250 women booked at the birth centre from 1989 to 1999. This study will form part of a PhD by Karin Gottvall, one of my doctoral students at Karolinska Institutet, Stockholm.

BREASTFEEDING

Two months after the birth 93% of women in both trial groups were breastfeeding exclusively (Waldenström & Nilsson 1994a). One year after birth, women in BCG said they had breastfed, either exclusively or partly, for an average of 8.6 months; women in SCG breastfed for 8.5 months. The breastfeeding rate at 2 months in the Stockholm area at the time was 76%. These figures demonstrate that birth centre care had no effect on the duration of breastfeeding and that the women in the trial, regardless of group allocation, were more motivated to breastfeed than the average population. Our study on women's background characteristics had also shown that women who participated in the trial had more positive attitudes to breastfeeding in early pregnancy than women who were not interested in birth centre care (Waldenström & Nilsson 1993a).

Other experiences of breastfeeding were also similar in the two groups. The only difference observed was that BCG women reported more breastfeeding complications at 2 months, such as sore nipples (36%, compared to 30%, p=0.03) and milk stasis (26%, compared to 19%, p=0.002), although the incidence of engorgement and mastitis did not differ statistically in the two groups. This difference may have been a result of reporting bias, the close relationship with the midwives encouraging greater openness and willingness to report problems, or it may have been because the birth centre midwives were less experienced in breastfeeding support. Their qualifications were primarily in antenatal and intrapartum care and they might not have been as focused on breastfeeding support as their colleagues on the postnatal wards of the hospitals were.

SATISFACTION WITH CARE

Women allotted birth centre care were more satisfied with antenatal, intrapartum and postpartum care than those allotted standard care, according to a questionnaire 2 months after the birth (Waldenström & Nilsson 1993b). Table 14.3 shows that the largest difference between the groups was in the women's assessment of the psychological aspects of their care, which related to the midwives' responses to women's feelings and emotional needs. The largest difference between the two groups was in the assessment of antenatal care. Almost two-thirds (63%) of BCG women said that their antenatal care had strengthened their self-esteem, compared with only 18% in SCG. This difference is interesting, considering that there was less continuity of midwifery care during the antenatal period in the birth centre group and yet this is believed to have a great influence on women's satisfaction with their care. In standard antenatal care in Sweden, women usually see the same midwife throughout pregnancy, but in the birth centre serious attempts were made to increase women's chances of knowing the midwife who would be present at the birth, which meant seeing a larger number of midwives at the antenatal check-ups. Parental classes were also deliberately led by a different midwife from the woman's principal antenatal care midwife. When evaluating a

Table 14.3 Women's satisfaction with antenatal, intrapartum and postpartum care (Waldenström & Nilsson 1993b). Mean values on 7-point scale: 1=very unsatisfactory; 7=very satisfactory

	BCG	SCG	Difference	P value
Antenatal care:				
Physical aspects	6.3	5.7	0.6	<0.001
Psychological aspects	6.5	5.0	1.5	<0.001
Comprehensive assessment	6.5	4.9	1.6	<0.001
Intrapartum care:				
Physical aspects	6.5	6.0	0.5	<0.001
Psychological aspects	6.3	5.5	0.8	<0.001
Comprehensive assessment	6.5	5.9	0.6	<0.001
Postpartum care:				
Physical aspects	6.1	5.0	1.1	<0.001
Psychological aspects	5.9	4.5	1.4	<0.001
Comprehensive assessment	6.0	4.9	1.1	<0.001

BCG=Birth centre group.
SCG=Standard care group.
Physical aspects of care included medical supervision and/or treatment; psychological aspects of care included professional response to women's feelings.

comprehensive 'package' of care such as birth centre care it is not possible to say which specific aspects of care explained an observed difference between the trial groups. Women's greater satisfaction with antenatal care in BCG may be related to a higher attendance rate at classes in preparation for childbirth and parenthood (83%, compared with 64% in SCG), to the way women were cared for by the midwives, or to the fact that the three phases of care were provided in the same home-like premises.

For women transferred during labour it was difficult to get a comprehensive measure of intrapartum care. They were usually more satisfied with the care provided at the centre than the care in the ordinary delivery suite. For the analysis we chose to use these women's measures of intrapartum care *after* transfer, which meant that intrapartum satisfaction scores for BCG were underestimated (Table 14.3). In spite of this, BCG women were more satisfied than SCG women.

The transfer system is often mentioned as a great disadvantage with birth centre care. When the women themselves were asked in an open-ended question to list what they considered the major disadvantages, no one mentioned antenatal transfers and 31% in BCG listed intrapartum transfers as the major disadvantage compared with 42% in SCG (p<0.001). The BCG women who actually gave birth at the centre and those who were transferred were analysed separately: 96% and 71% respectively expressed a hope that they might have birth centre care for a future birth. We concluded that transfer in labour was a problem, but that most BCG women regarded the system as a measure that ensured medical safety, rather than a disadvantage.

Women in BCG were more satisfied with postpartum care, in spite of the fact the length of their stay was shorter than in SCG (1.7 and 2.8 days respectively). The percentages of women who received domiciliary visits after birth were 71% and 36% in BCG and SCG respectively. For those who received home visits, the average number of visits was 1.2 in BCG and 1.9 in SCG.

An outcome such as satisfaction with care may be very sensitive to bias caused by disappointment with being randomised to standard care when the preferred choice would have been birth centre care. We tried to control for such bias by asking women about their reactions to their allocation. One month before term 59% of women in the standard care group were disappointed, which fell to 29% 2 months after birth. We controlled for this 'disappointment bias' by conducting a sensitivity analysis. The findings remained essentially the same and did not change the conclusions of the study.

WOMEN'S EXPERIENCE OF CHILDBIRTH

The childbirth experience is a much more complex outcome than the experience of care received. It may be affected by the content and quality of the services, but also by factors such as the woman's own attitudes, personality traits, the relationship with the partner and delivery outcomes. In the present study (Waldenström & Nilsson 1994b), women were asked 2 months after birth about different aspects of their experience, such as pain intensity, attitude to labour pain, involvement in the birth process, anxiety and satisfaction with own achievement. These questions were followed by a question asking for an overall assessment of labour and birth.

The primiparas in BCG and SCG had the same average score of 5.1 on the pain intensity scale, which ranged from 'no pain at all' (1) to 'worst pain imaginable' (7), in spite of the greater usage of pharmacological pain relief in SCG. The multiparas in BCG, on the other hand, assessed pain as more intense than the SCG multiparas–5.1 and 4.5 respectively (p<0.001). This difference may be related to their prenatal expectations of pain, BCG multiparas expecting pain to be more intense than multiparas in SCG. Women's attitude to labour pain 2 months after birth, measured on a 7-point scale ranging from 'very negative' (1) to 'very positive' (7) did not differ statistically between the trial groups.

There was no statistically significant difference in women's overall assessment of labour and birth when expressed on a 7-point scale from 'very negative' (=1) to 'very positive' (=7) (primiparas–5.5 in BCG compared with 5.3 in

SCG; multiparas–6.3 in BCG compared with 6.1 in SCG). Birth centre care did not reduce the incidence of traumatic birth experiences, but it increased the proportion of women who felt that they had had a 'very positive' birth experience to approximately 10%. However, this difference was not statistically significant and could therefore have occurred by chance. When looking at the specific aspects of childbirth, positive effects of birth centre care were mainly observed in the experiences of first-time mothers. Primiparas in BCG were more satisfied with their own achievement and felt more involved in the birth process than primiparas in SCG. Both primiparas and multiparas in BCG felt a greater freedom to express their feelings during labour and birth than did women in SCG. Levels of anxiety during labour and birth did not differ between the trial groups.

FATHERS' EXPERIENCES

In both the birth centre and in standard care expectant fathers were encouraged to join their partner at the antenatal visits and to participate in childbirth education classes. Exact information about the expectant fathers' participation in antenatal classes was not available, but almost all men join their partners for these classes in Sweden. The attendance rate at antenatal classes among BCG women was higher than in the SCG (83% compared with 64%). The men were encouraged to be present during labour and birth in both models of care, but fathers usually stayed with their partners during the whole postnatal stay in the birth centre, while most fathers went home after the birth in standard care. The policy of early discharge in the birth centre also made a difference for the fathers, compared with standard care (in which mothers and babies were taken care of by hospital staff during the first few days). During labour and the postnatal stay in the birth centre the fathers often took responsibility for practical issues like preparing meals and caring for the baby. In standard care, midwives and other staff were more involved in these activities. Altogether, expectant and new fathers in the birth centre were more involved in, and took

greater responsibility for, events around pregnancy, birth and the newborn baby than did fathers in the standard care group.

The men in the trial filled in similar questionnaires to those the women were given in early and late pregnancy and 2 months after the birth. Altogether, 1143 men were included in the study (87 of the 1230 women were single)–576 had partners randomised to BCG and 567 to SCG. The men in the two groups did not differ statistically regarding background variables such as age (mean age was 33 years in both groups), total duration of education (means were 14.5 years in BCG and 14.7 years in SCG), proportion of native Swedes (85% in both groups) and proportion of first-time fathers (51% in BCG compared with 47% in SCG) (Waldenström 1999a).

Table 14.4 shows that fathers in BCG had more positive experiences of intrapartum and postpartum care than fathers in SCG: attitudes by staff were assessed as more positive, the fathers felt they were treated with greater respect, and during labour the midwife was more supportive of their needs as partners.

The fathers' experiences of labour and birth were measured in a similar way to the mothers' (Waldenström 1999a). No statistical differences were found between men in BCG and SCG in overall experience of the birth or in any of the specific aspects of labour and birth (such as anxiety, the experience of being involved in the birth process, and freedom to express feelings) or in the assessment of the value of their own support to their partner. Men in both groups felt equally that their attendance at the birth had a positive impact on their relationship with their partner and on their immediate feelings for the newborn. The birth was a positive experience for most men, irrespective of model of care.

In the study of women's experiences of childbirth, birth centre care seemed to have a greater positive impact on first-time mothers. A similar pattern was not seen in the fathers. All aspects but one resulted in similar outcomes between the trial groups. The only difference was that birth centre care seemed to have greater impact

Table 14.4 Fathers' satisfaction with care (Waldenström 1999a)

	BCG	SCG	Difference	P value
Intrapartum care:				
Intrapartum care overall (1=very poor; 7=very good)	6.4	5.8	0.6	<0.001
Staff attitudes to father (1=very negative; 7=very postive)	6.4	5.9	0.5	<0.001
Respect shown to father by staff (1=very little respect; 7=very much respect)	6.1	5.5	0.6	<0.001
Support of father by midwife (1=none at all; 7=much support)	5.9	5.1	0.8	<0.001
Postpartum care in hospital:				
Postpartum care overall (1=very poor; 7=very good)	6.0	5.1	0.9	<0.001
Staff attitudes to father (1=very negative; 7=very postive)	6.2	5.2	1.0	<0.001
Respect to father shown by staff (1=very little respect; 7=very much respect)	5.9	5.0	0.9	<0.001
Postpartum care including home visits (1=very poor; 7=very good)	6.0	5.5	0.5	<0.001

BCG=Birth centre group.
SCG=Standard care group.

on first-time fathers' immediate feelings for the newborn in BCG than in SCG, when assessed on a 7-point scale ranging from 'very negative' (=1) to 'very positive (=7) (mean score in BCG was 6.5, compared with 6.3 in SCG, p=0.03).

Birth centre care did not seem to have any long-term effect on the fathers' adaptation during the first 2 months. Measures of physical and mental well-being, experience of fatherhood, involvement in infant care and utilisation of parental leave did not differ statistically between the trial groups.

As with the women, the men in the trial differed from the general population of expectant fathers in Stockholm. They were older and better educated than men who were not interested in participating in the trial (Waldenström & Nilsson 1993a) and their involvement in practical care activities indicates that they were more family-oriented than the average Swedish father. Fathers in the trial had spent an average of 3.4 hours (BCG) and 3.3 hours (SCG) with their

baby over the preceding 24 hours, when asked 2 months after birth; Swedish fathers in general devoted an average of 7–8 hours per week to household chores or childcare, according to a study published in 1987 (Hwang).

SECONDARY ANALYSES

Additional studies have been undertaken, based on data from the birth centre trial. At an early stage of the project we were concerned about possible adverse effects of immersion in water during labour, after the membranes were ruptured. Pharmacological pain relief was not available in the birth centre and we were all very open to alternative, less invasive methods of relieving women's pain. Baths during the first as well as the second stage of labour had become very popular among home birth advocates, in birth centres and also in some hospitals. At the time, little was published on the pros and cons of immersion in water during labour and of giving birth in water.

The birth centre guidelines did not allow elective water births because of the lack of evidence of its safety, but we felt fairly confident that immersion in water during first stage labour was safe when the fetal membranes were intact. However, we were uncertain about how safe it was after the membranes were ruptured. We therefore conducted a study in which we compared 89 women who took a warm bath after spontaneous rupture of the membranes at term with 89 women with the same time interval from spontaneous membrane rupture to delivery, but who did not bathe (Waldenström & Nilsson 1992). No statistical difference was observed between the groups with respect to infections, asphyxia or respiratory problems in the newborn infant, or maternal signs of amnionitis. However, a tendency towards more complications was observed in the bathing group. Babies born more than 24 hours after rupture of membranes had significantly lower Apgar scores at 5 minutes in the bathing group. As a result of this study and the sparse literature at the time, we modified the bathing policy at the birth centre from a rather enthusiastic to a more cautious approach.

My interest in understanding what factors affect women's experience of labour and birth resulted in another publication based on the data (Waldenström 1999b). The outcome variable was women's assessment of labour and birth overall, as measured in the questionnaire 2 months after the birth. The explanatory variables were collected from the pregnancy questionnaire, hospital records and the 2-month questionnaire. Regression analysis was conducted by including all the explanatory variables that were associated with the experience of childbirth when tested one by one. In the regression model, only five variables remained statistically significant: the woman's feeling of being involved in the birth process and midwife support were associated with a positive experience; anxiety during labour and birth, pain and having a first baby were associated with a negative

experience. A second regression analysis was conducted in which only variables measured independently of the principal outcome were included (excluding those in the 2-month questionnaire). Parity remained a significant predictor in this model, but the others were replaced by augmentation of labour, caesarean section, instrumental vaginal delivery and nitrous oxide, which were all associated with a negative birth experience.

Still another study of the experience of childbirth has been conducted. The aim was to explore whether a traumatic birth experience at a woman's first birth has any effect on her future reproduction (Gottvall & Waldenström 2002a). Data on primiparous women's overall assessment of the birth from the 2-month questionnaire in the collapsed trial groups were linked with the Swedish National Birth Register, which included information on these women's subsequent births and the time interval to the second birth, during a follow-up period ranging from 7 to 10 years. When controlling for a wide range of possible confounding factors, we found that a traumatic experience (1 and 2 on the 7-point scale of overall experience of labour and birth) was associated with fewer subsequent births and a longer interval to the next birth.

TRANSFER FROM RESEARCH PROJECT TO ROUTINE CARE

By July 1993 the project period had come to an end and the centre was transferred from being part of a research project to routine care. This process took place amid a certain degree of turmoil, which may be hazardous for me to describe because of my own involvement. The following description is therefore my personal view of what happened.

The birth centre was paid a lot of attention during its first years, in the media, among professionals, such as midwives and obstetricians, and by politicians. The centre did not have any major problems recruiting 'parents to be', and the scheduled time for visitors was always fully booked. Visitors, besides potential candidates for the project, were professionals and sometimes politicians from different parts of Sweden or from other countries. A professional film team produced two films from the centre. One followed a few couples through labour and birth and is being used in childbirth education classes in Sweden and in some other countries to illustrate natural childbirth. The other film, which was made for Swedish Television, illustrated natural childbirth and described the birth centre concept by interviewing parents and midwives at the centre. This attention was a great asset because it facilitated the recruitment of women to the birth centre trial, but it also caused problems within the Department of Obstetrics and Gynaecology in the hospital. There was a feeling among some of the medical and midwifery staff that there was too much focus on a unit which was actually only a minor part of the Department, one which only cared for a minority of all the women who gave birth, and which even transferred women out of the unit if any complication occurred.

The birth centre was part of the large Department of Obstetrics and Gynaecology and depended on good collaboration with it, especially when transferring women during active labour. Most of the time it worked out well, but not all the time. One reason for this was that some of the staff outside the centre were not in agreement with the birth centre concept. Critical attitudes related to concerns about safety, the lack of pharmacological pain relief, the transfer system or to the fact that the midwives practised very independently.

Another reason was the independence of the birth centre. Even though it was a unit within the Department, headed by the Head of Department, the birth centre was part of a research project, with its role specified in detail and with no possibility of changing this during the period of evaluation. Besides, the project had not evolved from within the Department and most of the staff were new.

Another factor was the premises. Part of the birth centre concept was to provide a calm environment that would make the expectant parents feel welcome and secure. As a consequence, we tried to limit the number of people in the centre to the parents and birth centre staff and we had the doors locked in order to prevent other staff in the Department from passing through the centre (unfortunately the centre was a shortcut between two blocks of the Department). All these factors contributed to the feeling that the birth centre was not 'owned' by the Department in the same way as other units were. This atmosphere of 'them and us' united the birth centre team, with positive effects on the working climate within the centre but with some negative effects outside. Several attempts were made to overcome these problems, such as joint meetings where staff from the birth centre and the delivery ward met and discussed mutual issues, but during the project period these meetings were not as well attended as we would have wished.

At the end of the project period the future status of the birth centre was discussed. All the midwives wanted to continue to work in the centre, and so did I. I wanted to continue for another 1–2 years in order to build up a midwifery research and development unit, with the birth centre as the clinical component. During the project period we had no midwifery students at the centre, and I envisaged the birth centre as a unique opportunity for students to see what natural childbirth was about. I therefore wanted to develop collaboration with the midwifery programme in Stockholm. It was also an opportunity to give midwifery research on normal childbirth a clinical base. As no funding was available for a separate position, focused on education and research, the only way to implement my ideas was to apply for the position as Charge Midwife at the centre.

It was decided that the birth centre should continue according to the same principles and in the same way as during the project period, but all positions were re-advertised. All the midwives, who had been working at the centre for almost 4 years, applied and I applied for the position as Charge Midwife. Half of the midwives were not re-employed and my application was unsuccessful. The new midwives were all less experienced than those they would replace. The decision was a shock for all of us, and those birth centre midwives who were re-employed did not feel they could accept the new positions, in solidarity with their colleagues (who were to be replaced to other wards within the Department). The informal explanation given for the decision was that the original group needed to be split up.

The decision attracted a lot of public attention. The 'consumer group' of parents at the birth centre, which was very strong, organised a large demonstration outside the hospital in support of the birth centre midwives, and the newspapers, local radio and television reported the event. However, the decision could not be changed. This was a traumatic experience for all those involved, which took years to overcome.

1993–2001

The birth centre continued, with almost all the staff replaced and with the same medical guidelines, except for the introduction of electronic fetal heart monitoring as an admission test and the exclusion of pregnancies over 42 weeks. The intrapartum transfer rate went up from 19% during the project period to 28% between 1994 and 2001. At the same time the proportion of first-time mothers decreased from 59% during the project period to approximately 40%, which is the same as the national figure. Considering the higher transfer rates in primiparas, the intrapartum transfer rate went up quite dramatically. The main explanation for this development was the adoption of a more cautious attitude to prolonged labours.

The changes in funding of antenatal care, which made the local antenatal clinics in Stockholm more reluctant to inform women about the birth centre option, and the less prominent media coverage affected the centre's admission rate. Closure of the birth centre was discussed several times between 1993 and 2000, for financial reasons related to insufficient numbers of admissions. However, the centre continued to operate, mainly because it was politically difficult to close it down. Whenever a rumour to close down started, parents rang the Head of Department and the political decision-makers and lobbied strongly to save the centre.

During the past 2 years there has been a dramatic shortage of delivery beds in the Stockholm region, caused by closure of two of the six maternity units in combination with a slowly rising birth rate. Pregnant women have been seriously affected by their lack of confidence that they will be admitted to the hospital of their choice when they arrive in active labour. Women at the birth centre, however, have always been certain that they will be able to commence labour at the centre. As a consequence, the admission rate went up and the pressure to close down for financial reasons decreased. A few women per month were also admitted for intrapartum and postpartum care only, without having had their antenatal care at the centre.

A couple of years after the dramatic transfer of the centre, our feelings of having been maltreated faded away and made room for gratitude that the centre still operated, with very minor changes to the original concept, as an option for pregnant women and their partners in the Stockholm region. One of the original midwives went back to work at the centre and I was invited by the Head of Department to present the research findings on a couple of occasions. Step by step we re-established collaboration and the Department decided to contribute to the funding of our study of the outcomes of all infants born to mothers admitted to the birth centre over a period of 10 years.

THE PRESENT STATUS

In 2001 the midwives at the centre were told once again, that the centre might close down. Faced with this threat, and having had difficulties in filling vacancies for a long time because of a general shortage of midwives in the region, the midwifery staff at the birth centre said 'enough is enough' and the majority submitted their notice to quit. The reduction of staff made it impossible to provide comprehensive care and over a period of several months the centre could only provide antenatal and postnatal care. The births had to take place in the ordinary delivery ward.

At the same time, a new birth option arose within the hospital. This option, named the

'Stork', was partly a response to a request from the politicians in Stockholm to come up with new ideas on how to solve the problem of the undersized services for labour, birth and the postpartum period. In their request, they specified that new units should be focused on normal childbirth, should be midwifery-led, and should include comprehensive antenatal, intrapartum and postpartum care. (These requirements were a true victory for the ideas underlying the birth centre concept.) The Stork was very similar to the birth centre in principle, but was three times larger and, if it could be funded, the birth centre could be incorporated within this new unit.

The crisis finally resulted in a decision to re-open the birth centre and to operate it to its full capacity until the opening of the Stork. The vacant midwifery positions were re-advertised, and half of them were filled with midwives from the project period! I was invited to speak at the re-opening ceremony in February 2002, which was a very happy event for all of us.

The Stork, which is scheduled to open in 2004, is a new challenge. It is estimated to have a capacity of 1200 births per year and will provide comprehensive antenatal, intrapartum and postpartum care for women at low medical risk. Three teams of midwives will care for their own group of women, within three separate wings, but during labour and birth midwives may sometimes also care for women in one of the other two teams. In contrast to the birth centre, the Stork will be equipped for pharmacological pain relief and with medical technology, which will make intrapartum and postpartum transfers unnecessary, except in cases of emergency caesarean section.

A new idea is that the Stork will be closely linked to the midwifery education programme in Stockholm and to research related to normal childbirth. There will be a focus on evidence-based care in practice and theory. In a way, the Stork is possibly a realisation of one of my earlier hopes, that the birth centre should be part of a research and development unit in midwifery. This time, the plans are well integrated and accepted by the Department of Obstetrics and Gynaecology in the hospital, and the planning has taken place in close collaboration with the obstetrician in charge of intrapartum care. Not all the decisions about the Stork have been taken yet, but the planning for the unit is ongoing. The major challenge is whether all the positive aspects of birth centre care, including low intervention rates, can survive within a larger context with close access to pharmacological pain relief and medical technology. It will take a few years before that question can be answered.

REFERENCES

Gottvall K, Waldenström U 2002a Does a traumatic birth experience have an impact on future reproduction? British Journal of Obstetrics and Gynaecology 109 (3): 254–260

Gottvall K, Waldenström U 2002b Does birth center care during a woman's first pregnancy have any impact on her future reproduction? Birth 29 (3): 177–181

Hwang P 1987 The changing role of the Swedish father. In: Lamb ME (ed.) The father's role: cross-cultural perspectives. Laurence Erlbaum, Hillsdale, NJ, p115–138

Waldenström U 1993 Midwives' experiences of working in a birth center. FoU-report 39, SHSTF, Stockholm (in Swedish)

Waldenström U 1999a Effects of birth center care on fathers' satisfaction with care, experience of the birth and adaptation to fatherhood. Journal of Reproductive and Infant Psychology 17: 357–368

Waldenström U 1999b Experience of labour and birth in 1111 women. Journal of Psychosomatic Research 47 (5): 471–482

Waldenström U, Nilsson CA 1992 Warm tub bath after spontaneous rupture of the membranes. Birth 19 (2): 57–63

Waldenström U, Nilsson CA 1993a Characteristics of women choosing birth center care. Acta Obstet Gynecol Scand 72 (3): 181–188

Waldenström U, Nilsson CA 1993b Women' satisfaction with birth center care. A randomized controlled study. Birth 20 (1): 3–13

Waldenström U, Nilsson CA 1994a No effect of birth center care on either duration or experience of breastfeeding, but more complications. Midwifery 10 (1): 8–17

Waldenström U, Nilsson CA 1994b Experience of childbirth in birth center care. Acta Obstet Gynaecol Scand 73 (7): 547–554

Waldenström U, Nilsson CA 1997 A randomized controlled study of birth center care versus standard care. Effects on women's health. Birth 24 (1): 17–26

Waldenström U, Nilsson CA, Winbladh B 1997 The Stockholm Birth Centre trial: maternal and infant Outcome. British Journal of Obstetrics Gynaecology 104 (4): 410–418

15

Birth centres in Italy

Verena Schmid

INTRODUCTION

How birth is organised in a society reflects female values and the values attributed to women. The creation of birth centres in Italy means that the process of birth will take on a different value to the one it has today. The meaning and place of birth centres in Italy can only be understood in their social context, and we will therefore be looking at the position of women and midwives in society as well as at the political development of health services in the past 30 years. We will discuss the position of physicians and of high-tech medicine in Italy, as well as the importance of midwives' education. The concept behind birth centres is deeply connected with the empowerment of social and female values, such as caring, respect for emotions and biological rhythms and with respect for medical care and technology when it is needed.

THE HISTORICAL BACKGROUND

In Italy the idea of the birth centre started with the 'Movement of Home Birth' in 1978. There was a move towards a new way of assisting birth, originating in Leboyer's message, which called attention to the sensitivity and vulnerability of the newborn baby, and in Odent's focus on the instinctive aspects of giving birth, on the importance of a protective ambience for women. It was influenced by Ina May Gaskin's manual of natural childbirth (Gaskin 1977), by feminist research on women's health and by Professor

Braibanti's teaching on physiology (he is a follower of Leboyer). All this, and a determination to succeed, opened the way for a new practice of midwifery. In those days it was seen as revolutionary in the eyes of medical obstetrics, but today it is a method which has been proved scientifically.

An important interdisciplinary conference held in Milan in 1985, 'The Culture of Childbirth', focused for the first time on the social aspects of birth. Meanwhile, there was an increase in the number of women who had experienced home birth as a moment of power and beauty. This small but powerful reality began to influence the medical establishment. The women's demand grew, and the process of humanising childbirth began, a process which slowly undermined the medical model of childbirth.

At the same time in Italy, modern life was increasingly detaching couples from their families–support for the woman/mother was dwindling. This directed women in two opposite directions: on the one hand there was a search for new solutions for the socialising of their experience; and on the other hand rationalisation of their disturbing biology led women increasingly towards delegation of their protection to the care of experts. Technology was offered and experienced as an answer to anxiety and feelings of inadequacy. Technology and birth centres seemed to offer alternative answers.

Already, in the second half of the 1980s, birth centres were being discussed and the first legislative bills were drawn up. In 1990 the first and only private birth centre in Italy was opened.

THE NATIONAL HEALTH SYSTEM AND BIRTH CENTRE LEGISLATION

MILESTONES

In 1978, within the context of reforming the healthcare system, each Region subdivided its territory into Local Health Departments ('Unità Sanitarie Locali' or USL). The same legal provisions abolished the institution of the district midwife, who had offered assistance at home and continuity of care. The midwife became an employee, working in the health department, and it was no longer possible for her to provide care at home or out-of-hours care. The woman changed from a *patient* and became a *user*, a consumer with rights. Giving birth outside the hospital system was possible only privately, at the expense of the woman and her family.

In the 1980s a users' movement arose to defend the rights of the patient, which included the rights of women in labour–basically, women were allowed to bring into the hospital a family member and the health-care operator who had followed them during pregnancy. Childbirth out of hospital was still not even considered.

'The Italian Groups for Home Birth' movement promoted bills to bring childbirth back into the home, under the healthcare system, and to open birth centres, and involved women's groups and politicians. A first law was approved in Lombardy in 1987, but it has not been applied till today. Other regional laws in five regions were formulated in its wake. Ongoing projects and their current position will be described at the end of this chapter.

In 1995 the Law of Informed Consent was passed. The relationship between physician/health-care operator and patient changed from a paternalistic to a democratic one, giving the 'client' greater opportunity for participation in their treatment. This was applied to home birth as well. A strong demand arose among women to be better informed, but the concept of truly informed choice remains as remote today as it was then.

ECONOMIC POLICY

In 1990, precipitated by the economic crisis in the health care system, USLs became 'ASLs' (Local Health Enterprises), with a managerial type of organisation and a new option to demand partial payment for services (by 'ticket'). The user had become a client with economic power, whose wishes and satisfaction had an economic value. Equality of services no longer existed, especially in obstetric services.

For example, epidural anaesthesia, amniocentesis and antenatal courses became ticket expenses. Health Enterprises, trying to save money, promoted de-hospitalisation and discharged women on the second day (and those who had had a caesarean on the fourth day), often without providing any further care at home.

Due to the severe economic crisis, Regions closed all maternity units with less than 500 births per year, concentrating childbirth in large centres. The many protests that ensued stimulated research into new, innovative services to replace the old ones. This resulted in the idea of promoting birth out of hospital and the concept of birth centres. The physiological nature of pregnancy and childbirth was recognised at the political level. The economic crisis led the Regions to overcome the powerful resistance of physicians and to embrace the concept of pregnancy as an aspect of health rather than illness. The midwife came back into favour due to the lower cost of her care, but without any personal economic benefit.

THE POLITICS OF BIRTH CENTRES IN ITALY

The home birth movement has produced a highly important social and political stimulus: by creating a reality of new experiences, it has raised the possibility of choice and, with this, the obligation to compare and evaluate.

The economic organisation of the Italian health system has meant that it has been possible to build birth centres that are independent of the national health care system, due to high management costs, and the high costs for users. Women have managed to bring the issue into law, however, tenaciously sensitising officials and politicians over the years with infinite discussion and a great deal of patience–it could be said that today's legislation is the fruit of infiltration from below. As this has not been a political project, knowledge is patchy and uneven. Many politicians have found in their hands a bill, either proposed or approved, the

meaning of which they had not an idea, having been totally ignorant of what a birth centre is. They tend to evaluate a project based on feminine values using a patriarchal value system. They entrust its realisation to the ASL, to the physicians. They adopt technological principles as safety criteria, rather than criteria for the promotion of health. This risks denaturing the project itself, establishing inappropriate modes and guidelines, and undermining its possible effectiveness.

The most critical point is the management of birth centres by midwives alone–physicians fear losing control, clients and power. They therefore want birth centres inside hospitals, but without providing for continuity of care, without any reorganisation of work into teams, and without medical reference to the social model of birth. We are therefore at the dawn of the era of birth centres, and of a women's healthcare model still in its infancy.

THE SOCIAL AND POLITICAL POSITION OF THE MIDWIFE

The midwife is trained as an auxiliary to the physician in the delivery room. Only since 1997 has the school of midwifery been separated from that of nursing, achieving recognition of a university diploma course in 2000. Teaching is conducted mainly by physicians, however, and is strongly oriented toward obstetric pathology. Practical training takes place exclusively in the hospital. The trainee midwife does not learn how to follow a normal pregnancy, how to differentiate physiology from pathology, how to conduct antenatal courses, or how to observe and treat a newborn infant. Nothing is taught about nursing and supporting the mother, nothing about care in the first months, nothing about consultation, nothing about contraception, adolescents, health and sex education, nothing on the many tasks of the midwife in promoting health, and nothing about her social role. She does not learn her profession during her basic training.

The independent midwife works alone and there is no support for non-hospital care.

Midwives who transgress are isolated and work under the pointing finger of the institutions (even the midwifery organisation), which are ready to denounce them at the first false step. Strong motivation is needed to work in this way and these midwives are often burdened with feelings of guilt and fear of punishment.

The midwife is also a woman, a woman who finds herself at a particular point in her own process of personal and social emancipation. She is frequently a woman who is subconsciously submissive, or strongly in conflict with man and masculine values. It is only a few midwives who open the conflict and deny the medical model of birth, placing themselves in a position of opposition. Most of them submit to masculine power and leave as a result of their frustration. The power exercised by physicians over women and over midwives is reflected by the number of caesareans: in the north, where the power of the physicians is wavering, the mean caesarean rate is 16–20%; in the regions of southern Italy the rate is 54% and there are hospitals with peak rates of 70–80%. Midwives are non-existent in their true role.

The industrial organisation of birth, with its segmentation, high numbers of births a day and its routine procedures, makes it very difficult to establish personal relationships with the women and to accompany them in their experience of birth, and job satisfaction is scarce. Midwives are absent from the social scene of the birth. The woman meets her only at the moment of labour. Political decisions on the midwife's behalf are always taken by physicians. Up until a few years ago the midwife was never directly represented in any institutional place–her political value is that of a specialised hospital nurse.

Faced with the prospect of launching an innovative project that restores to the midwife her true professional capacity, many fear the increase in responsibility, medico-legal blackmail, and the lack of security. They are not, in fact, prepared for their new role. Continuous education for midwives was totally ignored until about 2 years ago. There are many midwives who have taken no refresher course in the last 20 or 30 years, who do not read, do not use the internet and who do not know English. Very little specific literature exists in Italian. At present the only opportunity that exists to acquire specific professional tools for midwifery care is provided by the Scuola Elementale di Arte Ostetrica (SEAO), a private school founded by midwives with professional experience in out-of-hospital births, but this school alone is certainly not able to satisfy all needs, nationwide.

Highly adverse situations drive some people in the opposite direction–the strength that is required to live with such obstacles becomes transformed into the strength required to promote a totally innovative project. The midwife can regain faith in her own capability and a stimulus to study–in direct contact with women, in a relationship of continuous care. Gradually, through constant verification, she can then regain many professional tools. The birth centre represents a great opportunity and challenge for midwives and for women.

THE TRANSITION FROM INSTITUTIONAL TO RELATIONAL OBSTETRICS

The birth centre and the care it offers finds its reference in the social rather than the medical model of birth. Birth is primarily a life event and only exceptionally a medical event, but the transition from a technological model of childbirth to a social model is neither automatic nor simple. All points of reference change (see Box 15.1). Attention is changed from the search for signs of pathology to those of health; from instrumental diagnostics to maintenance of health; from exogenous to endogenous tools; from a directive to an empathetic relationship; from control to support; from giving advice to listening; from segmentation to holism. Care is no longer provided on an 'industrialised' basis, with the inevitable protocols of routine, but becomes personalised. Technology is no longer a tool of control and legal justification, but an aid to the well-being of a woman, its use determined by the woman herself. The operator is no longer

---

Box 15.1   Models of obstetric care

Institutional	Relational
Patriarchal model	Integrated model (incorporates different modes of care)
Childbirth seen as a medical event	Childbirth seen as a biosocial event
Mechanistic concept; physical event	Humanistic concept; psychophysical, spiritual and sexual event
Linear approach; evaluating constants; quantity; result-oriented	Circular approach; evaluating variables; quality; process-oriented
Absence of rhythm	Rhythmic (achieving balance between opposite polarities)
Use of technology as a tool of control and prestige, aiming at efficiency	Use of technology as an aid, a tool for effective care, aiming at well being
Pregnancy and childbirth seen as potentially risky, pathological, filled with unknown factors	Pregnancy and childbirth seen as a potential expression of power and health; reference points of women's security are inside the woman herself
Competencies, sense of protection and control are the province of the physician; security is seen as protection for the woman from her own emotions	Competencies, sense of protection and control are the province of the woman, herself; an emotional experience
Authoritarian	Informed choice
Segmentation of care, using the logic of industrial production	Continuity of care; life event
Adaptation and subordination of the woman	Central role played by the woman/couple
Intervention: aggressive, destructive; can augment pathology	Conservative, protective interventions, oriented towards re-establishing physiology, in relationship with the woman, involving her in therapeutic decisions
Interfering obstetrics	'Awaiting' obstetrics
Paternalistic, regressive medicine	Ecological, holistic, self-healing, educational medicine
Manipulation by operators; disabling of the able	Facilitation; enabling of the disabled
Science, opinion	Art, knowledge

the only competent person (exogenous, rational and empathetic competence)–it is the woman herself who is competent above all (endogenous and intuitive competence). Decisions are no longer taken by the operator, but are submitted to the woman for her considered choice, often a time-consuming process which requires support. Professional capability is focused on relationship skills and on the art of supporting. The principles of evaluation and intervention, both instrumental and pharmacological, can become holistic, involving emotional and behavioural or environmental aspects.

All of this requires the midwife, who is accustomed to working in a dependent role, in a medical system of obstetrics which focuses on (and often creates) pathology, to radically change her attitude. She has to become able to relate to others and to herself, to change her own professional identity. In brief, it requires her to work from within, as all modes of all health care in the social model of birth are characteristically feminine (see Box 15.2). The masculine modes are functional in emergency situations calling for fast decision-making; the feminine modes are for accompanying a healthy physiological process.

Box 15.2 Sexualised aspects of care

Masculine

Centred on: performance, functionality, speed, efficiency, results. Assigns no value to the process itself, mechanical, based on domination and aggression.

In childbirth: functionality, mechanisation. Aimed only at expulsion of the baby. Anxiety about performance. Requires adaptation and subordination of the women.

Feminine

Centred on: tenderness, affection, communication, dialogue. Assigns importance to the process itself, the quality of the experience. Tends to create bonds, feels emotions, is based on openness.

In childbirth: intimacy, gentleness, respect for biological and emotional rhythms, awaiting. Proposes options, allows expression of emotions, of pain. Provides support and protective environment.

Neither a masculine nor a feminine model alone can grant absolute security, a fact often obscured in the medical model of obstetrics. Appropriately integrated, however, they offer both security and quality of care.

But cultural and mental change is not enough. We need to create experiences of transition for the women, midwives and physicians, which allow them to explore themselves and lead to gradual acquisition of new tools of professional security. What is needed is specific training, in alignment with the new principles.

THE SOCIAL AND POLITICAL CONDITION OF WOMEN IN ITALY

The emancipation of Italian women has been very rapid. In moving towards independence, however, they are moving away from what is feminine and maternal and the fear of falling back into old patterns is still very strong. On the social level, femininity is still undervalued. It is therefore not surprising that childbirth continues to be interpreted according to masculine values, even by women themselves.

Emancipation in the personal, intimate sphere has not kept step with emancipation in the social sphere. This cannot take place through rejection or denial of women's history, but rather through a process of integration. In this way a woman is able to encounter, to recognise and to re-evaluate the furthest reaches of her femininity, to integrate

it into her social identity as well as into her society. The value of women in our society will be changed and the transformation of technological childbirth into humanised childbirth and eventually into free, sexualised and sexual childbirth, will be the consequence. The birth centre is the laboratory for this transformation.

DO WOMEN WANT BIRTH CENTRES?

As no survey has been conducted in Italy, we do not know the answer to this question. From various studies carried out in Italy and abroad we know, however, that a high percentage of women would prefer to give birth in a different place from the one that has been chosen for them. This divergence is linked in part to the unavailability of other facilities, in part to fear of 'doing the wrong thing'. Deep within women is a fear of social transgression, as women know through historical experience that this may be severely punished. Consequently, the woman protects herself, does not expose herself, especially where her child is involved. This atavistic fear can be overcome only by offering and socially reinforcing places of new experience, places free of prejudice. A private birth centre, created by 'alternative,' midwives is not reassuring in the face of such fear, while an institutional birth centre, if approved and supported, can quell this deep, unconscious anxiety. In this sense, a birth centre can meet the needs of a broad range of users only if it enjoys the full support of the institution, of the hospital department and of the other pertinent facilities, and if the midwives involved are fully supported by the institution.

WOMENS' DECISIONS

Women are confronted by other ambivalent attitudes that have to be addressed. As Briffault (1977) states in *The Mothers*, human beings have two natures, a biological one (instinctual) and a social one, which holds the group together. Conflict arises for a woman when the social model is in contrast with inner values. A masculine model of birth creates conflict with the inner biological, self-preservational nature of woman, and this can paralyse her in making her decisions. These conflicts are connected with the most intimate needs of women, such as intimacy, individuality, and the sharing of the experience of pregnancy and delivery with her family. There is a great need for social acceptance, for safety, and for care. There is often a need to express something of the sacred nature of an event, in a special place.

To make decisions about childbirth the woman must explore her own ambivalence and face possible silent disapproval, fear and uncertainty as to the outcome. She therefore needs scientific knowledge and the experience of others, on which to base her decision, as well as to be in contact with her needs and physical and spiritual resources. The continuity of care which is provided in a public birth centre is the ideal framework for accompanying women going through these decision-making processes, with all their implications.

OTHER NEEDS IN CHILDBIRTH

THE BABY'S NEEDS

Another strong need felt by parents who experience the birth of their baby at home or in a birth centre is the need to welcome their child into the world according to their own values, without extraneous interference.

This matches the baby's need to be welcomed, to be allowed to orient himself through his senses, to find his mother, her arms that hold him, her breast that replaces the lost placenta, her heart that beats for him, her gaze that welcomes him, her familiar voice that tells him, 'I will take care of you.' This is everything the baby needs. His first impressions will remain imprinted in him for a lifetime, due to the very high levels of adrenaline after childbirth, and will influence his perception of life.

THE PARTNER'S NEEDS

Men too experience strongly ambivalent attitudes towards pregnancy and childbirth today. A man's virility is seen to be endangered by too close a contact with profound feminine energies, and, deep down, he fears the terrain of birth. At the same time his role in the couple has changed. He is the partner of the woman in all areas of life in the context of the nuclear family and shares in her emotional life as well, once an area from which men were precluded. The couple's relationship itself is subject to varying dynamics, and ranges from one of deep communication to more formal relations. The man sees himself as socially obliged to confront pregnancy and birth as mediator and companion.

One of the man's needs which undoubtedly remains unfulfilled is that for support in this confrontation, as a person, not merely as an appendage of the woman. He needs to be guided towards a specific role interpretation, be recognised and strengthened in his generative power, be helped to navigate between feminine and masculine territories, without losing his identity. He needs to be affirmed in his role as the woman's sexual and emotional partner, as the father of the child being created, as the ecological power of the woman and the child. Only by strengthening each partner in the couple, man and woman in their specific roles, will it be possible to overcome the feelings of impotence and inadequacy that can trigger competition, revenge and mutual envy. The birth centre can welcome the couple and accompany them in their voyage toward parenthood.

TOOLS FOR MIDWIVES

TRAINING

Training is the basis of the midwife's process of emancipation. Ongoing training with active teaching provides the tools for the personal development necessary for change, puts the midwife in contact with the new conceptual references, offers her support in the process of change, and acts as a cohesive force in the group. Training is not limited, in fact, to aspects of health care, but also furnishes the midwife with the professional tools which enable her to function autonomously, to dialogue with other operators, to work in a team. A specific training model for birth centres include:

- Scientific methodologies (research, data collection, verification, computer science)
- Clinical care, holistic physiology and continuity of care, scientific evidence, procedures for emergencies
- Communication (self-affirmation, therapeutic relationships, managing emotions, informed decision-making, counselling)
- Specific policies for midwives (political and promotional strategies, power and potency, gender and power, medical and social models of birth, historical and cultural aspects)
- Legal aspects of the profession
- Pre- and postnatal courses (work on the body, group dynamics, methods of adult teaching, standards)

The fundamentals of midwifery training are rooted in physiology and centred on the woman, her experience and needs, on helping her in making and affirming her decisions. They are built around the midwife's professional experience, integrating the empirical and the rational but giving intuition a place. In short it is a holistic approach.

Active methodology allows each participant to express and elaborate on her own experiences, doubts and fears, to experiment with her own body (through bodywork experiences), to discover and implement her endogenous resources, to bring to consciousness her own intuitions, to strengthen herself in a group of peers with similar values. Training should be considered a laboratory of experimentation and experience.

SUPPORT

1. *Social support:* midwives who assume personal responsibility for birth centres must be recognised and supported by the institution and by society. The humanisation of birth cannot take place without midwives. Political and economic reassessment of this profession is essential.

2. *Operational support* is provided by the work team which surrounds the operational group: consultant physicians, midwives and doctors from the host department, other operators who form a network of support and consultation. Collaboration needs new bases–working in a team is an innovation. There must be periodic updating, periodic supervision, and confrontation within the work team. Midwifery care can be both objective and highly subjective and there are frequently no certainties–nor are the operators all-powerful. In moments of difficulty, therefore, support and collaboration among the operators and services are vital.

3. *Theoretical support:* midwives should study the scientific literature and reports of research in obstetrics and therefore need to subscribe to reviews and to the Internet.

4. *Organisation of the work:* team collaboration, continuity of care and periodic rotation with the midwives from the hospital department in the case of institutional birth centres are the salient features of birth centre working. Working in a team means waiving some degree of individuality in favour of the group but, in compensation, it offers the support necessary for such demanding work.

STEPS IN THE DIRECTION OF CHANGE

It is important to create transitional experiences first, moving gradually from the exclusively medical/technological model to the humanised model of birth. This may be done by the construction of rooms for natural childbirth; by assigning spontaneous, active childbirth to the direct and exclusive responsibility of midwives; by establishing a new working relationship with the physician; by taking over the screening of normal pregnancies and the care provided for new mothers, (all tasks which are not at present assigned to the midwife, with very few exceptions).

Some modifications can be made in the organisation of work, in the direction of greater continuity of care. 'Physiological' midwifery departments, run by midwives alone, can be created–'maternity wards', with teamwork organisation, with supervision and with a support figure in the host institution.

The final, major step to out-of-hospital birth centre then becomes feasible, working in a good relationship with the hospital facility. Supervision, as a form of support, and circular learning (experience → verification → deeper investigation → change → experience, etc.) should accompany the first year of experimentation.

DIFFICULTIES
New costs

Even when an open institutional culture allows midwives new planning capacity, many practical obstacles still remain to be overcome. The first is the pressure of time. As there is no tradition of meetings during working hours for discussion or planning and because the new services call for greater commitment, more resources in terms of time and money will be needed. If requests for these resources are not answered, the enthusiasm of the midwives who are pushing for change will lack sound foundations. Once birth centres have been created, it cannot be expected that the midwives will go on working for the same salaries when they are assuming much greater responsibility.

New work patterns

The organisation of work represents another problem: the midwives, accustomed to rigid hospital shifts, will have to become flexible and be available out of normal working hours. Instead of working individually and in a hierarchical mode they will work in a team. They will need to learn how to manage their new responsibilities for developing a relationship with the woman and for her health without the direct supervision of the physician. This is a little like deciding to leave one's family and live alone.

Opposition

There will be opposition from the physicians and hostility from many midwife colleagues who are not participating in the project. The midwife, previously in a subordinate position, now enters into the hierarchical system of competition and envy and this can lead to severe disintegration among midwives themselves. It is frequently the case that colleagues prove to be the greatest obstacle.

Bureaucracy

Another typically Italian problem is the *bureaucracy* and the highly complicated political and administrative organisation of the health care system. It is practically impossible to dialogue with a manager in a decision-making position. Institutional power can neutralise all innovative energy in this way. These obstacles exhaust the midwives' strength, faith and motivation.

The resistance of women

Still another difficulty lies in the lack of a change of opinion on the part of the women users. Italian women are followed by gynaecologists during pregnancy–the women are oriented towards apparently easy external solutions rather than new options and growth.

POSSIBLE SOLUTIONS

Despite the difficulties, where midwives do manage to offer new services for pregnancy, women arrive. It is the midwives' responsibility to rebuild the bridge between themselves and women, to promote and offer services which welcome women with the intention of restoring to them their generative and creative potency. It is only out of this alliance that birth centres can be created, and with them a new way of experiencing childbirth, of being a woman, a family. A fundamental step in this direction is for midwives to resume personally the screening of pregnancy, thus accompanying the women and creating the basis for a different kind of birth.

Training, as the indispensable basis for change, has as an objective not only new health care competencies, but also group work, communication, self-esteem and self-assertion, contractual capacity and solidarity. The involvement of a broader group of operators, including those who work in the host or neighbouring hospital department, of physicians and administrators, is indispensable to the creation of the necessary supporting network. The first projects will be highly experimental, requiring regular supervision. The first stages of their realisation will be accompanied by extensive cultural and promotional work.

BIRTH CENTRES PROJECTS IN ITALY

The first and only birth centre in Italy was founded in Milan, in 1990, thanks to a series of exceptional coincidences. It was the private initiative of a group of midwives who were already assisting home births. They found hospitality at the 'Home of the Mother and Child' a foundation established in 1945 to assist unmarried mothers in difficulty and who were unsupported by their families. The girls stayed in the home during pregnancy, gave birth there and could live there until the child was 3 years old. The facilities were therefore already set up for childbirth. The birth centre midwives were welcomed in exchange for their offer of care to the girls living there. After an eviction notice was served, however, the facility had to be closed. Meanwhile, a new group of midwives and mothers was formed and they found both new premises and the money required, which means that a new centre is to be opened soon. It

seems that Italians are nearly ready, socially and culturally, for the advent of birth centres.

In 1996 the Scuola Elementale di Arte Ostetrica (SEAO), a school for the ongoing training of midwives, and run by midwives, was established. Its purposes are to promote the new holistic model of obstetric care, to personalise midwifery care, and to proclaim the right of midwives to learn their profession from other midwives. It introduces, on both a practical and a theoretical level, the essential concepts of midwifery care: choice, continuity of care, control of women and woman-centred care. Up until then these had been the exclusive appurtenance of the few home birth midwives. All the teaching midwives at SEAO are experienced with home care and continuity of care. The school is active throughout Italy. It publishes a professional review *Donna & Donna, Il Giornale delle Ostetriche* ('*D&D*'), the only one in Italy, to spread awareness of the issues involved in midwifery care.

Since its foundation, the subject of birth centres has been the focus of its attention. In 1997 a whole issue of *D&D* was dedicated to this subject, serving as an inspiration for the regional law of Emilia-Romagna. It contained the design for an ideal architectural project for a birth centre based on feminine values (*www.catpress.com/donnaedonna*). In 1998 the school formulated a specific training project for Health Enterprises (ASLs) which had approved the setting up of a birth centre. The bases for the training project are European and American international standards, a philosophy for birth centres inspired by the experience of home birth and a system of midwifery care centred on the woman. The objectives are to offer sound methods along with working principles that will allow the birth centres to produce results that are superior to those of hospital care. Up to now this training project has been implemented by two ASLs, Bologna and Ancona.

The school has also actively contributed to the preparation of regional laws on birth centres and to bills proposed at the national level. In 2000 it organised a European symposium, concentrating the whole existing experience and promoting birth centres to midwives, politicians and administrators and to women, in response to increasingly deeply felt needs.

The school would like to establish a birth centre itself in future, both as an example and as a place of training for midwives. At present the birth centre project acts as driver, promoting a general change in childbirth care and a more professional role for midwives.

THE BOLOGNA EXPERIENCE

In 1997 health service development groups of the Bologna Health Enterprise proposed and assigned six midwives to set up a birth centre project. In consultation with SEAO they drew up plans for a project, directed by midwives but with the collaboration of consultant physicians. It was approved by health care officials in spite of resistance from physicians. A training programme, involving the basic group, the community midwives, the hospital midwives, the gynaecologist and consultant neonatal physicians was carried out from 1998 to 2000. A site outside the hospital was selected and reconstruction work started. The midwives began to use the tools acquired in training: the community midwives began to perform antenatal care (overcoming the protests of physicians); the hospital-based midwives began to assist active childbirth and to create a family atmosphere in the delivery room. At first they met with resistance and opposition from those colleagues not involved in the training programme, but later on they collaborated with them to start an antenatal course. Encouraged by their newly discovered competencies, they gradually established a programme of continuity of care. The birth centre is not yet ready, but the process of change is irreversible, women have realised this, and the demand is growing. The midwives are no longer willing to give up their competencies and if the ASL fails to prepare the facility, they have decided to move in another direction.

THE ANCONA EXPERIENCE

In 1990 a women's association promoted a regional law for birth centres, which was finally approved and financed in 1997. Since the approval of the law, an elected Women's Forum has exerted pressure to establish a birth centre, but no group of midwives in the Marche Region was ready to realise this new service. Finally, under strong pressure from the Region, the Ancona Hospital decided in 2000 to promote the birth centre project. This hospital boasts a 60% caesarean section rate and childbirth is managed in a conventional manner–in the lithotomy position, with shaving, enemas and maximum medicalisation. It was decided in a hierarchical manner who would participate and which physicians should offer their services as consultants, and the hospital is responsible for the training process.

Only five midwives, with no professional experience of providing care in a birth centre, are motivated to participate. The site for the birth centre is annexed to the hospital, but has a separate entrance and structure. The work of restructuring has been delayed by the ASL. The midwives fear that their goodwill will be abused by the ASL, which they suspect may obtain funds from the Region without any intention of carrying out the project. They are therefore increasingly losing motivation. The impact with the new model of care is hard to absorb, and there is no place for experimentation. However, the Women's Forum is watching every step taken by the Ancona Health Enterprise and pushing for the realisation of this project. The undertaking is arduous, but the voyage has been started.

A SMALL-SCALE PRIVATE INITIATIVE

An independent midwife from Varese (Milan), who works in the area of home birth, in 2001 set up a small private birth centre in her new house. She is in this way reviving the methods of the district midwives in the first half of the nineteenth century, who sometimes had women come to their homes for childbirth. This method reduces the fixed costs of care provision. The social aspect of the birth centre is limited, but the family aspect is highlighted–instead of a large group, there is a small group. But this is also a way of launching a project quietly, allowing it to grow within a social context as a reality already nourished by experience.

CONCLUSION

We find ourselves faced with a few initiatives arising in entirely different circumstances. The birth centre is a highly experimental element. It is not only a new place in which to give birth and to be born, but it also works as a 'lighted fuse' pushing towards change in social and political values with an enormous power–feminine power. The politicians know this and fear it. When I presented the birth centre project to a political official of the Region of Tuscany, he told me clearly: 'home childbirth, yes; birth centres, no–their impact is too strong'.

The existing birth centre projects still need to mature culturally and socially, but they are driving towards that maturation, a long, but fascinating process.

REFERENCES

Briffault R 1977 The Mothers. Atheneum, New York

Gaskin I M 1977 Spiritual Midwifery. The Book Publishing Company, Summertown, Tennessee

16

Madame de Béarn's birth centre in France

Judith Wolf
Jane Flint

INTRODUCTION

In France in 2001 more than 99.5% of women gave birth in hospital. Home births are rare. No other option for place of birth is offered. This situation has arisen as a result of a succession of government decisions concerning public health and also because birth and pregnancy are generally perceived as risky processes (Akrich & Pasveer 1996)[1]. The concept of 'safety' depends to a large extent on how the birth event is perceived, and because of the safety issues, and because a high-tech acute unit offers medical and technical expertise, small birth centres (those with fewer than 300 births per annum) have been closed. Hospital maternity units are therefore tending to grow larger, with annual birth rates of several thousand, at the same time becoming more and more medicalised.

However, in the Dordogne region of southern France, there is a small establishment which is the antithesis of these huge maternity units. This birth centre is the work of one woman, Madame de Béarn. Madame de Béarn is 83 years old. She has delivered more than 9000 babies and continues to practise midwifery today. The house in which she has lived and worked for more than 50 years, the Villa Sainte Thérèse, is in

---

[1]Pregnancy and birth are considered as natural processes in the Netherlands, but in France they are considered normal only after the event. Naturally this view gives to fundamentally divergent ways of treating pregnancy and birth. The concept of 'safety' depends to a large extent on how the birth event is perceived.

Sarlat-la-Canéda, in the Périgord region. When she moved there in the 1950s, she took over what was Sarlat's official maternity clinic, the place where local women came to give birth. Today her home has become the only independent birth centre in France, welcoming women (and their partners) who don't want a 'medical' birth and who sometimes travel hundreds of miles to have their babies there. However, its existence is precarious and rests entirely on Madame de Béarn's shoulders. French legislation does not actually recognise the status of 'birth centre'. Condemned by the authorities, the birth centre has continued to function thanks to action by parents and those who, in supporting Madame de Béarn, support greater freedom of choice in childbirth.

FROM CLINIC TO BIRTH CENTRE

MIDWIFERY PRACTICE IN 1950s RURAL FRANCE

In 1949 the clinic which Madame de Béarn took over had six beds and approximately 150 births a year (twice the number of deliveries at Sarlat's maternity unit). At this time half of all births took place at home. Madame de Béarn talks of occasions when she had to deliver babies in fields or even in the mother's 'cart': 'They'd felt the first contractions and they didn't have time to get down from the cart! But that's as good as anywhere, after all!' During the days following the birth she would go round to see if everything was all right: 'I would see the baby, a few days later, lying in the grass next to the grandmother...it was great...they were at the same rhythm you see.'

From the early 1950s Sarlat's maternity unit grew and the delivery rate increased–birth became a medical affair. In a few years home birth disappeared almost completely[2]. At the same time, antenatal care was transformed: after the war, the creation of the Mother and Infant Protection Service and the creation of Social Security in 1945 facilitated 'medical' maternity care. Henceforth, antenatal care became obligatory, becoming a condition of payment of antenatal benefits which were created at the Libération. Once the costs of the birth and the hospital stay were being reimbursed, things quickly changed and women got used to going into hospital to give birth. Midwives lost their specialist skills and their autonomy; submitted to the hospital hierarchy, they became more and more dependent on doctors and obstetricians.

CHANGE IN STATUS OF THE VILLA SAINTE THÉRÈSE

For several years, Sarlat's maternity unit and the Sainte Thérèse clinic functioned side by side. Soon the hospital's delivery rate had reached 200 per annum and consequently Madame de Béarn's client numbers dwindled.

On August 13th 1986, a court order was issued which stated that the clinic did not adhere to the standards imposed on health establishments (by a 1972 law) and the clinic was ordered to close. Here begins the story of what was to become a birth centre. At the request of a number of child-bearing couples, Madame de Béarn continued to practise and the clinic became the Sainte Thérèse Parental Birth Centre.

So, was Madame de Béarn's practice illegal from then on? Ambiguity arises from the fact that French law allows independent midwives to practise anywhere, yet there is no law governing a birth centre which does not claim to be a health establishment. This is a legal void[3]. In carrying out births in a place which does not exist in the eyes of French law, Madame de Béarn is acting a-legally. For some years the government turned a blind eye to her activities. In 1997,

---

[2]Up until the Second World War most women in France gave birth at home. In 1952, 47% gave birth at home; by 1968 this figure was only 4%.

[3]On this point, various administrative and government authorities have stated explicitly:
'In French law, a "collective home" does not exist; the law recognises only "home" and "health establishments."'
(Letter, February 6th 1998 from the Dordogne Health Authority, to the President of the Sainte Thérèse Parental Birth Centre Association)
'The name "Parental Birth Centre" with no legal reference, does not fit into any category of establishment or Sarlat's health structure, so is the only one of its kind in France.'
(Letter, 23rd January 1998 from Bernard Kouchner, Secretary of State for Health, to a Dordogne MP)

however, the DDASS (the local health authority) began proceedings against Madame de Béarn for ignoring the order to close in 1986. Initially Madame de Béarn won the case because she argued that a birth centre was not a health establishment and did not therefore need to adhere to the regulations for this type of establishment. But the DDASS appealed and this time Madame de Béarn was found guilty. The court of appeal concluded that the birth centre was continuing the activities of the clinic, just using a different name. Madame de Béarn went to a final court of appeal, which only confirmed the judgement of the first one. Today the only remaining legal option is the European Court.

In spite of these prohibitions by the authorities, and contrary to all expectation, the birth centre survives yet.

THE ROLE OF MADAME DE BÉARN'S SUPPORT ASSOCIATION

Since 1986 Madame de Béarn has been able to continue practising because of the support and active participation of parents who formed the Sainte Thérèse Parental Birth Centre Association.

The birth centre survives financially because a client and father, Eric Despretz, bought the house, allowing Madame de Béarn to remain there and to live rent free. It is also funded by the fees paid by clients for board and lodging[4], annual subscriptions from active members of the Association[5] and donations. On the practical side, parents participate voluntarily in the day-to-day running of the centre (meals, cleaning, reception etc.). One of the peculiarities of the home, and one which distinguishes it from birth centres in other European countries, is that it is called a 'Parental Birth Centre'–it is managed entirely by parents. Both clients and volunteers 'adopt' the house as if it were their own and it is their goodwill which enhances the warm and welcoming atmosphere.

[4]Board costs 200 francs per day per adult antenatally and 250 francs postnatally. This price includes a room and three meals.
[5]Subscription to the Association (renewable every year) costs 200 francs, 15% of which is given to the National Parents' Federation, 'Naissance et Libertés'.

The alliance of this elderly, wilful midwife, determined to practise her profession to the end, and families determined to have a natural and demedicalised birth is conflicting, complex, and yet fruitful. It is an unlikely combination, yet at the same time a poignant one. There is something profoundly human about the fragility of this unplanned enterprise which has managed to function so effectively.

However, support for Madame de Béarn and support for the birth centre model are two separate concepts, sometimes even divergent. The two cross over without merging. However, because Madame de Béarn is at the head of the only birth centre in France, one cannot exist without the other. Numerous birth centre projects are underway in France. Some have been planned for years yet none so far has seen the light of day, simply because of the lack of government support. The only certainty is that Madame de Béarn is getting older and can no longer stand as a credible representative of birth centres. It is becoming more and more evident that Madame de Béarn and her supporters are not always pursuing the same objectives. In October 1999, a few days after the court sentencing, the Association decided to disband. Nevertheless, one of the most interesting aspects of this story is without doubt that this combination has permitted the creation and development of a unique establishment, one which has been maintained for almost 15 years.

The end of the Association did not mean the end of support for Madame de Béarn. A few people continue to help on an individual basis. She never gives up: 'The moment you think a battle has been lost, that is the point when you must carry on, otherwise it's not a battle but a submission. Only when you think nothing else can be done, that's where the real battle starts.'

THE WORKING BIRTH CENTRE

THE HOME

The first thing to strike you on entering the birth centre is that it is a family home. Outside, the key is always in the lock, telling you that this house is constantly open. Then you quickly notice labels telling you where everything is, inviting you to take possession of the house, to feel at home. There are children's drawings, sculptures, paintings on the kitchen cupboards and children's toys in the garden. You get a sense of history in this house. Laurent, a father who has participated in the life of the centre for 4 years, explained that even couples who come for only a few days feel at home and take part in the daily routine:

'At the beginning the couples who come here have only one goal: they just want to give birth. But little by little the atmosphere of the house encourages everyone to help one another, and everyone enjoys taking part, whether it be in the kitchen, in the garden, doing some painting or DIY...practically everyone leaves their mark on this house.'

A FAMILY EVENT

At the birth centre priority is given to a personal welcome–pregnant women are welcomed as individuals and are never reduced to the status of 'patients'. For Madame de Béarn it is not simply a pregnancy, it is a couple or a family who are expecting a child. A pregnant woman is not welcomed alone–partners, children, relations, friends and even pets all have a place in this house.

Pregnancy and birth are not viewed as exclusive events, rather as events which occur in a social and family context. This viewpoint is illustrated by the fact that, whenever she can, Madame de Béarn likes to go and visit a couple in their own home, in their day-to-day environment, even if she has to travel many miles. She likes to do this to gain a better understanding of them. She also regularly invites pregnant women or couples to visit her at the birth centre and have lunch with everyone. Children and grandparents are also welcome. These lunches are greatly valued by clients as an opportunity to meet other pregnant women and couples, to share in the childbirth event. Moreover, there are certain things which simply may not be discussed in an antenatal consultation but which can be much more easily expressed in this informal

atmosphere. For example, once when having lunch with Madame de Béarn and Fanny, who was seven months pregnant, Fanny suddenly turned to Madame de Béarn and said, 'Guess what? My mother is pregnant!' Madame de Béarn said to her, 'You seem staggered!', and Fanny was able to talk about this unexpected news which she had been given the day before, and share that she was somewhat disturbed at being pregnant at the same time as her mother.

Madame de Béarn considers that a birth involves the whole family. She does not separate the biological aspects of birth from the family and social context–birth involves a change in relationships between all those surrounding the child. It is not unusual for Madame de Béarn to have delivered several generations of the same family: she has been present at the births of thirty-year-old women whom she brought into the world. This was the case with one couple who were both born at Madame de Béarn's birth centre. It was there that they gave birth to their two daughters. They said: 'When our parents came to attend the birth of their grandchildren, we were welcomed warmly as a family. It was also a way for our mothers to relive their birth experiences.'

THE BIRTH

Madame de Béarn prefers to involve the whole family in labour and birth, allowing fathers, brothers and sisters to take part. During one discussion, we asked her what happens at these 'family' births, 'When children are present at the birth of a little brother or sister, do they want to hold the baby straight away?' she replied:

'No, not really, no. They are very quiet during the delivery. Afterwards, some cry, which is very good. You can usually tell whether they're going to be jealous or not. When they haven't yet seen the baby, they can't show their opposition or their joy, you see. So I always say to the mother, 'You just need to let them get on with it.' Sometimes after the birth they want to be with their mother, so I take off their shoes and place them next to the mother and baby. But I let them show what they're feeling immediately. A child which doesn't show any reaction means that something is stuck. When the baby comes out, the emotion is very strong…before the birth they say nothing; it's only when they see the baby that they show it. This emotion is very strong and it's an emotion that their father feels too. …The emotion is physical….

I have seen children who help their mother to push much more effectively than their father. They say, 'Push mummy!' in a far less intimidated way than the father. When it's not their real father, if their mother has remarried, then they really take over from the father. That's funny, isn't it! Afterwards I show them the placenta which really interests them. If it's fallen apart I put it back together to show them. I tell them, 'See, you were like that.' And often they ask me if they can touch it.'

Madame de Béarn may emphasise the family aspect of birth, but she also insists on respecting each woman's own rhythm. The promotional leaflets for the birth centre are explicit on this point: 'Priority is given to the natural process of birth, to the freedom of position, to allowing every woman to take her time and give birth to her child at her own pace and to respect each individual experience.'

Women who give birth at the centre are effectively free to use any position they choose. They can stay in the bath until fully dilated, they can move around as they wish, get into any position as they feel the need (lying down, sitting, squatting, supported from behind by their partner etc.). Madame de Béarn adapts to each woman, to each couple. For example, she says one woman delivered her baby curled up in a corner, while another went out into the garden to give birth leaning on a tree. As long as there are no problems, Madame de Béarn leaves each woman to give birth at her own pace and does not intervene in the natural process.

Respecting the rhythm of every woman means not inducing labour if it has not happened by the expected date. We learned from one woman who turned up at the birth centre that twins are not necessarily born on the same day. It was her birthday: she had been born 30 years earlier at Madame de Béarn's and had come on some sort of pilgrimage. She was a twin–she had been born on a Saturday and her brother was born the following Monday.

Madame de Béarn also remembered that she had delivered several members of this family and the young woman proudly added, 'Yes, all my cousins were born here.'

AFTER THE BIRTH

It is after the birth that the family atmosphere of the birth centre becomes important: all the women interviewed declared that it was wonderfully beneficial to be surrounded by their families at this time. Madame de Béarn is very attentive to new mothers. Lola, who has had two babies at Madame de Béarn's birth centre, felt this strongly:

'She always says that a baby is well if the mother is well too. So, after the birth she is careful about infection and it is always very clean. She also makes sure that the mother rests and eats well. I remember having a row with her because I was breastfeeding my daughter. At the first feed I hadn't eaten and she said to me, 'You're exhausted and the milk won't be rich enough for her.''

Food is one of the strong points of the birth centre and meals are convivial events which are particularly appreciated by families.

Madame de Béarn does not neglect the babies either. Lola says that she had taught her a lot on this subject:

'The best thing she taught me about babies was to handle them a lot, not to treat them like fragile little things. You'll never guess how she picks the babies up–she holds the sacrum and the head, like everybody does, but it's so quick: they certainly feel their bodies and the space around them! Babies are not pampered, yet at the same time there is great respect for the body…She doesn't cosset. Basically, she combines a heap of talents: she has the ability to really care for us and our child before, during and after the birth, and I believe that's a rare thing.'

Madame de Béarn's personality contributes to the warmth and friendliness of the birth centre. One particular characteristic is her capacity to welcome those who are seen as 'different'. She accepts them as they are. She is curious, yet open-minded; nothing human is really strange to her. When meeting new people (and her life is filled with countless meetings) she becomes a chameleon, she accepts, adapts and tries to understand what drives the people she accompanies during their birth experience.

THE QUESTION OF 'MEDICALISATION'

It is commonly believed that birth centres offer a 'demedicalised' birth. This term is somewhat inadequate. In fact, as soon as birth was accompanied by a midwife it became medicalised, because the profession of midwifery was a medical profession. Birth centres run by midwives are therefore not demedicalised. One cannot say either that Madame de Béarn is necessarily a supporter of demedicalisation. She had herself begun to study medicine but her studies were interrupted by the Second World War. After the war, an exhausted mother of two children, she switched to midwifery training which was shorter (4 years in France). Madame de Béarn does not reject the contribution of medicine in her practice. When she was in charge of the clinic she had obstetric medical equipment, including a monitor, an incubator and a resuscitation table. When she looks after pregnant women, she does all the usual necessary examinations. And, if need be, she will not hesitate to transfer a woman to hospital if labour is not progressing[6]. Women who have had to have a caesarean often come back to the birth centre for a few days. Madame de Béarn may share with families a vision of birth as a whole event, but every aspect of her practice seems to be rooted in a vigilant attention to physiology. One cannot therefore say that she advocates a demedicalisation of birth–she simply considers that the majority of births do not need obstetric intervention.

In contrast to the high-tech environment of acute units, the birth centre employs no monitoring (but does have a sonic aid, a small machine to listen to the baby's heartbeat), no drips (though injections are given if necessary) and no epidural anaesthetic. Furthermore, Madame de Béarn is not limited to allopathic medicine; she is open to alternative approaches such as homeopathy and herbal medicine. Women (and men) who have had their babies with Madame de Béarn praise her for her knowledge, her 'good sense' and her intuition, which results as much from experience as from solid medical expertise.

One may conclude that birth centres and medicalisation are not necessarily opposites. A birth centre seeks to preserve the possibility of birth not being exclusively medical.

WHO CHOOSES TO USE MADAME DE BÉARN'S BIRTH CENTRE?

Users of the birth centre are characterised by the fact that they have all made a choice to go there. Nobody ends up there by accident. It is important to note that all pregnant women are welcomed by Madame de Béarn. Nobody is refused entry to the centre. Primarily, users share a conception of birth which is in the minority in France: they consider birth a physiological, not a medical event which does not necessarily need to take place in a hospital environment. Pregnancy and birth are normal life events which, in the majority of cases, require warm-hearted support as opposed to medical intervention. However, it would be wrong to say that the only thing these people have in common is their refusal to give birth in hospital. Their approach, in fact, rests on two interrelated concepts, the first one relates to the idea of 'natural' and the second, to resistance and freedom.

NATURAL

The concept of 'natural' (repeated constantly in the witness letters sent to support Madame de Béarn during the court case) is based on a certain vision of life which stretches beyond its

---

[6]The nature of the relationship between Madame de Béarn and the hospital in Sarlat is not discussed here because hospital midwives and other staff were not interviewed as part of this research. According to Madame de Béarn there are conflicts but we are unable to provide more detail.

relevance to childbirth. To live 'naturally' certainly includes giving birth simply and without hindrance, by oneself and without anaesthetic, listening to one's body and letting the event unfold in its own rhythm. Madame de Béarn would call this 'becoming a mammal again for several hours'. The majority of women who give birth at the birth centre breastfeed their children for several months, sometimes even for years. Breastfeeding is considered an essential.

This concept is also about having a certain relationship with the environment. This relationship can be defined as 'ecological' and reveals itself in a number of ways. For some people, their profession may be related to the environment. Others are conscious of the products they consume; some are vegetarian; some eat food they grow themselves. Finally, many accord great importance to their lifestyle, generally preferring to live in the country than in towns (sometimes described as 'neo-rural', i.e. families who have made a choice to leave the town to go and live in the countryside, sometimes changing their job in order to do this).

For people who live out their choice of 'returning to nature', Madame de Béarn is particularly attractive: on the one hand because she allows families the choice to welcome the birth in a warm, family environment which is demedicalised (or rather, 'de-technicalised'); and, on the other hand, because she is the archetypal matron, the midwife, the wise woman who 'has always done it this way', the authenticity of her actions therefore guaranteed.

If birth with Madame de Béarn is a family story, it is equally a story of women. Over the centuries the management of maternity care has been taken out of the hands of women and put into the hands of doctors. With Madame de Béarn, birth is in the hands of women. She is an elderly midwife who manages a birth centre alone and has delivered generations of women. Through her we are able to rediscover the birth event, anchored in ancestral history, as it was before the arrival of men on the obstetric scene.

Madame de Béarn is equally a figure of resistance: she was a member of the Resistance during the Second World War and today she continues to practise her profession clandestinely. Laurent summarised this:

'Courage is her domain. This woman is a warrior, a lion. Her life has been a fight and this is what has always attracted people to her, people who have felt pretty much outside of tradition and outside of what "they" want to impose on us.'

This brings us to the second concept which attracts parents to the birth centre. This can be described, according to circumstances, as a desire for freedom, the attraction of resistance, or commitment to a cause.

RESISTANCE AND FREEDOM

To come and give birth at the centre is not just a case of viewing birth as a natural and physiological act: clients must recognise their right to realise their beliefs and be willing to commit themselves. Amongst other things, the birth centre's history is a story of resistance to public authorities and militants have gathered around Madame de Béarn. However, not everyone sees themselves in this way: some do not want to use their experience at the birth centre for any kind of 'glory'; some are not involved in the Association and feel that they are not 'militant material'. Others, on the contrary, openly accept that their support for the birth centre is a commitment, a political act. This is notably the case for Eric Degen and Edouard Schalchli, who have both been presidents of the Association and for whom 'the action of the Sainte Thérèse Parental Birth Centre Association supports national and European demands for women's right to choose their place of birth' (Association Maison de Naissance Parentale Sainte Thérèse).

Whatever the degree of their political engagement and whatever form it takes, in coming to the birth centre people manifest their right to choose their place of birth. What these people all demand is the choice not to be forced to conform to a single model. The refusal to conform is common to all, although it reveals itself in different ways. It is a question of being in control of one's own life. Couples express their demand for control by choosing their birth experience to be a family event and by not allowing themselves to be dispossessed of it. Users of the birth centre are united by their desire to be architects of their own lives, to experience important life events actively rather than passively and by their willingness to fight to defend their rights.

THE MEDICALISATION OF MATERNITY UNITS IN FRANCE

Though this is the only birth centre which exists in France, the birth centre concept seems to be attracting the attention of an increasing number of professionals and clients. One might therefore question the foundations of our mainstream practice in the care of pregnant women and, moreover, in the treatment of birth as a whole. More widely, we need to rethink the position of the maternity unit in our society (Knibiehler 1999).

The French Government is in favour of replacing small health establishments with large hospitals. The reorganisation of the health network began several years ago and was controlled by special organisations such as the ARH (the Regional Hospitals Agency), which controls the closure of small units. By 2001, the target date set by Government, all the small maternity units (those with an annual birth rate of less than 300) had to be closed.

Birth mainly takes place in hospital in France and tends to be treated as a medical procedure. Maternity units are based on the hospital model, pregnancy regarded as an illness. As soon as pregnancy and birth are taken over by 'professionals' in a medically specialised environment a pregnant woman becomes a patient. Maternity is no longer a family and social event, rather a bodily change to be medically controlled. The maternity establishment exists as a specialist obstetric hospital service, which functions like any other hospital service. White

collars have taken over the territory of pregnant women.

The hospital environment is not a place where pregnant women feel comfortable: there is no space for themselves (such as a playroom for children, a reading room, or even a library), a space where they can be something other than a 'waiting' patient–a wait which may last many hours. Each space in the hospital (waiting room, consultation room, treatment room, ultrasound scanning room etc.) is defined by its medical function and in these surroundings pregnant women can only play the passive role of the 'patient'. Why is it not considered normal for older children accompanying their pregnant mother to have their own space, instead of being confined to a chair with a tray of toys, as in a GP waiting room? Why can't the maternity services welcome parents as human beings who are going through an emotional experience, instead of treating them as patients enduring a medical procedure? When a father wanting to be present at his baby's birth is asked to leave the delivery room (perhaps when the epidural is administered or if he wants something to eat), where can he go? He must go into the corridor or the waiting room–places completely excluded from the event. Why can't a room be made available for partners? Such a space could also be used for visitors who do not want to be confined to the bedroom (just because this so resembles a 'hospital visit', the 'ill person' confined to bed).

There is a total absence of alternatives to the strictly medical management of pregnancy and birth in France. Few would agree that the maternity unit supports childbirth in a social environment. It is generally regarded as the medical place for the birth *procedure*, where biological aspects are considered without reference to the social, 'existential' and symbolic aspects of birth. Medical requirements are given utmost priority while the whole non-medical dimension of birth is left in the shade. These family, emotional, psychological and social dimensions all find their place at Madame de Béarn's birth centre.

REFERENCES

Akrich M, Pasveer B 1996 Comment la naissance vient aux femmes. Les techniques de l'accouchement en France et aux Pays-Bas. Collection 'Les empêcheurs de penser en rond'. Synthélabo Groupe, Le Plessis-Robinson

Association Maison de Naissance Parentale Sainte Thérèse. Dossier. Available at: *http://www.ctanet.fr/naissance-liberte*

Knibiehler Y (ed.) 1999 Repenser la maternité.Collection 'Panoramiques', Corlet edition, Condé-sur-Noireau

FURTHER READING

Althabe G, Fabre D, Lenclud G (eds) 1992 Vers une ethnologie du présent. Editions de la Maison des sciences de l'homme, Paris

Knibiehler Y 1997 La Révolution maternelle depuis 1945. Femmes, maternités, citoyenneté. Perrin Paris

Les Dossiers de l'Obstétrique 1999 Revue d'informations médicales et professionnelles de la sage-femme. Les maisons de Naissance. April, Number 271

Thébaud F 1986 Quand nos grands-mères donnaient la vie. La maternité en France dans l'entre-deux guerres. Presses Universitaires de Lyon, Lyon

Wolf J 2001 La maison de naissance de Madame de Béarn, Presses de l'Université Paris VII-Denis-Diderot, Paris

17

Birth centres in Germany

Elisabeth Groh

INTRODUCTION

Obstetrics in Germany has undergone a lot of change over the last 20 years. The ever-increasing invasion of technology into childbirth led to widespread dissatisfaction. As a result of this the first 'birth centre for a self-determined birth' was opened in 1983 in Berlin. Since then, about a hundred birth centres have been founded throughout Germany.

The birth centre movement, as well as women's consciousness, has influenced the development of hospitals. Labour and delivery units are changing into cosy, comforting places, where women can feel safe and supported during labour. Birthing stools, slings to hang in and water pools are available, though they are not as widely used as one would wish. The overwhelming amount of work, hospital routines and old habits often prevent midwives and doctors from changing to new ways. Education of parents as well as medical staff will be needed before old-fashioned ideas about childbirth can change.

About 98% of all births in Germany take place in a hospital; only 2% are out-of-hospital births, which include birth centre births and home births. Birth centres in Germany operate on a midwife base and offer personal, individualised care throughout pregnancy, birth and the postpartum period for healthy women with normal pregnancies. We believe that pregnancy and childbirth are natural processes in a woman's life and need emotional, social and physical support. If, in some cases, further medical treatment becomes necessary, women can be transferred to the care of a doctor.

WHOM IS A BIRTH CENTRE FOR?

A birth centre provides holistic care in pregnancy and childbirth as well as postpartum care for all healthy women. Birth centres in Germany have criteria which exclude women with a history of pathological conditions, such as:

- previous caesarean sections
- breech presentation
- twins
- premature births (<37 weeks of gestation)
- post-term labour (>42 weeks of gestation).

We very much encourage fathers, siblings and the woman's wider family to participate in the birth of a new family member. This has been proved to have many advantages. It offers expectant mothers a safe and comforting social haven during what can be a novel and sometimes anxious time of adaptation to all those changes that come with the birth of a baby. Fathers get more involved in the process if they feel that they are really wanted and necessary. There is no better emotional support for a labouring woman than her partner and it can be a very enriching experience for both partners. Siblings, regardless of age, usually cherish the life event of the birth of a baby brother or sister. All they need is a familiar person with them to attend to their needs and answer their questions. It also helps to strengthen bonds between all the family members if the event is shared.

WHAT A BIRTH CENTRE OFFERS

A birth centre can provide care from the day of a positive pregnancy test until the end of breast-feeding. German midwives offer a wide range of classes, antenatal care, counselling and support. Birth centres support the freedom of informed choice. Ultimately, there is no 'correct way' for a woman to give birth. A woman can only know

what she wants if she has all the information available to help her decide what she might or might not need in order to give birth successfully and happily. For some, this might be a large hospital with a neonatal intensive care unit attached; for others it might be a birth centre; and for some it might be their own home. It all depends on the couple's focus and their personal definition of what safety means to them. It is important that women are helped to make the right choice, based on sufficient and unbiased information about their options.

Most birth centres offer orientation evenings once a month to inform couples about the birth centre option. If couples are interested an initial counselling session will follow in order to rule out any medical reasons which would preclude a birth at the birth centre. A midwife takes an in-depth look at the medical history, previous pregnancies and births and at the woman's present condition. Women can then choose to be cared for by their obstetrician or by a midwife. (While working at the Frankfurt Birth Centre for 10 years, we found that most women like to alternate their care between the two.) German health insurance will cover the cost of a physician as well as a midwife.

Women are usually seen every 4 weeks until 30 weeks of gestation, then every 2 weeks to full term. Antenatal care at a birth centre enables women to get to know the midwives who will actually be present at the birth; most doctors now only work in their own practices and no longer work in hospitals. German maternity law recommends that women have three ultrasound scans, in weeks 12, 20 and 30, which are done by a physician. In practice, however, most women not only have a scan at every visit to their doctor, but they also believe that they need to have one in order to have a healthy baby. Midwives at a birth centre take a different, more personal approach. When a birth centre midwife performs Leopold's manoeuvre to evaluate the size and position of the baby many first-time birth centre mothers say: 'Nobody has ever put hands on my tummy before.' What a sad expression of how pregnancy in our times is perceived–indirectly, through ultrasound and the measurement of laboratory parameters rather than directly, through physical touch and examination. Getting women involved and educated about the exciting process of a baby growing in their womb is a main focus of our work.

Naturally, birth centres also provide the necessary laboratory services, such as blood typing, rubella and hepatitis titres, HIV testing and many more, according to German maternity law. They also offer counselling during pregnancy for problems like heartburn, varicose veins, water retention, high blood pressure, sleepless nights and breech position, advice on the natural induction of post-term labour and seek to answer the many other questions that can arise during the course of a pregnancy.

Listing the classes that German birth centres offer is rather difficult as they are all different in terms of size, staff and facilities. Nevertheless, the following programme, from the Frankfurt Birth Centre, can be used as an example:

- Childbirth preparation classes (for couples/women/primipara/multipara)
- Care for a newborn for expectant parents
- First aid on infants
- Postpartum exercise class
- Pelvic floor exercise class
- Breastfeeding group
- Baby massage
- Haptonomy
- Homeopathic treatment for infants
- Vaccination: pro and cons
- Acupuncture for pregnant women
- Postpartum ayurvedic oil massage.

Midwives in German birth centres see their position during a birth as an accompanying one. Every birth is different and so are the needs of every woman. We strive to provide individualised care rather than imposing a rigid, inflexible routine. This can be accomplished by the midwife and the woman getting to know each other prior to labour, and by having one midwife take care of one woman throughout the birth. Every woman receives one-to-one care. As a safety feature, many birth centres have a second midwife present when the baby is actually born, so that both mother and baby may be cared for if necessary.

Right after the birth the baby is assessed using the Apgar scoring system and immediately given to the parents. Provided that mum and baby are in good condition, both midwives then leave the new family to get to know each other and enjoy those precious first moments with their baby. Bonding is vital for healthy family development. The young mother is helped with the first breastfeed and is encouraged to feed her baby often during the first 3 days. After the mother has been examined for possible perineal tearing and any necessary suturing has been done, she is present at the first check-up on her baby, which is done by midwives.

The new family stays at the birth centre for approximately 3–5 hours after the birth, when they are discharged into the care of a midwife at home. Ideally this would be one of the birth centre midwives, but if they live further away it would be a colleague from the area. A few birth centres offer the woman the option of staying overnight or even for a few days. This is, for the most part, not paid for by health insurance, however, which makes it rather difficult for parents to afford. In fact, many clients at this stage are still waiting to be reimbursed for the facility fee, which they have to pay in advance. This includes rent for the premises, overhead costs, material and laboratory supplies, and an on-call fee for midwives. The more persistent parents are, the more chance they will have of getting their money back. All other midwife charges are fully covered by health insurances.

Midwives and other staff also benefit from the birth centre concept. Many midwives in German birth centres are freelance and they are able to schedule their own appointments, classes and on-call times, which gives them more freedom and therefore better job satisfaction. The majority of birth centres also have regular team meetings when they reflect on their work, aiming at constant improvement.

"Guidelines for Birth Centres" describe main structure and necessities to open up and run a Birth Centre. It also contains values that differentiate the treatment in a Birth Centre such as personal individualized, one to one care and stresses the open mindedness for different races, beliefs and mentalities.

SUPPORT SYSTEMS FOR BIRTH CENTRES

From the early 1980s to the present day the birth centre movement has seen enormous changes. What started out as small groups of women and families in a few cities, determined to provide a better and more humane way of giving birth, has now become a movement of great diversity.

The main idea behind each birth centre still remains the same and they all share the belief that women should have the right to choose the place and conditions for the births of their babies. In the early years local women's rights groups, families, midwives and other groups such as the 'Association of childbirth preparation' (the Gesellschaft für Geburtsvorbereitung or GFG) helped to promote the idea of birth centres and supported many of them as they were set up.

It soon became clear that it would be advantageous to link birth centres in some way, in order to share knowledge and experience and to support new birth centre initiatives. Based on the successful structure of the NACC (National Association of Childbearing Centers) in North America, and with their help, the 'European Network to promote the idea of birth centres e.V.' was founded in Halle, Germany in 1993. At this time the only members were from Switzerland and Germany. Many other countries, including France, Spain and Italy also had birth centre initiatives but their birth centres were still not up and running as a result of legal problems, or were under immense pressure from the authorities. Although aiming to meet every country's needs, the European Network membership was fundamentally unbalanced. The outcome of this dilemma was the founding of the 'Association of Swiss Birth Centres' (the IGGCH) and the 'German Network of Birth Centres e.V.' (Netzwerk der Geburtshaeuser in Deutschland e.V.).

The European Network was restructured and is currently run by a Board of Directors of three midwives. It runs a website as a way of connecting birth centre movements around Europe. The website contains valuable information on each country and their obstetric services, as well as details of a contact person. It is very important to have a connection between birth centres in Europe, even though it seems at the moment that they are concentrating on their own problems and legislation rather than looking at the greater, European picture. Maybe now, after the implementation of one currency, Europe will grow closer and the European Network will find its place as a connecting point between all the birth centres in Europe. For more information, or to contact members of the Board of Directors, visit the website at *www.birthcenter-europe.net*.

THE GERMAN NETWORK OF BIRTH CENTRES

Founded in 1999, the German Network now has 45 members and represents the needs and the aims of birth centres in Germany. It is run by three midwives as the Board of Directors and has its headquarters in Bonn. The main goals of the German Network are to:

- connect birth centres and other out-of-hospital birthing institutions in Germany
- support and help the founding of new birth centres
- Promote the idea of birth centres to the public and to health insurance companies.

The duties of the Network office can be described as:

- looking after their members
- preparing for the Annual General Meeting
- overseeing the planning of the Annual Convention
- issuing a newsletter for members every 3 months
- distributing the network manual, *How to start a birth centre*.

The manual on how to establish a birth centre contains information on facilities, equipment, team structures, organising finances and a guide to negotiating with health insurance companies. It also describes some of the experiences of other birth centres.

The German Network offers regular practical seminars on setting up a birth centre which cover all the information contained in the manual as well as guidance on legal issues.

One of the German Network's main activities is negotiating with health insurances companies in order to gain recognition and hence coverage of the facility fee. In order to enable the Network to define quality and safety in birth centres, a quality management system has been developed and is currently implemented as a pilot project in five birth centres in Hessen.

For more information on the German Network of Birth Centres or how to get in touch with them visit the website *www.geburtshaus.de*

QUALITY MANAGEMENT

Two years ago the members of the German Network decided to design a quality management system that would be valid nationwide. The impetus came from birth centres themselves. Midwives were looking for a systematic way of screening structures and processes in their centres to enable them to lay stable foundations and to clarify responsibilities. The quality management system will also play an important role in the future in gaining recognition by health insurance schemes.

The German Network supports variety in the way different midwives work *within one institution*. A birth centre ought to be a place where midwives can use their high quality skills with sensitivity, creativity and intuition. We don't strive to standardising procedures but would much rather coordinate the best possible work methods for a particular team. It is also of major importance to develop and stabilise teamwork within the birth centre, for example through staffing arrangements, reflective practice and risk management.

Our goal was to develop a set of guidelines for all birth centres to enable them to establish their own quality management system. We did

this with the support of many groups and organisations, including:

- birth centres midwives
- German midwifery associations (BDH and BfHD)
- The Quality in Out-of-hospital Obstetrics Association (QUAG e.V.)
- health insurance companies (e.g. AOK, VdAK)
- The Medical Council of Health Insurance
- Dr Michallik Consulting Association (to develop a concept suitable for the special features of the birth centre work).

The content of these guidelines follows the European Standard EN ISO 9001: 2001, so that it will be possible to certify all birth centres at a later date.

According to the International Organisation for Standardisation (ISO 9001: 2001) three main characteristics have to be examined to get an overall view of an institution:

- structures
- processes
- results.

Structures are fixed and include organisational structure, equipment and personnel. The things an organisation does in order to fulfil its aims are called *processes*.

Results will show whether specific goals were achieved and expectations satisfied, and include measurements of parameters such as client satisfaction and profitability.

Birth Centre processes can be separated into three different types (see Fig. 17.1):

1. All genuine midwifery skills can be considered as *executive processes*, which lead directly to fulfilment of the aims of the birth centre.
2. *Supportive processes* describe all events assisting midwives in their work.
3. Coordinating and directing processes form what we call *management processes* and operate at a level above the two.

Our goal is to develop a quality management system which supports creative solutions to

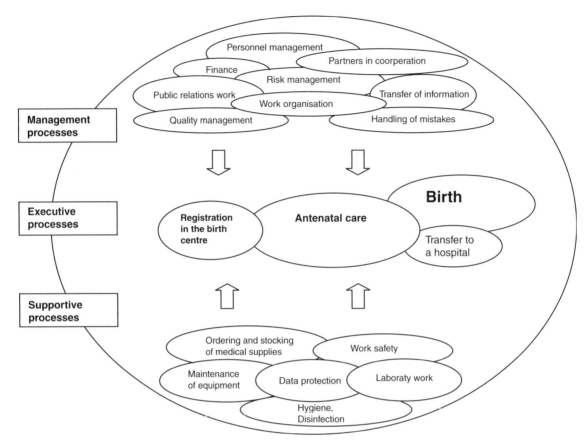

Figure 17.1 Birth centre processes.

questions such as these:

- How can we make our team a stable one, able to manage conflict?
- How can we structure our risk management system in order to be able to concentrate calmly on the actual care?
- How should work be organised in order to allow for a good balance between working time and leisure time?
- How do we go forward financially?
- What are the shortcomings of our birth centre?

The introduction of the quality management system will be a long process. Only the efforts of all the people involved will result in a successful realisation of this system. The project was supported idealistically as well as financially by midwives, Associations, QUAG e.V.,

health insurance companies, the medical council of Health Insurance and the Ministry of Social Affairs in Hessen, Germany.

Contact Johanna Hoepner-Fruehauf, executive project manager for the German Network of Birth Centres e.V. via e-mail: *johanna.hoepner-fruehauf@t-online.de*

CONCLUSION

Pregnancy, childbirth and the postpartum period are not times of illness, but natural processes in family life. The extent to which we are willing to share power with women and their families will determine how far we will go in changing our birthing culture into a humane and friendly one. Autonomy for mothers and genuine partnership between expectant parents and caretakers should become the norm of maternity care.

The question of safety remains unanswered. If 'safety in childbirth' means a satisfying, healthy outcome for both mother and baby, then it is of major importance to educate parents about their options and to get midwives, doctors, birth centres and related staff working together.

The process of birth works best if interference is kept to a necessary minimum and to let nature take its course.

We all need to create a system in which babies can be born in an environment that provides support, medical knowledge, empowerment and the freedom for women to choose how and where they want to give birth to their babies.

REFERENCES

European Network to promote the idea of birth centres e.V.: *www.birthcenter-europe.net*
German Network of Birth Centres e.V.: *www.geburtshaus.de*

Johanna Hoepner-fruehauf, executive project manager for the German Network of Birth Centres e.V.: *johanna.hoepner-fruehauf@t-online.de*

18

Birth centres and the American spirit

Andrea McGlynn

INTRODUCTION

Birth center midwives must possess the spirit and expertise of an entrepreneur in matters relating to practicing out of the hospital and running a business. (*Ernst, 2001*)

Other chapters in this book have demonstrated the myriad benefits of and the urgent need for birth centres–in any country. The over-medicalisation of birth and the inadequacy of hospital care for healthy, childbearing women is unfortunately a worldwide phenomenon. The United States of America (USA) must take a fair share of blame for this dominant culture, but it is not alone. This chapter on American birth centres will not reiterate the shortcomings of the medical establishment or the advantages of birth centre care, as these are common to obstetric care systems in any country. Instead, it will focus on features that are unique to the birth centre movement in the USA, especially the educational and organisational infrastructure that supports midwives in moving it forward.

Like most things in the United States, it is very difficult to generalise about American birth centres. Fifty states can mean fifty laws on the very same topic; neighbouring regions within states can differ demographically as much as do countries in Europe. This means that 'a birth centre is not a birth centre is not a birth centre' in the USA. However, they all share a common purpose, filling what was once a gaping hole in the health-care delivery system. Birth centres in the USA also share a common culture, and it is this purpose and this culture that have defined the birth centre movement since its inception. America's health care system, business mentality, consumerism, and fervour for regulation are all key to understanding birth centres in the USA in their proper context.

THE AMERICAN HEALTH CARE SYSTEM

In a country of 281 million people, 3.9 million women aged 15–44 years gave birth in the year 2000 (Bachu & O'Connell 2001, US Census Bureau 2000). Almost all mothers and babies pass through America's vast and complex health care system that consumes over 13% of the country's gross domestic product (OECD 2000). Private health insurance pays for the majority of health care services. In 2000, 72% of the population had some form of private insurance. Although the government provides health insurance for certain categories of the population, including the military, senior citizens, and some of the poor, 14% (39 million people) are not covered at all (Mills 2001).

There is a wide range of health care services available in the USA, from the most scientific to the most alternative, the highest tech to the highest touch. The USA spends almost double what the United Kingdom spends on health care yet the American people as a whole, are less healthy than the people of most European countries (Wanless 2001). There is no systematic process for matching need to provision and maternity care is a prime example of this: 'Why is it…that we have emphasized hospital-based maternity care increasingly in university medical centres which are tertiary care institutions, when 80–90% of all maternity care is, in fact, primary care?'(Lee 1993).

The birth centre concept answers the call for order in the chaos that is maternity care, representing a shift from routine medical intervention to a holistic approach to normal childbirth. In 1997 the National Association of Childbearing Centers (NACC) website stated: 'In a wellness

orientation to pregnancy and birth, birth centers…eventually will help to reduce the number of costly hospital beds and expand primary care services…. Birth centers will help to develop a system of care based first on the needs of the family.'

A BUSINESS MENTALITY

There is much talk of the 'almighty dollar' in the USA, the world's biggest economy. Cultural consultant, Richard Lewis (1999) asserts that the aim of Americans 'is to make as much money as they can as quickly as they can, using hard work, speed, opportunism, power (also of money itself) as the means towards this.' Most Americans involved in the delivery of health care are very business-minded and recognise that even not-for-profit agencies are not viable unless they pay strict attention to the bottom line.

The birth centre movement has been no stranger to the language of business. The demonstration childbearing centre established by the Maternity Center Association in 1975 could not have succeeded without negotiating a special contract with Blue Cross Blue Shield, the largest health care insurer, for payment of services provided (EKM Ernst, personal communication, 2002). In 1993 Lucy Holmes Johnson, President of the Maternity Center Association, exclaimed, 'Entrepreneurs, backed by large corporations and insurance companies, tell us of their plans to make the birth center as ubiquitous as McDonald's.' From the American perspective, it is only ambition such as this that can realise the vision for birth centres, especially in terms of increasing access to the unique services they provide.

Cost-effectiveness is central to this vision–but also, good business. As early as 1982, Bennetts and Lubic began to draw attention to the fact that the Maternity Care Association charged approximately $1000 for comprehensive services while hospital fees in the same locale ranged from $2500 to $5000 (Bennetts & Lubic 1982). Throughout the 1980s this trend continued (Scupholme et al 1986) and in 1995 Stone and Walker performed a comprehensive cost-effectiveness analysis, comparing a birth centre to a hospital for low-risk deliveries. They found that, on average, hospital costs were 38% greater than those for birth centres.

CONSUMERISM

At the other side of the commercial relationship is the consumer, who, in American society, is not the mere recipient of a free economy but its driver. American Personal Consumption Expenditures rose from $70 billion in 1930 to $6728 billion in 2000, with a parallel rise in the power of the consumer (US Bureau of Economic Analysis Statistics 2002). Under the influence of Ralph Nader, this development has been identified as nothing short of 'the creation of "consumer sovereignty" in a seller-dominated economy' (Bollier 1992). Women's health was no exception to the consumer movement. Sydney M. Wolfe, MD, a public-interest physician, voiced a popular protest to 'the surgeon's seemingly endless capacity to cut into women's bodies, removing "useless" uteruses through millions of unnecessary hysterectomies, surgically delivering "perfect babies" through cesarean sections'. Regarding childbirth specifically, the 1960s saw the creation of the consumer organisation, the International Childbirth Education Association (ICEA 2001) and the American Society for Psychoprophylaxis in Obstetrics, which became Lamaze International (Bing 2001): 'Since the beginning, the prepared childbirth movement has been a consumer movement. Its ideas and philosophy were accepted by large numbers of women and men who asked their obstetricians to support a birth in which they could be active participants.'

Natural childbirth, family-centered maternity care and breastfeeding became explicit consumer demands by the 1970s, and the women's movement articulated the ways in which medicine was beginning to alienate women (Lubic 1979). The Maternity Center Association (MCA), at that time a health agency in New York City, received feedback from families who were discontented with childbearing services. The depersonalisation, surgicalisation and high cost of maternity care resulted from routine obstetric behaviour that overlooked 'the satisfactions prized by families' (Lubic 1979). This led to the establishment of the MCA's Childbearing Center (CbC). Birth centres were not a brand new concept at that time (the first birth centre was built in 1945 in New Mexico), but consumer demand in the 1970s prompted their proliferation and they soon numbered in hundreds (Rooks 1997).

REGULATION

American society is very much characterised by a fervour for regulation. This is essential in the light of the multi-layered federal, state, and local governments and the fragmented, privatised health care industry. In 1998 the Code of Federal Regulations filled 201 volumes, nearly a 50% increase since 1980 (Office of Federal Register 2000). From 1996 to 2000 18% of the 287 new regulations pertained to health alone (Regulation.org). In fiscal year 2000, 54 federal departments, 130 000 federal employees and $18.7 billion were used to write and enforce federal regulations (Warren & Weidenbaum 1999). This snapshot of regulation does not even begin to profile other levels of government, each with their own laws and regulations.

By the early 1980s over half of the 50 states had birth centres, but few states had regulations and reimbursement by health care insurers was difficult to obtain. This meant that even insured families were having to make out-of-pocket cash payment for services. The health care facility and the provider must be licensed by the state before insurers will consider payment for services. Many also require that the facility be accredited. In 1981 MCA formed the Cooperative Birth Center Network (CBCN) to try and identify the problems encountered by birth centres springing up across the nation. It was soon realised that if birth centres were to become part of the health care system, a foundation for insuring quality care would have to precede any major growth (Rooks 1997, EKM Ernst, personal communication, 2002). The CBCN became the National Association of Childbearing Centers (NACC) in 1983. NACC worked with a multidisciplinary task force in the American Public

Health Association to develop the guidelines for state regulation of birth centers, *Guidelines for licensing and regulating birth centers* (APHA, 1982). This facilitated the writing of regulations in the 72% of the states that now license birth centres. Six states are exploring regulations and none have started in seven.

But regulation does not stop at licensing. A typical birth centre will be subject to no less than 15 categories of regulation, including zoning rules, building and fire codes, business licenses, laws regulating professional practice, laws pertaining to corporate and organisational structure and operation, as well as federal, state and private insurance requirements for reimbursement of services. These standards form the basis for national accreditation by the independent Commission for Accreditation of Birth Centers (EKM Ernst, personal communication, 2002).

Accreditation goes beyond licensing: this process applies national standards in assessing the quality of the facility, the staff and the programme of care. It looks at the fiscal operations and financial viability, the outcomes of care and the level of client satisfaction. Accreditation, a familiar concept for hospitals, is also a strong message to consumers who have few ways of assessing quality. It is a voluntary process by which a centre aspires to achieving a mark of excellence and increased assurance of payment for services. S.B. Peck, representing the insurance industry, said: 'As the health insurance industry aggressively encourages consideration of new alternatives for care and treatment, it simultaneously is concerned that the care provided is of high quality.' He suggested that, with accreditation, insurers would be likely reimburse for birth centre care (Peck 1986–87). Fifty birth centres are now accredited by the Commission (Kunz, personal communication, 2002).

Regulation is both the beginning and the result of a successful movement in the USA–it is difficult to survive without regulation, but regulations are not created until there is something to regulate. Regulation can facilitate the development of birth centres but it can also become so politicised by forces desiring to eliminate competition that it actually restricts the development of the concept. However, for all that regulation demands of individuals and institutions, the general consensus is that what it provides in terms of recognition, validation and even promotion is invaluable.

AMERICAN BIRTH CENTRES

At present there are 160 birth centres in the United States (Kunz, personal communication, 2002). Although they are all different, the birth centre concept can be defined (NACC 1955):

The Birth Center is a home-like facility, existing within a health care system with a program of care designed in the wellness model of pregnancy and birth. Birth centers are guided by principles of prevention, sensitivity, safety, appropriate medical intervention, and cost-effectiveness. Birth centers provide family-centered care for healthy women before, during and after normal pregnancy, labor and birth.

Local birth centres, in communities ranging from rural to urban, serve many populations. The birth centre in the urban South Bronx of New York City is designed specifically to promote self-reliance, enhance self-esteem and strengthen hope in inner-city families. Holy Family Services Birth Center is located on the Texas–Mexico border. Most clients are immigrants or migrant workers and rarely have insurance or the means to pay. However, no one is turned away because of an inability to pay: 'Care is provided in a God-centered atmosphere of love, compassion and family involvement to all.' (NACC).

In its 1999 survey of all known birth centres in the USA, NACC (2000) reported that of the 48% of birth centres that completed surveys:

- 87% are staffed by certified nurse-midwives
- 17% had licensed midwives or certified professional midwives
- 6% had family physicians
- 11% had obstetricians
- 25% had more than one type of provider.

Birth centres offer preconception, antenatal, intranatal, postnatal, newborn and well-woman gynaecological care. Some also offer home visiting and general community health services. The Reading Birth and Woman's Center offers home, hospital and free-standing maternity care and it also runs a programme that includes breast and cervical cancer screening for low-income women (NACC).

Birth centres may be reimbursed under contracts from as many as 30 different insurance companies. A few birth centres only accept direct payment from clients or, if serving the uninsured, rely on subsidies through grants, donations or charitable sources. Ruth Lubic, a certified nurse-midwife and anthropologist, founded the demonstration Childbearing Center on the upscale East side of Manhattan. She then founded the Morris Heights Center in the South Bronx to demonstrate that birth centres could create a place where disadvantaged inner-city families could become empowered through their childbirth experience. For this she received the prestigious MacArthur Genius Award. She used the generous 5-year award to expand the birth centre concept, opening a one-stop family centre in Washington's most deprived neighbourhood. It took almost 7 years to build the trust of the community and the coalition of agencies and providers that participate in this ambitious project. An abandoned supermarket was donated by a philanthropic Washington businessman, but it took $785 000 of District of Columbia city grants and nearly $1 million in private contributions to restore it to house the birth centre, social and welfare services, and newborn and toddler day care. (Loose 1998). The concept is being replicated in several cities across America (EKM Ernst, personal communication, 2002).

Rooks et al (1992a, 1992b, 1992c) conducted the National Birth Center Study (NBCS), which generated and analysed extensive data from a major prospective, descriptive study of 84 birth centres and almost 18 000 women seeking birth centre care. Of the 11 814 women admitted to birth centre care, combined rates of intrapartum and neonatal mortality (1.3 per 1000 births) were not higher than rates from studies of low-risk hospital births. The incidence of infant low birth weight for preterm deliveries at birth centres

was one-fifth of the national rate and low birth weight rates were also significantly less than national rates for term and post-term infants. Episiotomies were performed on 23.2% of birth centre clients, compared to rates of 35–78% in similarly low-risk women in other studies (Rooks et al 1992c). Only 4.4% of birth centre deliveries resulted in caesarean section, fewer than in any other low-risk population studied during the same decade (Rooks et al 1992c). The NBCS concluded that 'there is no evidence that hospitals are safer' (Rooks et al 1992c).

Over 92% of clients in the NBCS responded that they would choose a birth centre again, and 98.6% said that they would recommend their birth centre to a friend. When asked about the charges for birth centre care, 96.8% of respondents stated that they were reasonable (Rooks et al 1992).

'Birth centers offer a savings in cost and minimize the rate of cesarean section. Some centers serve rural populations that are too small to support a hospital obstetrical unit. They may be located in residential areas and can be designed to suit the needs of particular communities. Because they are small and generally non-bureaucratic, they may overcome social and emotional barriers that contribute to the poor use of care facilities by some groups of women.

Few innovations in health service promise lower cost, greater availability, and a high degree of satisfaction with a comparable degree of safety. The results of this study suggest that modern birth centers can identify women who are at low risk for obstetrical complications and can care for them in a way that provides these benefits.' (*Rooks et al 1989*).

Payment for services rendered is central to the birth centre concept in the USA. Birth centres and midwives demonstrate improved outcomes and client satisfaction with their time-intensive and education-intensive care, but they constantly have to prove that they merit payment for services which are of an equal or higher standard than those provided by more mainstream hospitals and physicians. According to the National Committee for Quality Assurance, the accrediting body for insurance companies, there are no restrictions on the reimbursement of birth centres (NACC 1995). The case for reimbursing birth centres is logical–the care is cost-effective, not only on a case-by-case basis, but also in terms of the greater health care economy. If only 100 000 births were attended in birth centres, the annual savings could be almost $314 million. In addition, for every 1000 women that birth centres save from having a caesarean birth, savings could be $7.4 million (NACC).

AMERICAN MIDWIFERY AND BIRTH CENTRES

An understanding of what certified nurse-midwives (CNMs) are is necessary as they provide the majority of birth centre care, they initiated the birth centre movement and they continue to guide its development and implementation throughout the country. The American College of Nurse-Midwives (ACNM) defines nurse-midwifery practice as: 'The independent management of women's health care, focusing particularly on pregnancy, childbirth, the postpartum period, care of the newborn, and the family planning and gynecological needs of well women' (ACNM 1992).

In 1999 CNMs attended 287 298 live births, accounting for 7.2% of all births and 9.4% of normal spontaneous vaginal deliveries in the USA (Ventura et al 2001). While surprisingly low compared to other countries, this rate has more than doubled in the past 10 years. Studies have demonstrated that midwives' outcomes and costs for care compare favourably to those of physicians (Rooks 1997). CNMs are less likely to utilise technology, their patients spend less time in hospital and are more likely to be satisfied with their care (Rooks 1997). However, because 99% of all births in 1999 occurred in hospitals (National Center for Health Statistics 1999) and because physicians usually determine hospital protocols, maternity care usually follows a medical model.

In 1999 the NACC stated:

A birth center is the practice of midwifery.... Midwifery care may be provided by any qualified provider who practices a wellness and holistic approach to pregnancy, birth, and women's health care. Midwifery care focuses on the promotion of health and the development of individual responsibility. Midwives take time to listen to women...midwives believe that childbearing is normal and that a woman and her family should create the birth experience that will be meaningful to them. Midwifery is a collaborative practice that involves midwives...nurses...obstetricians... pediatricians and other specialists as needed. Midwifery honors and respects the wisdom and dignity of all women.

The birth centre movement is the only large-scale response to the barriers to midwifery practice throughout the USA and to the demands of consumers seeking alternatives to routine obstetric care. The birth centre is the vehicle by which true midwifery care can be institutionalised (in the best sense of the word) and midwives can be used to their greatest capacity in serving women and their families (Ernst 2001).

Contrary to popular misconception, midwives in the USA are not obstetric nurses. CNMs in the USA are educated in nursing and midwifery to be autonomous practitioners, they have advanced postgraduate training, and most have Master's degrees. CNMs must pass a national certification examination which is administered by the independent corporation, the ACNM Certification Council (ACC). Nurse-midwifery is legal in every US jurisdiction and CNMs must fulfil specific licensing requirements in each state (Rooks 1997). In 1997 the ACNM created a new and professionally equal category of midwives called 'certified midwives' (CMs) who are subject to the same standards of practice, professional regulations, stipulations on continuing education and ethics as CNMs (ACNM 1997). For the sake of simplicity, the term 'CNM' is used to refer to both categories throughout this chapter.

In addition, 'certified professional midwives' and 'licensed midwives' practice direct-entry midwifery that does not require nursing training. In recent years their leadership has worked diligently to bring the direct-entry education and practice into the mainstream, but they do not enjoy the same privileges of wide recognition, regulation and reimbursement (EKM Ernst, personal communication, 2002). Registered nurses, practical nurses, health care assistants and doulas are also integral to many maternity teams, including those in birth centres.

BIRTH CENTRES IN MIDWIFERY EDUCATION–CNEP

The birth centre movement in the USA has found an important place in the midwifery education curriculum. The Community-based Nurse-midwifery Education Program (CNEP) at the Frontier School of Midwifery and Family Nursing pioneered the concept that birth centres could not grow without more CNMs–CNMs trained in the practice and operation of birth centres (Ernst 2001). To achieve the goal of training more CNMs, CNEP, having recognised that there were many nurses who wanted to be midwives but who could not relocate for their education, designed the first distance-learning programme. To prepare CNMs for practice in and operation of birth centres, a four-credit course on this subject was made central to the curriculum. On an academic level, the birth centre curriculum is a theoretical template for educating midwives about the politics, policies and payment mechanisms that determine the delivery of health care, often a weakness in clinical training for health professionals.

CNEP's three-class series on birth centres has been referred to as a 'mini-MBA or mini-MPH' (Ernst 2001). It begins with a detailed history of birth centres, the evidence-base for birth centres, the various models of care, reimbursement methods and the regulatory texts that dictate professional licensing and birth centre legislation. The capstone of the curriculum is preparation of a proposal for a birth centre in the student's community: this includes a community assessment to determine the health and social demographics of the area, a survey of primary source documents for birth centre and hospital regulation, and an assessment of niche or need in the form of a survey of all groups of providers and consumers to determine readiness for midwifery and birth centres. Faculty teach students how to calculate requirements for staffing, space and supplies and their corresponding costs so that in their final proposal students are able to project utilisation, staffing, income and expenses in order to budget for the first 3 years of operation.

Another goal of midwifery education is to make midwifery care and midwives visible in the health care system:

Midwifery had never had a place of practice. The acute care hospital was the physician's place of business–a place for medical care. Nurse midwives have tried to fit into the medical place but…midwifery had little autonomy in the acute care setting and even less identity for women seeking choices in their care. Thus the free-standing birth center gave midwifery a face. (*Ernst 2001*)

The ultimate goal of this training is to contribute to the improvement of maternity services overall. There are still very few birth centres (the out-of-hospital birth rate has yet to exceed 1%) and by no stretch of the imagination do all women have access to a birth centre option in their communities. It is critical that future midwives cultivate the drive and develop the skills to create more birth centres.

The last survey of all graduates from the CNEP programme completed in 2000, reported that 6.7% of the respondents work in free-standing birth centres (PW Stone, personal communication, 2002) and, nationally, 8.2% of all CNMs who attend birth do so at both hospital-situated and free-standing birth centres (Kovner & Burkhardt 2001).

THE NATIONAL ASSOCIATION OF CHILDBEARING CENTRES

NACC was founded to support the development and promotion of birth centres (NACC 2002). Indeed, a national organisation is needed to steer the birth centre movement through the quagmire of commerce and regulation in American society, so that birth centres can assume a significant role among maternity services. NACC provides practical assistance to those who are planning, managing or working in birth centres. Functioning as the trade association of the birth centre movement, NACC serves as a clearing house of resource materials (Bauer 2000, Ernst 1995, Stapleton 1996). Its services include:

- *Membership*: available to established and developing birth centres, organisations, individuals and others interested in supporting the development of the concept.
- *Accreditation assistance*: NACC produces and sells materials that help birth centres prepare for accreditation, including templates for continuous quality improvement programmes.
- *Regulatory guidance*: information is available on how to analyse and/or develop regulations for birth centres.
- *Consultancy*: experts in the birth centre field who are affiliated with NACC can be consulted regarding issues specific to birth centres and general legislative/regulation queries.
- *Data collection*: NACC conducts regular surveys of birth centre operation and, with help from the Centers for Disease Control, has completed the UDS (Uniform Data Set) computer programme to facilitate the collection of a wide range of data (from the reasons for women choosing the birth centre to outcomes of care).
- *Standards*: NACC has compiled national standards of excellence for birth centre operation and services.
- *Resource materials*: policies and procedures, business planning and marketing materials give birth centres the option of adapting generic materials for their individual setting rather than starting from scratch. Birth centres can also personalise NACC's slogan and logo for marketing purposes.
- *Newsletters*: produced for NACC members three times per year and include articles, editorials, classified ads, announcements and updates.
- *Conferences*: Several times a year NACC sponsors 'How to Start a Birth Center' workshops around the country. There is also a yearly conference and annual meeting.

- *Information packs*: these contain a wide variety of materials and introduce readers to the birth centre concept (distributed to providers, payers and the public at large).
- *Collaborations*: NACC has cooperated with, mediated between and advocated for many organisations, including the American Public Health Association, private companies, accreditation bodies and government offices.
- *Research*: in addition to the national studies mentioned previously, a 10-year study on vaginal birth after caesarean section in birth centres is in preparation for publication.
- *Education*: NACC serves as a resource for consumers, authors and students.

CONCLUSION

As a proportion of the health care economy of the United States, the birth centre movement is admittedly small, yet it is growing and the numbers of women who have received birth centre services, the dollars invested in this progressive form of health care, and the size of the infrastructure behind it are all truly impressive, especially when compared to the birth centre profiles of other countries. Because of the overwhelming size of the medical establishment and the inequalities in the health care system in the USA, there is a feeling that, in international circles, American maternity models are not viewed as applicable or worthy of study. This does not seem to apply to American models of industry, entertainment or technology, which are all minutely scrutinised and often eagerly adopted by other countries. Much of what has been accomplished in the United States with respect to midwifery care, especially the birth centre model, should be noted internationally. The United States has abundant resources to share and our experience of establishing birth centres is no exception. Even if the culture of birth centres in the USA is uniquely American, the lessons learnt, the data gathered, the educational initiatives and the national resources are all available for universal examination and, where appropriate, can be adapted for use in other cultures.

REFERENCES

American College of Nurse-Midwives 1992 Definition of a certified nurse-midwife and definition of nurse-midwifery practice. American College of Nurse-Midwives, Washington, DC

American College of Nurse-Midwives 1993 ACNM standards for the practice of nurse-midwifery. American College of Nurse-Midwives, Washington, DC

American College of Nurse-Midwives 1997 A Tip Sheet for ACNM State Legislative Contacts Number 4, ACC Certified Midwives. Available at: *http://acnm.org/legis/display.cfm?id=161*

American Public Health Association 1982 Guidelines for licensing and regulating birth centers. Position Paper 8209. American Public Health Association

Bachu A, O'Connell M 2001 Fertility of American Women: June 2000. US Census Bureau, US Department of Commerce

Bauer K 2000 Birth centers online is your resource. NACC News 14 (1): 3

Bennetts A B, Lubic R W 1982 The free-standing birth center. CBCN News 1 (2–3): 11–12

Bing E 2001 Lamaze childbirth: then and now. Lamaze International. Available at: *http://www.lamaze.com/birth/preparations/articles 0,9474,167852_209025,00.html*

Bollier D 1992 Nurturing the consumer-side economy. In: Bollier D Citizen action and other big ideas, a history of Ralph Nader and the modern consumer movement. Available at: *http://www.nader.org/history/bollier_chapter_2.html*

CBCN 1982 Information for establishing standards or regulations for free standing birth centers. CBCN News, 1 (2–3): 1–2

Cole E 1986–87 The role of accreditation. NACC News, 4, 25–26

Ernst E K M 1982a The human side of legislation . . . . CBCN News, 1 (2–3): 22–23

Ernst E K M 1982b Editorial: Rights and responsibilities. CBCN News, 1 (2–3): 1–2

Ernst E K M 1983 The human side of reimbursement. CBCN News, 1 (4): 21–22

Ernst E K M 1995 Highlights of two decades of developing the birth center concept in the US. NACC News, 10 (4): 8

Ernst K 2001 Who wants to be a midwife? International Journal of Childbirth Educators 16 (1): 12

US Bureau of Economic Analysis Statistics Information Please. (copyright 2000–2002), Gross Domestic Product or Expenditure, 1930–2000. The Learning Network Summary of US Bureau of Economic Analysis Statistics. Available at: *http://www.infoplease.com/ipa/A0104575.html*

International Childbirth Education Association 2001 Available at: *http://www.icea.org/*

Johnson L H 1993 Consumer address: the birth center vision: a rebirth for women, families, society. NACC News, 8 (3): 3

Kovner C T, Burkhardt P 2001 Findings from the American College of Nurse-Midwives' annual membership survey, 1995–1999. Journal of Midwifery and Women's Health 46 (1): 24

Lee P 1993 A Visionary return to Washington. NACC News, 8 (3): 1

Lewis R D 1999 When Cultures Collide. Nicholas Brealey Publishing, London

Loose C 1998 A battle won, a center born. The Washington Post, September 30 1998

Lubic R W 1979 Barriers and conflict in maternity care innovation. (Doctoral dissertation) Columbia University, Teachers College, New York, p 29

Mills R J 2001 Health Insurance Coverage: 2000. US Census Bureau, US Department of Commerce

National Association of Childbearing Centers 1998 Standards for Birth Centers. National Association of Childbearing Centers

National Association of Childbearing Centers 1995 Removing payment barriers. NACC News 10 (1): 6

National Association of Childbearing Centers 2000 NACC survey report of birth center experience. National Association of Childbearing Centers

National Association of Childbearing Centers 2002 Birth Center Info. Available at: *http://www.birthcenters.org/*

National Center for Health Statistics at Centers for Disease Control 1999 Attendant, place and timing, and use of obstetric interventions of US births change over past decade. December 2 1999. Available at: *http://www.cdc.gov/nchs/releases/99facts/attendant.htm*

OECD 2000 A System of Health Accounts, Version 1.0, OECD, Paris.

Office of Federal Register 2000 Key Regulatory Facts & Figures. Available at: *http://www. regulation.org/keyfacts.html*

Peck S B 1986–87 The health insurers perspective on birth center accreditation. NACC News 4: 26–28

Regulation.org. Key Regulatory Facts and Figures. *http://regulation.org/keyfacts.html* (Accessed: 2002, May 19)

Rooks J P 1997 Midwifery and childbirth in America. Temple University Press, Philadelphia

Rooks J P, Weatherby, N L, Ernst, E K M 1992a The national birth center study: Part I–methodology and prenatal care and referrals. Journal of nurse-midwifery 37 (6): 361–397

Rooks J P, Weatherby N L, Ernst E K M 1992b The national birth center study: Part II–intrapartum and immediate postpartum and neonatal care. Journal of nurse-midwifery 37 (6): 361–397

Rooks J P, Weatherby N L, Ernst E K M 1992c The national birth center study: Part III–intrapartum and immediate postpartum and neonatal complications and transfers, postpartum and neonatal care, outcomes, and client satisfaction. Journal of nurse-midwifery 37 (6): 361–397

Rooks J P et al 1989 Outcomes of care in birth centers. New England Journal of Medicine 321 (26): 1804–1811

Scupholme A, McLeod A G W, Robertson E G 1986 A birth center affiliated with the tertiary care center: comparison of outcome. Obstetrics and Gynecology 67 (4): 598–603

Stapleton S 1996 The NACC Uniform Data Set. NACC News, 11 (5–6): 1

Stone P W, Walker P H 1995 Cost-effectiveness analysis: birth center versus hospital care. Nursing Economics 13 (5): 299–307

US Bureau of the Census 2000 State and County QuickFacts. http://quickfacts.census.gov/qfd/ US Bureau of the Census, Washington DC (Accessed: 2002, April 14).

Ventura S J et al 2001 Births attended by certified nurse-midwives are on the rise. Quickening (32) 6: 1

Wanless D 2001 Securing our future health: taking a long-term view. interim report. HM Treasury.

Warren M, Weidenbaum M 1999 The rise of regulation continues: an analysis of the budget for the year 2000. Center for the Study of American Business Regulatory Budget Report 22

19

A lesson in naivety: Casa de Nacimiento

Linda Arnold

THE VISION

I founded the birth centre, Casa de Nacimiento in 1985 in El Paso, in the belief that birth is a normal physiological function of the human body, that it should be a family event and that women should have options to choose how, where and with whom they birth. At that time nationwide, choices of providers were generally limited to general practitioners and obstetricians. There were a few women acting as midwives at home births, but education and experience were limited. More women wanted to become midwives, but needed a place to learn. I believed that in opening Casa de Nacimiento I could meet these goals by providing a clean, safe, caring environment to birth and to learn about birth.

El Paso, Texas is situated on the Mexican border, separated from its sister city of Juarez only by a relatively small river, the Rio Grande. Seen from the air, there is little to differentiate the two cities. El Paso has a predominantly Hispanic population, most people being considered as 'working poor', as well as people from Mexico who want to use United States services in almost every commercial sphere, including its health care. Its per capita birth ratio is one of the highest in the country, making it an 'excellent' site for the birth centre I envisioned.

Midwifery has always been legal in the state of Texas and governed by the Texas Department of Health Midwifery Board. The city of El Paso regulated its midwives and their practice standards by a City Ordinance. The governing body was the El Paso Lay-Midwifery Commission. This commission set the standards of practice and the risk criteria used by midwives in the city. The community had already been supporting birth centres operated and staffed by direct-entry, 'lay' midwives. However, there had been contention between the doctors and the midwives. I knew that my knowledge, skills and background were excellent, and that I would be able to pass this on to the clients we would serve, and to the aspiring midwives that the birth centre could train. This knowledge made me confident that I would be able to gain credibility in the community and win over the physicians so that client-centred births could become the norm. By my definition, 'client-centred births' are those in which the clients' needs supersede the political and financial agendas of the medical community, and my aim was that of working towards better outcomes for the women and their babies.

THE PREPARATION

In 1975 I began working for Dr Hai Abdul who was my preceptor and mentor. The hospital he practised at was unwilling to do labour bed births and very critical of any accidental bed births. He encouraged me to begin to look for another hospital which would allow labour bed births and which would consider establishing home-like birth rooms where labour bed deliveries could be done. Several hospitals refused but finally a small community hospital with a need for increased revenue recognised that it would be a sound decision for them economically. We then noticed that although some women did not feel safe at home, they did not want to go to the hospital to deliver either. The need for a freestanding birth centre became apparent. I found a building that would suit our needs and we set up a fully functioning obstetric unit with a classroom and two birth rooms. I worked with Dr Abdul in his practice of 70 to 90 births a month for over 3 years, gaining not only skills as a midwife but also the skills which are necessary to start a birth centre. I then moved and began a private practice in a rural setting. After 8 years of home births

I then made the decision to move again, this time to a site where I could open a birth centre, work out of one place and be able to train aspiring midwives. I felt that I had the experience and confidence to make my vision come true.

In the spring of 1985 I arrived in El Paso to begin my quest. I happened upon a real-estate agent who taught me about the history, demographics and politics of this city but also listened carefully to what I thought my needs were. So, as we drove a grid, beginning in the central city at the border and working slowly, street by street, up towards the mountain, we talked and noted all the properties that were available or appeared to be abandoned. The agent sifted through the list that we had made and we began to actually look at the properties. Several things then became apparent–I realized that the location would have to depend on accessibility, visibility, city zoning regulations, bus routes and parking availability, and not just on the actual building architecture. After 2 weeks of diligent searching we found an old cinder block building, 4000 square foot, which had formerly been used by an advertising agency, facing Interstate 10. It had been sitting empty for 2 years with windows broken and a leaky roof and had no showers or baths. It was like a maze, with no lights and dangling wires hanging from the ceiling. It would take a good imagination and a lot of work to make it into a functioning birth centre. My agent negotiated a lease with an option to buy, 4 months rent-free for cleaning and repairing, no first- or last-month prepayments and a reduced rate during the start-up time.

In 2 months Casa was ready for its grand opening, a large portion of its space had been refurbished with examination rooms, birth rooms, a laboratory, and a waiting room. Casa was not like the other birth centres in El Paso–it was large, clean, well decorated and well equipped.

MIDWIFERY IN AN EL PASO BIRTH CENTRE

To practice legally in the city I had to get an El Paso lay midwifery permit. The El Paso Lay Midwifery Commission mandated that the clinical experience for this permit had to be gained in the city, regardless of any previous experience. To my surprise, one of the physicians and the certified nurse midwife on the Midwifery Commission invited me to spend a month doing clinical rotations with them at the county hospital, which had about 600 births per month. They had opened a door for me in a way which was unprecedented. This same hospital was the one which received most of the transfers from birth centres, the one whose security officers escorted midwives out when they came in with their clients to the hospital! The clinical rotation they set up for me allowed me to meet all the necessary requirements and to take and pass the next scheduled exam, a much faster process than going to births with the two friendly midwives in town. I thought at the time that they had set this up for me because they knew that I was highly qualified and would be an asset to the community.

In a matter of 5 months, Casa's client load had increased from zero to 30 births per month. I hired two Hispanic women to help in the office, translate and work with the clients, but I needed qualified staff midwives. Hiring a midwife was difficult–they would need a high level of experience, commitment and stamina, as well as an El Paso lay midwifery permit. Out-of-state midwives began to consider relocating to El Paso and obtaining a legal permit to practice there. Occasionally, friendly local midwives helped out at Casa to ease the load when things were busy.

I had envisioned Casa taking midwifery students from the very beginning. Two of the apprentices that I had in my private practice followed me from Idaho to Texas. Gradually, more aspiring midwives came to Casa to train and gain experience. These students have been an essential part of the workforce necessary to care for Casa's clients.

Casa was busy all the time, with appointments, deliveries and students. The media and the government were fascinated by us. Reporters came from as far away as Japan and Brazil to interview and photograph Casa. I appeared on business programmes and morning talk shows. The US State Department brought tours of physicians in to see this birth centre, a phenomenon that had been created and run with few financial resources but with great results, using it as an example for possible duplication in other countries. Here was a free-standing birth centre on the border with Mexico which provided full maternity services for women in the community for $450 to $600, staffed by direct-entry midwives who could provide care for low- to moderate-risk clients without the need for medication or surgical procedures. This birth centre was using no government funds, such as welfare, loans or grants, and yet it was prospering.

PERSECUTION

Before 2 years had passed, Casa had approximately 60 to 70 births per month, with a client load of about 225 women. At about that time, however, it appeared that the medical community of El Paso turned and became hostile toward Casa. The other birth centres had closed down and there was another new centre opening in El Paso, but Casa was now the largest birth centre in the state of Texas. Even by conservative estimates, Casa's 60 births per month were taking about three and a half million dollars annually from El Paso medical providers. I never imagined that prejudice against midwives and the economics of a free-standing birth centre could so inflame a medical community. Everything that we did was scrutinised by the city's Midwifery Commission. This commission was made up predominantly of physicians who controlled the midwives and their practice using the El Paso City Ordinance regulations and their power to suspend and revoke midwifery permits.

Meanwhile, with all this attention on the birth centres in El Paso, and more centres opening across the state, Texas decided to begin mandatory licensing of birth centres by the Texas Department of Health, Certification and Licensure Division. Regulations were drawn up by Department staff physicians and nurses. They had never done out-of-hospital deliveries, run a birth centre or had an active practice. Some of the rules and standards of practice represented positive efforts to improve the quality of care and provide protection for the clients and practitioners, but others amounted merely to harassment. Department representatives would go through birth centres' premises and records, searching for anything that might be construed as a violation of safe practice or of some regulation. One small mistake on a chart could easily be blown up into multiple violations and become an indefensible mistake. During those first years many birth centres closed as a result of the constant intimidation and their inability to afford the legal battles required to keep this state licensing agency at bay. Additionally, the pressure and stress of such defensive practice was more than most could endure. The state had endless financial resources and at least 50 to 60 lawyers to counter any defence mounted by a small birth centre and its lawyer.

By 1989 Casa had become embroiled in the Department's feeding frenzy that had already closed many birth centres across the state. There was close collaboration between the medical community, the Commission and the Department in their efforts to close Casa. That year a staff midwife at Casa transferred a woman by ambulance to a nearby hospital, with the baby in a breech presentation and a cord prolapse that she was handling appropriately. Upon their arrival at the hospital the attending physician ordered the midwife to remove her hand and get out and threatened to have her removed by security if she did not. She did as she was told and left in tears. All we found out was that the baby was put on life support, then was pronounced dead. This started a chain reaction that resulted in a legal battle that lasted for years. The attending neonatologist hired a lawyer to sue Casa on behalf of the clients for $25 million. Neither Casa nor I have ever carried malpractice insurance so this legal battle had to be taken on by my private lawyer. In the United States, once you are sued you can legally obtain all medical records. These records showed that no one continued to keep the baby off the cord. Instead, the attending emergency room physician called (from the

hospital emergency room) the City County Health Director (who was the chairman of the Commission) to tell him that they finally 'had' the midwives at the birth centre for attending a high-risk presentation. Thirty-five minutes later the woman was taken upstairs from the emergency room and a caesarean section was performed. The baby was born in severe distress and was resuscitated. They later pronounced the baby brain-dead and kept him on life support until they sold and removed his organs for use at two teaching hospitals in other parts of the country. This act of malpractice by the hospital emergency room physician and staff allowed Casa to bring the hospital and physician into the lawsuit.

There were three other lawsuits filed against Casa at this time that came to a total of over $45 million. The conspiracy continued with attempts to discredit the birth centre and its midwives by calling in the media to witness them filing their lawsuits in court or by making defamatory statements which claimed that we were burying babies in the alley. Interestingly, none of these lawsuits were ever tried against Casa–they were all dismissed. The breech, $25 million lawsuit against Casa concluded with the hospital and the emergency room doctor settling out of court with the family for their malpractice. Casa, the obstetrician and the neonatologist were dismissed from the case.

These same medical 'professionals' who initiated the lawsuits against Casa also made complaints to the Department, which then began to investigate them in full earnest. They made unannounced visits to the birth centre, with two or three people flying to El Paso every 3 to 4 weeks from Austin. They would go through our files, interview staff and inspect the premises. They compiled a list of 61 allegations against the birth centre in less than a year. The Department then served Casa with notice that it intended to close the birth centre. Casa requested an administrative hearing before the Department to defend itself from the allegations, most of which were trivial in nature.

I learned that the administrative hearing was to be conducted by a lawyer employed by the

Department, who would act as the 'hearing examiner',–in other words, the judge. The hearing was therefore to take place with the lawyers for the Department presenting their case to another lawyer for the Department, who acted as the judge! Meanwhile, Casa was continuing as normal, but I was concerned about whether Casa could possibly get a fair 'trial' at this hearing. We were not guilty of these charges, but it was us against the Department. Once the hearing began it took 13 days of testimony, spread out over 3 months, with the state officials flying back and forth between Austin and El Paso. The Department spent tens of thousands of dollars in its case against Casa; Casa's legal fees exceeded seventy thousand dollars. The results of the hearing were astounding–the hearing examiner found only six minor violations out of the 61 original allegations. He recommended to the Department, in a lengthy and detailed report, that Casa should not be closed because the violations he found were so minor.

Under normal circumstances the Department would follow the recommendation of its own hearing examiner, who had conducted the proceedings and heard the evidence. However, in this case the Department overruled the hearing examiner and ordered Casa to be closed. The lawyers for the Department immediately faxed a restraining order to Casa, ordering its immediate 'closure' without giving us the advance notice allowed in law. The birth centre licensing regulations, as they were written, stated that a licence was required for 'births', so antenatal and postpartum care did not need a licence. We needed to act quickly and creatively so that the clients would not become alarmed. I made the decision that any clients in labour would be informed and offered a home birth and that all other care would go on as normal. This 'sneak attack' by the Department's lawyers meant that Casa was 'closed' for a total of 3 days, until our lawyer could file and obtain a 'stay' with the State Court in Austin. Fortunately, only one woman went into labour and delivered at home. The 'stay' would temporarily stop the Department's closure of Casa until the Court could rule on the evidence and proceedings. Finally we got the

break that we needed–once the case was in the State Court, the Department's lawyers could no longer represent the Department against us. Instead, the Department was represented by lawyers from the State Attorney General's Office. Once the State's lawyers reviewed the proceedings, they were surprised by the Department's actions. The lawyers from the Attorney General's Office contacted our lawyer and expressed deep concern that they would be embarrassed to go before the Court to try to close Casa for such trivial reasons. They asked us to agree to dismiss our stay and they would then agree to dismiss the closure order. We accepted gratefully. It had been a life-changing ordeal, but we had survived.

The Commission had to save face somehow as the Department had essentially lost its case. After another highly visible hearing it was decided that they would withdraw my personal midwifery permit for 1 month because I had not made sure that my staff midwife had transferred a client with a breech presentation in a timely manner. The Commission continued to try and discredit midwives in this community. This was easy for them because the doctors on the Commission were the receiving physicians for transfers and they had access to our most difficult cases and their records. The physicians on the Commission became careless in their pursuit, however. They began to abuse their privileges quite flagrantly, placing themselves above the law in their efforts to bring further charges against midwives. I learned of the new charges to be brought against me in an open meeting of the full Commission at which the findings of a secret subcommittee were adopted and there was open discussion about my criminal prosecution and licence revocation. This time, however, I decided to defend myself, as I had done against the State, and take up an offensive position. I appeared at the public meeting with my lawyer, two well-known criminal defence lawyers from El Paso and a professional videographer with his camera running. My lawyers advised the Commission and the City Attorneys, who were present to assist the Commission, that the subcommittee's findings were in violation of the law. The Commission and its members then recognised their precarious position, with everything they said and did being recorded on videotape, and decided to adjourn immediately without taking action. The El Paso City Council decided soon afterwards to dissolve the El Paso Lay Midwifery Commission and leave the regulating of midwives to the Texas Midwifery Board.

I have reflected deeply over the years about why members of the Commission initially helped me to obtain my midwifery permit, so that I could open Casa, and why these same people later became Casa's most vociferous critics. The only conclusion I have been able to reach is that they initially believed that Casa would do well and push the other birth centres out. Once Casa was the sole surviving birth centre, they thought that I wouldn't have the strength and determination to fight off all the lawsuits, the medical community and the state and city authorities. They had drastically underestimated this midwife's determination to survive.

BRIDGING THE GAP

When I came to El Paso, I left a community that was not totally supportive of home births. However, over time I had acquired the respect of a significant portion of the medical community there. That respect created good working relationships between medical providers and myself which greatly benefited the clients: I was able to choose the provider with the particular gifts or specialties that could best serve an individual client. There was no jealousy between us–we worked together hand in hand to serve the needs of the client. I was perhaps naive in my belief that accomplished, qualified providers could work together here in El Paso with a similar respect for one another's skills and services. Since my arrival here I have become disillusioned and probably a little cynical as a result of the struggles that Casa and I have had to endure. I no longer believe that, as a whole, the medical community here in El Paso focuses on

the client as an individual, with specific physical, emotional and social needs. There may be some who do, but they are few.

Recently, I received a phone call from a young paediatric resident. She explained that her sister (in another city) wanted to deliver at home with a midwife. She had decided that she wanted to come to Casa and observe how we assisted childbirth. This was the first time in all our years that a member of our medical community cared enough to learn about us and what we did at first hand. I assigned her to follow one of my best staff midwives and explained that she was to be allowed to observe and participate, where appropriate, in all the services we provided. She was courteous and considerate to all, she asked appropriate questions and helped with even the most menial of tasks. She was able to see and understand that not all deliveries and babies needed all the interventions that she had been taught. She came to understand better why her sister wanted less intervention, by delivering with a midwife, and that it could be safe. With this new understanding and respect for our place in the birth process, she wanted to share her side of birth and babies with our midwife. She arranged with her supervisors at the hospital to bring in a 'visiting medical student', our staff midwife. A few short weeks passed and our midwife was at the hospital doing rounds with our new 'secret friend', the paediatrician. Our midwife was able to move throughout the shift without question as the visiting 'medical student'. She was able to observe and learn about the 'other side', including caesarean deliveries, neonatal intensive care and the interventions that can save lives. What a tragedy that we cannot support each other openly and bridge the gap in maternity services in this community.

Nearly 17 years have passed since I began the mission. Countless people have contributed to Casa over the years. There are so many without whose help Casa might not have survived. My family and friends helped to support me as Casa was born. As Casa grew and developed, other midwives, staff, students and financial and legal professionals helped it to stand on its own feet. The birth centre survived great trials and grew stronger and better for those trials. Casa is still running today, having delivered up to 90 births per month, over 8400 babies, including our babies' babies and our own children and grand-children. Casa has been a place of clinical train-ing for over 300 midwifery students from around the world. These students have gained some of the finest clinical experience available. Some of the very best of our students have been coming to Casa for many years and they have become a vital part of Casa's family, history and workforce. Casa is a fine example of a high-volume birth centre which serves its community with quality maternity care at affordable prices.

20

Birth centre midwifery down under

Kate Griew

INTRODUCTION

This chapter explores what it means to be a birth centre midwife in Australia. With a trend towards improved facilities, more appealing labour wards and models of care that provide continuity, it is pertinent to distinguish between birth centre and other forms of midwifery. The greatest resource in addressing this subject is midwives who have worked in birth centres since their inception. The first Australian birth centre opened in 1978 (Ryan 1997) and there is a wealth of midwifery experience to draw from. This chapter reports on insights that birth centre midwives have shared regarding their work.

Historical, socio-political, economic and organisational factors that form the background to the opinions of the midwives interviewed are outlined. The midwives showed depth of understanding about the nature of their work, their engagement with the women they care for, the development of clinical skill within the field, and the integrated nature of the 'birth centre experience' for both the women clients and the midwives who work in birth centres. In recognising areas of philosophical and practical discord between midwifery models, the midwives identified a clinical specialty in the field of birth centre midwifery. In doing this they demonstrated that they valued their colleagues in other areas of midwifery.

THE BACKGROUND

Consumer dissatisfaction with existing med-icalised maternity care drove the movement to establish birth centres in Australia. Governments, under pressure to expand birthing opportunities and include a home birth option, improved funding to birth centres instead. Birth centres have since been promoted as being 'half-way' between home and hospital birth. However, the majority of birth centres exist in urban set-tings, within the ambit of public hospitals. They may form a section of the labour ward, a self-contained unit in the hospital or in the hospital grounds, or, rarely, may be located indepen-dently of a hospital (Senate Community Affairs References Committee 1999).

Despite a number of government-funded reports recommending the development of birth centres to provide care to women (Health Department NSW 1989, Health Department Victoria 1990, Health Department WA 1990) there is scant evidence of continued expansion of funding (Senate Community Affairs References Committee 1999). Funding has been provided through state, commonwealth governments and, more recently, from mainstream public health resources.

Public birth centres are accountable to the institution or area health service under whose auspices they fall and therefore the forces that govern that institution or area. There is no sepa-rate regulation of birth centres at either state or national level. The political and administrative climate, the support or hostility of midwifery staff, management, obstetric and paediatric per-sonnel, institutional policy and protocol and the cultural beliefs and practices in the local com-munity and in maternity care all impact on birth centre operation. These factors explain signifi-cant variations in inclusion and exclusion criteria and in clinical protocols between birth centres.

Birth centres provide care for less than 5% of pregnant women in Australia. Data collection systems in a number of states do not distin-guish between birth centre and antenatal clinic/labour ward care, which makes it impossible to gather exact figures (Senate Community Affairs References Committee 1999). Maternal and neona-tal outcomes and measures of consumer satisfac-tion show impressive results. Birth centres provide safe, cost-effective and woman-centred care. However, limitations on, and opposition to, birth centres do exist. Funding difficulties and obstruction by those who have an interest in medicalising rather than normalising preg-nancy and birth are the most apparent (Senate Community Affairs References Committee 1999).

Birth centres revolve around a philosophy that pregnancy and labour are healthy life events for most women. The aim is to facilitate active, nat-ural birth with minimal intervention through the provision of physical, emotional and social sup-port and preparation. A woman is encouraged to participate in all aspects of her pregnancy. Antenatal care provides continuity and the cen-tres provide a relaxed, home-like environment for women to labour in when the time comes.

Women are likely to have met their midwives and be familiar with the centre's layout prior to arrival in labour. If they haven't met the midwife they know that their carer will support an active birth with minimal intervention. Waldenström (1998) reports that birth centre clientele in a Swedish study reported no less satisfaction when the intrapartum carer had not been met before. She speculated that the reduced impor-tance placed on having a 'known midwife' in this environment might relate to continuity in attitude and philosophy amongst carers.

Generally, birth centres provide an antenatal and intrapartum service for pregnant women who are deemed 'low' or 'low to moderate' risk. If deviations from a healthy pregnancy are detected, care might be transferred to, or shared with, a hospital-based antenatal or specialist clinic. In a number of institutions the need for any medical review is considered reason enough for permanent transfer of care. If complications arise during labour the woman usually trans-fers to a labour ward for continuation of care. Transfer rates during pregnancy or labour vary from under 30% to nearly 50%. (Senate Community Affairs References Committee 1999). Postnatal care is provided through birth centre midwives, the hospital's wards or midwifery discharge teams.

Protocols may allow for self-referral or may rely on medical screening to determine suitability if a woman states a desire for birth centre. Inclusion depends on the woman's awareness of this option and on staff involved in the medical screening process being sympathetic to a birth centre approach. A number of Australian birth centres accept private 'obstetric' clients, whilst at some centres no private obstetricians work with the centre. At others, women may share care with their own general practitioner.

Up to 85 women may access a centre per month but, generally, monthly numbers are significantly smaller than this. Because an expectation exists that women will have encountered their midwife prior to labour, the number of midwives in a team tends to be limited. Care may be provided by midwives working a 24-hour rotating roster. Pre-booked antenatal appointments and education sessions are provided through a clinic in or outside the centre. In some centres, small teams look after a predetermined number of women throughout their pregnancy and birth. In this situation midwives are on-call for women in labour, provide pre-booked antenatal care and education sessions and receive an agreed salary package. A number of small teams may operate through one centre.

THE PERSPECTIVE OF THE BIRTH CENTRE MIDWIFE

It is birth centre midwives themselves who are the authorities on the question, 'What makes a birth centre midwife?' In a study designed to look at this question material was gathered from a series of interviews and small focus groups with 13 midwives who have worked in Australian birth centres. Participation was voluntary. Midwives were asked the same questions (see Box 20.1). Certain questions generated extensive discussion. Interviews and focus groups were audiotaped, transcribed and the content was analysed and grouped thematically. What follows is a summary of the information

---

Box 20.1 Interviews with birth centre midwives–the questions asked

- What do you most like about working in a birth centre?
- What are the biggest challenges about working in a birth centre?
- What are the differences between labour ward and birth centre midwifery?
- How do you feel when a woman you are caring for transfers to labour ward during labour?
- If you are not involved in a 'caseload' practice already, what would be your response if your place of work transferred to a situation where you cared for a woman wherever she birthed?
- Do you think the geographical distance between labour ward and birth centre is important to the women and/or the midwives or in determining outcomes in any way?

---

gathered from this material. Data was grouped into four main themes: social and emotional; communication and language; clinical; and organisational. These themes are outlined and illustrated with excerpts from the interviews and groups. Confirmation and further discussion of the identified themes was obtained through informal discussions with a further 12 (mostly birth centre) midwives who had not participated in the initial data collection. In the brackets following the excerpts from interviews I have included the number of years that the midwife has worked in birth centres, with 'TM' denoting previous team midwifery experience. Names have been changed to protect the anonymity of the midwives interviewed.

The midwives who participated in the interviews had had between 6 months and 16 years of experience in birth centres and between 3 years and 21 years of experience as midwives. A number had worked in as many as five different birth centres. The midwives had worked in eight birth centres throughout Australia. A number had worked in other continuity-of-care programmes, four in 'team midwifery' and two in independent practice providing home births. Two of those who had worked in team midwifery had worked in teams that operated through birth centres. Many had worked or trained overseas.

Two midwives had moved continents to work in Australian birth centres. All the midwives had worked in labour wards, the longest period being for 14 years. It should be noted that there were clusters of midwives who had had similar years of experience in birth centres.

SOCIAL AND EMOTIONAL CARE

Interacting on a social level with women afforded a depth of connection that the midwives had found difficult to achieve in more traditional care settings. They felt more able to provide emotional care and support in the context of having exchanged values, aspirations and social details. They regarded the ability to form strong connections as a privilege that helped create a greater sense of equality or partnership. In Pairman's research participants coined the term 'professional friendship' to describe the relationship between midwives and women involved in continuity-of-care model care. She noted that these relationships could produce empowering and emancipatory benefits for both midwives and their clientele (Pairman 1998). The midwives interviewed here reinforced this.

'The women knowing us—you've got this social aspect with her' (Jodie, 2)

Midwives identified the importance of women feeling known as individuals. This replicated the findings of Coyle et al (2001a, 2001b) about mothers' perceptions of birth centre care.

[The women know that] they'll be valued ... they're not just numbers. (Jill, 1)

[The midwives] don't feel so much like you're invading them, 'cos you know them and there's some sort of relationship that's been established. (Jill, 1)

The midwives reported feeling 'much more on an even footing with the women' (Beau, 1, TM).

One midwife noted that despite strong rapport which could be built up in the labour-ward situation, the nature of the rapport was different:

When you've never met her before it's harder to establish that social connection. The main thing you base your relationship on is what's before you, the physical things of labour, and policy, rather than knowing the woman. (Ingrid, 1)

She compared the two areas and suggested that the greater proportion of social interaction in a labour ward was between colleagues rather than between midwives and women.

Trust was a recurring theme throughout. It took four forms. In the context of social relationships within birth centres the midwives talked about women's development of trust in their midwives:

You have to treat them in a way that enables them to trust you. (Julia, 11)

They want to know that you know what you are doing. (Loretta, 2, TM)

The midwives also discussed women's trust in the process of pregnancy and birth:

She has to trust her own body to get through this. (Ingrid, 1)

Their bodies do know what to do. (Jill, 1)

Part of that is trusting birth as a natural process, not feeling that they need to hang on to a medical system, a doctor. (Carla, 3, TM)

The development of trust also influenced clinical practice and will be discussed later in the chapter.

Knowing the women: 'Knowing where they're coming from' (Jill, 1)

Women's commitment to a birth centre approach helped the midwives participate in women's care. Knowing the women were committed to a similar philosophy removed some of the barriers encountered in other settings:

You know you're not pushing them into having *your* birth experience ... when it comes to pain relief, you know they're already there, rather than you wanting them to have a natural birth—they really want one. (Jill, 1)

I feel more able to make suggestions ... that they won't feel pushed or coerced .... It's easier to work when you're not feeling like you're holding back on something. (Jodie, 2)

I have to own that I have an expectation of the clientele, that they're expecting a certain type of experience and role.... They want support and low intervention ways of managing labour. I think that it makes caring for them in this context a little bit simpler...you gear your care that way. (Lil', 5)

I know a lot of my confidence has come from the fact that this is what women have wanted. (Loretta, 2, TM)

Offering follow-up for women was seen as important, regardless of the outcome of the pregnancy and birth:

You really need to go back a few days later and see how they're doing. (Ingrid, 1)

...having a postnatal group where the women have a chance to come and debrief and check out what happened.... 'Cos I think...while they're in hospital they're on a high from the birth and it's 3 months down the track that they're starting to ask questions about, 'What if I'd done this or that?'... One thing I have learned is there is no way you can anticipate how people feel about their experience. (Julia, 11)

Emotional Care: 'Having some empathy' (Julia, 11)

Many midwives focused on emotional issues that arise while providing care for women. They discussed factors that impact on women's experiences of pregnancy and birth. These factors included cultural understandings around birthing, socialisation as women and individual experiences as women or in childhood:

I'm more aware of my own agenda and how that may impact on women. (Beau, 1, TM)

You have to read between the lines a lot...there are a number of psychological skills that you probably need to work in this environment. Treating each person individually rather than saying, 'You've come into this category so we must do...'.(Julia, 11)

When I'm practising clinically, a lot of what I do is...emotional work, exploring her fears...her emotional history. (Carla, 3, TM)

...having a baby is such a social thing...you can try and set the scene for her. (Ingrid, 1)

The midwives approached these issues compassionately, with a belief that birth centres may offer space and time for a woman to manage emotional concerns that may occur during pregnancy or labour. One midwife recounted a traumatic birth she had attended. She felt strongly that the woman was a survivor of sexual abuse:

I needed to stay with her, her partner had...disassociated at this stage. (Lil', 5)

Midwives agreed that a birth centre often provides an appropriate, safe environment for women survivors.

There was recognition that there are limits to what even the most productive relationships between midwives and women can achieve:

She looked at me...she said, 'It never goes away, does it?', and that was the only acknowledgement...and there's no way you can delve into it without risking her safety. (Lil', 5)

I mean, you can only do so much–she can only meet you half-way. (Carla, 3, TM)

...no matter how intuitive you are we all miss some. (Julia, 11)

...at the end of the day she has to trust her own body to get through this. (Paula, 1)

...you can't debrief a woman from the first day she was born, all the stories she's been exposed to. (Ingrid, 1)

Knowing each other: 'The team was a big part of it' (Melissa, 7)

Being part of a group of midwives that share, 'much the same philosophy, the same approach' (Melissa, 7) was seen as a benefit of working in a birth centre. Regular reference was made to 'like-minded views about midwifery (Jodie, 2). This was seen as a huge advantage of working with birth centre colleagues:

...it's lovely...to hand over [and]...know that they're not going to be rushing into interventions...which you can't always be assured of in the situation of a labour ward transfer. Quite often you're handing a woman over at a very vulnerable stage but if she has confidence in the person she's moving on to then it doesn't interfere in the whole process. (Ingrid, 1)

There is a close team feel, a humour. (Beau, 1, TM)

Developing a greater trust in the process of pregnancy and labour was part of the midwives' like-mindedness:

I've changed... realising that the women who come to the birth centre are well and their babies are well, so you act on that trust. (Jill, 1)

I have much more faith in women's ability to birth naturally. (Beau, 1, TM)

[You] trust that something is going to happen even though you don't have your hands on, you're not stuck in the middle of it trying to do things. (Ingrid, 1)

There were also a few reports of struggles amongst colleagues:

I think when you're working with a small team... there'll be tension around styles of practice and personality, the irritations that happen. In bigger teams they can be calmed over because you have more people around to diffuse it.... Even though I have 'moments' with some of my workmates, I trust their midwifery and know that they... will back me in caring for a woman. (Rachel, 6)

COMMUNICATION AND LANGUAGE

You work with the women more; you work with each woman differently. (Jodie, 2)

The style of communication used by the midwives was emphasised. The midwives saw their role as tailoring information to make it accessible to individual women, observing, listening and supporting women to make their own decisions. Interactions with women and supporting partners were described as less directive and more personal. Midwives reported heightened observational skills as a result of working in birth centres:

you're... the one that's giving them the information that's allowing them to make decisions for themselves, not leaving them floundering or asking them to make decisions that they shouldn't have to make. (Julia, 11)

...she's making the decisions, but you're working with her. She's telling you what she wants to do, rather than following policies that are not necessarily geared to individualised care. (Loretta, 3, TM)

I think I probably listen more to what the women say. Even though I thought I used to before, I realise in comparison that I didn't. I take much more notice of things like noises, and signs that were always there but I... didn't rely on them as much... I tended to rely more on doing VEs rather than just stepping back and watching. (Jill, 1)

The environment enables you to *truly listen* to women and what they want, what they're saying. You always work safely but you're not 'forced' to adhere to such procedures as admission CTGs, regular VEs etc. You're able to work much more easily *with* women. (Beau, 1, TM her emphasis)

Many midwives commented that their documentation contained a less clinical, more accessible vocabulary than they had previously used in labour ward practice. In one birth centre that was tightly governed by the obstetric protocols of the hospital, rather than applying the constraining rules verbatim, the midwives carefully documented what they were witnessing that they considered reassuring of progress. They saw this as a way of justifying their practice, educating other staff regarding alternative ways of operating and protecting themselves against criticism.

Language: 'It hasn't occurred to them to try and use ordinary language' (Jasmine, 16)

The midwives observed that they now used less 'medical' language. Many criticised the use of medical jargon, arguing that it promotes a medical view of pregnancy and birth. Anspach (1994) argued that through the linguistic construction of an occupational register, through socialisation to a medical perspective and depersonalisation, practitioners become compelled to put their faith in the power and accuracy of medical science and suspend their belief in clients' subjective experience. To refuse to participate in dominant linguistic practices can discredit the speaker or challenge the dominant cultural beliefs of those around them. Midwives provided examples of the use of non-medical alternatives as reinforcing the construction of pregnancy as a physiological process. Some midwives saw this as a form of subversive activity:

Up there [the labour ward] it's full of medical jargon ... on labour ward you tend to get the feeling that you're in control of the process, the woman is just passively involved ... you talk about things as 'confined' or 'delivered' as opposed to 'giving birth' or 'having the baby'. There's a lot of jargon. Down here [the birth centre] it feels a bit more normalised. We say 'baby' instead of 'fetus'. In labour ward ... you're talking about 'doing things' to people. (Loretta, 2, TM)

Many of the midwives were critical of the language used by labour ward midwives:

I mean, 'delivered' is bad enough but 'confined' is outrageous. (Chris, 6)

... saying something as simple as 'birth' rather than 'delivery' ... instead of saying 'the cervix', saying 'your cervix', recognising the woman owns it, rather than trying to be detached. (Jill, 1)

Using 'birth' as a verb for a start! (Julia, 11)

One midwife suggested that linguistic differences might reflect institutional demands on a unit. She thought that where there is greater skill-mix, volume and activity there is, perhaps, a greater need to adhere to standardised communication patterns. She noted that in the birth centre:

... language is probably less instructional for a start ... [it's not] 'you will do, must do, can't do, I want you to', etc. It's more, 'Here are the options, the information, you could try, what do you feel about that?' ... reinforce that it's *their* situation. Women learn to expect choice. (Julia, 11)

Another midwife speculated that language operates to create a cohesive and authoritative occupational group:

You are really protected by language. You can stand behind it. Sometimes I think we feel vulnerable as a midwife, like did you get it wrong? ... There's a huge group of women ... different backgrounds ... we've all got to fit in and get on. And if you're a midwife who stands out ... you're the one who uses words like 'birth' ... I don't know if words make us feel like we belong a little bit ... if we all used words like

'confined', maybe it makes us feel like professionals. Whereas if we say 'no' to words, what are we? (Loretta, 2, TM)

CLINICAL PRACTICE AND SKILLS: 'There's more autonomy and more responsibility' (Beau, 1, TM)

In addition to particular motor skills and the emotional components of care, recurrent themes raised by midwives regarding clinical practice concentrated on: the development of autonomous practice; trust in the process of pregnancy and birth; the development of trust in their own abilities, and the importance of making judgements and taking action when it was necessary. Although the involvement of other personnel was often viewed as an intrusion, some midwives regretted that they got little opportunity to witness their colleagues' practice:

... you need to have good midwifery skills ... be good at palping ... managing ... all those emergencies. You need to be able to recognise a problem or when you or the woman needs help ... reading those signals, between the lines. (Julia, 11)

Probably for me the biggest challenges were clinical decisions ... when somebody doesn't want to move out and you feel clinically that they should. And I guess the ultimate scare is the flat baby, the big PPH when you are on your own, that's pretty challenging .... getting used to new practice ... like waterbirths. (Melissa, 7)

... less people, less fingers in the pie, less people poking their noses in the door wanting to know what's going on. (Melissa, 7)

You are managing the case well and truly ... in a delivery ward you're incorporating other people into it. (Carla, 3, TM)

I like using the full range of my skills. I like being able to do everything from booking right through to delivery. I like being able to take responsibility for my actions, making decisions and taking responsibility for them, not having to ... control. I like having to be up to date and I think you have to be in this job. (Loretta, 2, TM)

You're more autonomous, more flexible in your approach ... I've done a fair share of abnormal births and I like the fact that it's basically working with women who are normal, healthy for a change. So I'm not having to do things... I like seeing the differences, the wide variety of normal.... It's good in this birth centre... because it's incredibly flexible.... That's quite freeing. But you also feel that support there if you need it. (Loretta, 2, TM)

...you're always answerable to whoever's in charge [in the labour ward], you always have someone with you. (Julia, 11)

The midwives frequently commented that the actions they *didn't* perform were of equal significance to those that they did:

It sounds ironic, but allowing yourself the ability to do nothing.... Not doing is as important as doing, and realising when it is appropriate to get in and do something if something needs to be done... you're not going to be doing the woman any favours for standing back and doing nothing when something is warranted. On the other hand, you need to stand back and give her the chance to get on and do it on her own. (Ingrid,1)

I sit back and wait a lot more. I'm more patient... I leave the baby and mum and family to have more time on their own. I take a more background role. (Beau, 1, TM)

Developing trust in their own abilities and judgement was of prime importance in the midwives' work in birth centres:

Trusting your judgement! It's a comfortable situation to be in, to always have someone else to refer to. Here you have to stand on your own. By all means we collaborate, but you have to be able to say, 'Yes, I feel this baby's breech.'... and be able to stand with that. And you actually do get more competent as you go along, you value your own decisions. (Ingrid, 1)

You learn to believe in yourself and your findings, not always turning to the nearest person for advice, so you have to trust your judgement and decisions. (Beau, 1, TM)

Now I definitely trust myself more and what I know... my own judgement... and trusting the women more too. (Loretta, 2, TM).

...you... get more confident in yourself and in the women. (Melissa 7)

Monitors: 'It's delightful not to have monitors' (Melissa, 7)

The presence and type of fetal monitoring equipment was significant in distinguishing labour ward from birth centre midwifery: '[In the labour ward] everything is based around the CTG, whether it's the first admission in labour or unrelated to labour.' This midwife had said that she knew she was ready for a change from labour ward practice–'I never wanted to do a CTG again' (Julia, 11).

The presence of monitors impacts negatively on the care a midwife can provide:

...you have to change your practice a fair bit... the women become a lot less mobile. Most women who transfer are going to need monitoring of some sort so that interferes... it feels more restricted. (Jill, 1)

...so many decisions are based on a trace. Yet we have no idea... whether they are justified or not. And more and more it's telling us that it's not, isn't it? And you just have to have confidence that people can labour without monitors and still have very healthy babies and good outcomes. (Melissa, 7)

The absence of monitors gives the midwives more opportunity to pay attention to the women:

'I think I pay a lot more attention when a woman's not on the monitor' (Loretta, 2, TM).

Complementary therapies

Midwives commented that complementary therapies were used more commonly by clientele in birth centres. While accepting women's choices to use different therapies they also perceived a need for further development in this area of birth centre midwifery. A number of midwives had undertaken further study in particular therapies.

'Generalism' versus expertise: '...it's about your comfort zone and moving outside of it' (Melissa, 7)

An interesting distinction arose in discussions regarding transfers and continuity of carer. Certain midwives valued continuity over all other concerns while others preferred to operate within a discrete area. Many midwives viewed themselves as 'birth centre' midwives with a distinct field of expertise. All the midwives reported that a birth centre position required flexibility of midwifery skills, especially in the case of transfers and they recognised the expertise of their labour ward colleagues in working with women experiencing 'complicated' labours:

It's not that I'm anti-medical, I know sometimes it's the right thing. It's that I've found that I'm much more comfortable with the non-medical. (Jill, 1)

If I had ... a massive APH, a bradycardia ... and I was only 32 weeks ... I'd much rather see someone in the labour ward who was used to working there, who was clued in to what needs to be done in that situation.... I don't think that that is my speciality.... So, I admire the expertise of people who deal with 24-weekers ... and I also admire the expertise of midwives who can sit back and ... support this process, letting a woman have her baby herself. (Ingrid, 1)

It's quite a skill for those labour ward midwives to make a labour ward birth. I mean, considering everything they've got up against them, all those time pressures, and those idiot doctors who are trying to get experience ... looking for problems ... it is a great skill to give a woman a great birth experience in those conditions. That's what they are really good at. They do it well. (Jasmine, 16)

If you want to work in a birth centre you have to have a focus on natural birth and normal delivery. I don't think you can be swapping between the two. I think you need a dedicated group of midwives working there. I wouldn't like to see it diluted ...' cos I think it takes a different philosophy on care doesn't it? If you always work on labour ward you see a lot of problems all the time ... start anticipating problems. Whereas here, it's much more normal, healthy ... and we've got this huge range of what's normal from our experience of working here. (Loretta, 2, TM)

Another midwife argued that a caseload model of care that included working in both a birth centre and in a labour ward diluted philosophy and practice:

It does change the whole notion of, if you're using birth centre as a philosophy around natural birth, birth centre/labour ward caseload model is not consistent with truly birth centre, it just acts like it, providing women with a nice environment as opposed to a natural birthing philosophy, that might work out or might not. I hadn't thought about it before but I think there is probably a philosophical difference, a division there. What happens ... is that you're looking after women and going for a natural birth and they need to transfer ... it's like it's out of my sphere of influence now. (Julia, 11)

Rather than seeing this as some sort of rejection of labour ward practice, this midwife identified the problem with such caseload practice as one of philosophical difference.

ORGANISATIONAL ASPECTS

The importance of both cooperative management and institutional support were identified. Many of those interviewed attributed their centre's continued success to a proactive midwifery manager, institutional support and respectful interactions with medical staff. In other centres, it was antagonism towards birth centre philosophy and practice that had produced a galvanising effect on their midwifery teams.

The preparedness of a midwifery manager to try new methods of care provision and to respond to staff initiatives encouraged high staff morale and good retention rates. Staff movements from birth centres were usually not related to dissatisfaction with the work. One midwife interviewed had specifically moved to work in a birth centre that provided small group practice, hoping that it would allow greater continuity with women. She had previously enjoyed working in a small centre that had generally allowed one-to-one care and in the interim had worked in a centre with a large monthly throughput. Another midwife said, however, that she missed the continuity of care for women that she had previously experienced in a centre that provided a small team approach.

A few midwives stated that one of the disadvantages of working autonomously was the missed learning opportunities that exposure to other midwives' practice would provide. They often talked difficult situations through informally, but they perceived a need to formalise this process of reflection in their centre.

Questions regarding the transfer of women from the birth centre to the labour ward and continuity of carers raised interesting and diverse opinions.

TRANSFERS

Although the midwives accepted that transfers are inevitable, most reported having had feelings of guilt when they were required. This had decreased for many over time. Self-doubt seemed particularly pronounced when the woman had transferred for pain relief alone:

I feel much less guilt than I used to…I used to beat myself up…If I'd done this maybe…. (Julia, 11)

That was really hard when I first started 'cos I put it on myself, that I'd done something wrong and the only reason she transferred is because I'd been working that day and if someone else had been looking after her she wouldn't have to. (Jill, 1)

If it's a long labour…then sometimes you feel guilty, like could I have done anything differently? Should I have done something earlier? Should I have suggested something? Sometimes you feel a bit of a failure…. (Loretta, 2, TM)

If the transfer was clinically indicated the midwives found it easier to reconcile:

Depending on what's happening for the woman, the situation…it's just more her options, her choices are being met. (Carla, 3, TM)

Sometimes you feel it's for the right reasons, if it's for thick meconium…an abnormal heart rate, then…that's fine…she needs to have some form of intervention, usually you feel quite relieved that it's there and that she'll get good care…. (Loretta, 2, TM)

Many sometimes felt disappointment:

Sometimes you feel a bit cheated by the world, like you wonder why that particular woman's needed to go…. You kind of think it's unfair (Loretta, 2, TM)

I'm more upset for the woman if she's disappointed. (Jodie, 2)

Midwives also identified more unpalatable feelings: the potential to be judgemental and to have mixed or negative feelings about transfers:

I try to come from the perspective that it's not my labour…obviously the woman's gone through a lot of things to get to that decision, and it's not for me to impose my feelings on it. I feel more disappointed for her if it's something out of her control. (Jill, 1)

Both good and bad: anger, irritation sometimes 'cos you think they could do it and they don't. Frustration! Sometimes you're pleased because you know it's the best thing for them. (Julia, 11)

The impact of additional personnel being involved in the care was seen as inevitable, but sometimes unsettling:

You've gone from a situation where you're in charge, to one where you're answering to someone else, it's difficult. (Julia, 11)

It's difficult moving…having to follow more rigid hospital protocols. There's more doctor input…It's a less conducive environment for labouring. It's more clinical. The staff are not necessarily like-minded. Your views and practice can be undermined. (Beau, 1, TM)

It's not that you want to be rid of the woman, it's that you don't want to be involved in all that politics of labour ward…it's easier to perhaps not be there. (Melissa, 7)

Midwives recognised that their having previously worked in the same labour ward made continuing care for women easier. Knowing the environment and the unit's protocols, and having relationships with the staff was advantageous. Some personnel exhibited criticism or hostility towards birth centre care and clientele. Some had unrealistic expectations of birth centre midwives, such as expecting a midwife to remain in the labour ward despite having other women labouring in the birth centre. For midwives who were not known to the staff in the labour ward, there was a sense of having to provide credentials:

Maybe if I'd come from [this hospital's] labour ward and I'd known all the staff better I might have felt more comfortable…it still was often a relief to come back. (Melissa, 7)

...you worry that people are going to think you should have done something different, 'cos still I trained in a very medical model, so you're still aware that people will think, oh you should have done an ARM or whatever. So you do think that perhaps you may be criticised a bit. (Jodie, 2)

...because I haven't worked up there...I'm still unfamiliar with the people and with things, equipment and supplies, so I still find it hard. (Loretta, 2, TM)

Negotiating a role in the situation where a midwife stayed in the labour ward with a woman also presented dilemmas. While most reported that they remained as the primary carer if required and if it was logistically possible, a number of midwives reported having stayed with a woman in a supportive rather than a midwifery capacity. Some preferred this role:

I do find it hard to work out my space and role in things in labour ward. I have come to realise that my skills are in the low-tech, normal, healthy, in support and talking women through things. I have learned to frame things in terms of the women needing the expertise of the labour ward midwives. And that my lack of quickness and efficiency in assimilating and coordinating the labour ward care makes it better for them to be involved. They seem to accept this candidness in the manner it's intended. (Jasmine, 16)

This midwife found negotiating a role with the midwives was more difficult:

I sometimes think that they're a little suspicious of my motives for staying. I wish they could understand it's for the woman–I have no desire to abandon the woman. I like to stay at least until they...have developed a rapport with the new midwife. I have tried doing things to help where I think I won't slow things down, but this sometimes appears to confuse both the development of rapport and raise issues about who's providing [primary] care. (Jasmine, 16)

'It's almost easier to become [a] support person in that situation and let another midwife take over the care,' added another (Jill, 1).

Other midwives stated that their role varied, depending on the woman's need and on staffing:

I'd be happy enough working with the monitors and the drips, but...[where] there were enough people to do those kind of things and it's not what that woman

need[s] at that time...we have to realise that there is that cut-off point where we serve a purpose or we don't serve a purpose, and you have to be flexible and listen and look. In that situation where if labour ward were short-staffed I certainly would have rolled in and been the midwife. Different things suit at different times. (Ingrid, 1)

Continuity: 'We're there to support, to guide.' (Ingrid, 1)

On the subject of continuity of carer, the midwives raised logistical, emotional and philosophical issues. They agreed that women, particularly those who feel vulnerable about transferring, generally value continuity. However, another common opinion was that a new perspective could positively influence a long or difficult labour:

I think fresh ideas can be good for someone too. And we can value our part too highly in a woman's labour; sometimes just a change of energy can actually help a woman. We like sometimes to feel indispensable, but that's not our role in labour...we are not actually the support people. As long as she has continuity of care, regardless of continuity of carer, she stands a great chance of gaining as much information from the next person that she meets as from me. And far be it for me to deny it to her. (Ingrid, 1)

There were comments precipitated by logistical concerns:

I'd...like that continuity.... The way it's set up, the hospital wouldn't let it happen easily. (Jill, 1)

...it's difficult, having...[as] many different policies as areas, to learn and apply to. (Jodie, 2)

Emotional responses included comments such as these:

To be totally truthful, sometimes it is quite a relief to hand over...you've tried everything that you can think of. (Melissa, 7)

I think there are benefits for the woman. You've got the same caregiver. Providing the woman is happy for that person to go. We're working on the presumption that the woman is happy about it, they're not likely to say, 'Hang on I don't like you, I don't want you to come.' (Julia, 11)

When the discussion turned to on-call arrangements, this midwife commented:

The burnout is the thing that bothers me...anything over that [12 hours with a labouring woman], I'm not convinced that there's any benefit or value for the woman...I don't think people are capable of sustaining it and start to make poor decisions, especially when it's busy.... If you're with someone and they're stressed out and you're trying to help them make decisions, then they're being made in tiredness. (Julia, 11)

Location of birth centres

There was agreement that the ideal geographical location for a birth centre was one which was separate from the labour ward. Being located within the labour ward, as some centres were, was seen as distracting and counter-productive to realising birth centre autonomy and philosophy. Some midwives felt that a location close to the labour ward would not affect the birth centre if the centre was the centre was governed separately:

I don't think any unit with an outpatient component should be above ground level.... I don't think a close proximity to labour ward should make a difference if you've got two separately employed groups of people within two separate areas–then easy access to labour ward shouldn't make a difference.... I think the problem occurs when you've got a birth centre and labour ward running in tandem with a common manager and staff that interchange. (Julia, 11)

For other midwives, who had worked in centres that were very close to the labour ward, there was more concern about remaining a separate entity. One midwife described working in a centre where there was a thoroughfare through the birth centre area:

There can be a woman wandering naked.... You don't have the confidence that no strangers are going to be walking past...where here we have this culture that wouldn't allow it. (Jasmine, 16)

Another midwife recounted her frustration while working in a birth centre (located at the end of a labour ward) which functioned as a corridor to the neonatal intensive care nursery. Medical staff insisted that the corridor remain open despite being able to access the nursery via other routes because '... they should get there as quickly as possible' (Chris, 6).

One midwife pointed out that, for some women, closeness is an issue in relation to ease of transfer should it become necessary, but that

'for others, it's important *not* to blend in–the sense of separateness is really important' (Jill, 1).

She believed that the midwives' lack of uniforms and the centre's different decor helped to create a separate identity.

Another midwife described working in a birth centre located in a wing of the labour ward:

We didn't have our own separate entrance. The women who called sometimes didn't even speak to the birth centre midwives 'cos we weren't in our office and the calls would go through to the delivery suite...we communicated a lot with delivery suite. (Carla, 3, TM)

She said that this situation was tolerable because there were cooperative relationships between the midwives from the two areas.

Midwives who had worked in hospitals with birth centres located in premises outside the main hospital building expressed a variety of feelings about this arrangement. In an institution with restrictive exclusion criteria and many external constraints, midwives considered the distance important in creating a boundary that was not crossed by medical staff. These midwives had to organise a transfer to labour ward for any medical involvement.

Another midwife, working in an institution with a similar geographical arrangement and forthcoming medical support in an emergency described how she felt:

We [used to be] in our own little hut, isolated from everything. And you knew if anyone had to come and help you they actually had to run up the hill. That worried you 'cos it took too long. Whereas [here] is good...it's only going to be a couple of minutes for help and your privacy doesn't get invaded.... So, once again, it depends on the midwife and her experience and perspective, and what you feel comfortable with. (Jasmine, 16)

In centres where midwives worked alone the relationship of the birth centre to the labour ward did impact on midwives' feelings, often depending on the rapidity of response in an emergency. Many midwives recounted initial fearfulness about taking a job in a birth centre where midwives regularly worked alone:

It was head stuff... you're on your own, but... the emergency buzzer's right there. You're not on your own. You're really not. It's just a matter of getting help and here it's just a matter of getting up to delivery ward or you can get help if you want it. (Carla, 3, TM)

CONCLUSION

Australian birth centres provide an alternative philosophy and practice for maternity care providers who are increasingly caught between physiological/social and pathological/medical models of pregnancy and birth. Philosophy and practice that normalise birth and which show high levels of safety and satisfaction are essential if targets to reduce interventions, particularly caesarean sections, are to be achieved. In Australia, drawing on the experience of birth centre midwives may help maternity carers to accomplish these reductions.

This chapter explored four interrelated themes that are related to birth centre midwifery: social and emotional care, communication and language, clinical practice and skills, and organisational issues. Further investigation into these themes may suggest strategies to improve midwifery care in this field, may also be transferable to other areas and disciplines, and could be valuable in educating the midwives of the future.

The midwives who generously shared their time and ideas in the development of this chapter outlined logistical concerns and challenges that impact on birth centre midwifery in Australia. They articulated an emotional and intelligent engagement with their work and with the women who access their centres. To work effectively in a birth centre a midwife must possess a broad but fine-tuned and balanced range of skills that cover the myriad experiences that surround pregnancy and birth. They should be flexible in their dealings with women and available emotionally for them as they face the demanding issues that can arise during parturition.

The midwives felt privileged to work in an environment that allowed them to incorporate their emotional knowledge with practical skills while working as partners in women's childbearing. They valued working with other midwives who they considered shared a philosophy of care. Those who experienced it appreciated institutional and medical support.

The high level of clinical expertise in the birth centres was attributed to the substantial degree of autonomy and responsibility the midwives held, and regularly witnessing women with healthy pregnancies and labours. The midwives had developed skills in dealing with the physical, social and emotional factors that impact on physiological birth. Being able to judge when healthy parameters are being breached was one of the skills that midwives confidently reported that they had learned and something they continued to remain vigilant about.

Birth centre experience promotes trust: trust in the process of pregnancy and birth, in women's abilities to self-determine, and in their own abilities as midwives. In cataloguing their own expertise those interviewed recognised the expertise of their colleagues in other areas of midwifery. The midwives valued skills that they had acquired in other areas whilst noting that many had been either shed or reconstructed during their time in birth centres. The argument that birth centre midwifery should be considered a unique, specialty field within midwifery was a convincing one.

ABBREVIATIONS USED IN THIS CHAPTER

APH: antepartum haemorrhage
ARM: artificial rupture of the membranes
CTG: cardiotocograph
PPH: postpartum haemorrhage
VE: vaginal examination

REFERENCES

Anspach R R 1994 The language of case presentation. In: Conrad P, Kern R (eds) The sociology of health and illness: critical perspectives, 4th edn. St Martin's Press, New York, p 312–332

Coyle K et al 2001a Ongoing relationships with a personal focus: mothers' perceptions of birth centre versus hospital care. Midwifery 17(3): 171–181

Coyle K et al 2001b Normality and collaboration: mothers' perception of birth centre versus hospital care. Midwifery 17(3): 182–191

Health Department New South Wales 1989 Maternity services in New South Wales: ministerial taskforce on obstetric services in New South Wales. Health Department New South Wales, Sydney

Health Department Victoria 1990 Having a baby in Victoria: final report of the ministerial review of birthing services in Victoria. Health Department Victoria, Melbourne

Health Department Western Australia 1990 Report of the ministerial taskforce to review obstetric, neonatal and gynaecological services in Western Australia. Volume 1: summary and recommendations. Health Department, Perth

Pairman S 1998 Women-centred midwifery: partnerships or professional friendships? New Zealand College of Midwives Journal (19): 5–10

Ryan M 1997 Birth centre-labour ward: do outcomes differ? (masters treatise) Department of Public Health, University of Sydney, Sydney (unpublished)

Senate Community Affairs References Committee 1999 Rocking the cradle: a report into childbirth procedures. Commonwealth of Australia, Canberra

Waldenström U 1998 Continuity of carer and satisfaction. Midwifery 14 (4): 207–213

21

Developing a midwife-led maternity service: the New Zealand experience

Sally Pairman
Karen Guilliland

INTRODUCTION

Over the last 15 to 20 years the New Zealand maternity service has been reshaped by successive changes in health policy and direction. The maternity service strategy throughout the last 10 years has led to the development and consolidation of a women-centred service in which the emphasis is on choices, access and meeting the individual needs of women and their families through the childbirth experience. The focus of the maternity service has shifted from maternity facilities and the needs of institutions and practitioners to childbearing women and their maternity care needs. This reshaped maternity service entitles every woman to have her own 'lead maternity caregiver' (LMC) and to choose her place of birth. The LMC provides continuity of care throughout the woman's childbirth experience, from early pregnancy through to 4–6 weeks after the birth of the baby. The LMC coordinates the woman's maternity care, in most cases providing all of the care, and accesses and integrates with other services if necessary. The LMC can be a midwife, a general practitioner or an obstetrician.

New Zealand midwifery, under the leadership of the New Zealand College of Midwives (NZCOM), has concentrated on developing a midwifery workforce that can take on this LMC role. The LMC role is ideally suited to midwifery, reflecting as it does the full scope of practice of a midwife, as defined by the World Health Organisation and the International

Confederation of Midwives (NZCOM 2002). Midwives have become the cornerstone of the maternity service in New Zealand. Today over 70% of childbearing women choose a midwife as their LMC and midwifery is a strong and autonomous profession.

The way that maternity services are organised and funded in New Zealand has meant that women and midwives have been able to achieve a level of autonomy in maternity care which in many countries is only possible in non-medicalised settings such as birth centres and at home.

However, strong midwives, a midwifery-led maternity service, partnership with women and professional autonomy are not enough, on their own, to challenge society's construction of childbirth and the continued dominance of the medical model of birth. The socio-political context of childbirth has an enormous impact on how midwives practice, what women understand about birth, how the maternity service develops and what it can achieve. In New Zealand both the midwifery profession and the government have underestimated the power of institutional medicalisation and the impact of the global anxiety around childbirth that is promulgated by the world's media (Health Funding Authority 2000).

NZCOM expected that a strong and autonomous midwifery workforce would be more likely to promote birth as a normal life event within the family context, regardless of the chosen place of birth. The government's vision for maternity states that 'pregnancy and childbirth are a normal life-stage for most women, with appropriate additional care available to those women who require it' (Ministry of Health 2002, p.11). Despite having this midwifery-led service, however, New Zealand's obstetric intervention rates, although showing a slower rise than elsewhere, are now similar to those of most western countries (Ministry of Health 2001).

There are, however, some hopeful signs: midwife LMCs do achieve better obstetric outcomes than the national rates (Midwifery and Maternity Provider Organisation, 'Midwifery outcome data', unpublished report, 2002) and the midwifery-led service has been extremely successful when

measured by broader public health and societal changes. For example, breastfeeding rates are high, immunisation rates at 6 weeks are high, informed choice and consent is predominant, consumer satisfaction is high, services are accessible and equitable for most women, Maori women and their babies have significantly improved their childbirth outcomes, the home birth rate has risen from 0.1% in 1989 to 6% in 1999, and costs per birth have been contained within a set budget (Health Funding Authority 1999a, 1999b, 2000, Ministry of Health 2001, National Health Committee 1999, Tracy et al 2002). However, the maternity service overall still reflects the global phenomena of medicalisation and unnecessary obstetric intervention and it will take more than midwifery autonomy to turn this around.

From this strong foundation of midwifery autonomy and midwifery-led maternity services, NZCOM is now turning its attention to developing strategies to decrease unnecessary obstetric intervention and the impact of global medicalisation on midwives and on midwifery care. Of prime importance is the recognition that the place of birth has a strong influence on the outcome of midwifery care. Homes, primary birthing units and birth centres provide contexts in which women and midwives can experience childbirth with less obstetric influence and where physiological birth is more readily achievable. In order to decrease the obstetric intervention rate in childbirth, midwives and women have to regain their trust in birth as a normal and healthy life event. Midwives need to be supported to promote home birth and the use of primary birthing units and to encourage women to choose these options with confidence. It is timely to consider the place of birth centres, particularly in urban areas, as part of these overall strategies.

Through its focus on structural changes to the maternity service aimed at enabling women-centred care, New Zealand has developed a social model for maternity care that is based on midwifery, placing midwives as the key providers in the maternity service. However, New Zealand society's expectations of the maternity service are still dominated by the medical model of childbirth and the challenges presented by a midwifery-led maternity system have done little to break this down. New strategies for challenging the dominance of the medical model of childbirth include focusing on the place of birth and redefinition of care in childbirth as a primary health service provided in the community. This chapter traces the development of the midwife-led maternity service in New Zealand, highlighting both the opportunities and threats faced by midwifery and the strategies used to deal with these.

ABOUT NEW ZEALAND

New Zealand is made up of two main islands situated in the South Pacific, somewhat closer to Antarctica than to the Equator. It has a population of 3.8 million people, over 70% of whom live in the top half of the North Island. The annual birth rate varies between 56 000 and 57 000. New Zealand's economy is based on agriculture and consequently there is a large number of rural communities. Some of these communities are small, relatively isolated and inaccessible, due to mountainous terrain and unpredictable climate changes.

New Zealand's indigenous people are Maori and they came to New Zealand around a thousand years ago. Their communities were small and based on a tribal (iwi) system and developed enduring cultural connections to the land. British settlers colonised New Zealand in the early 1800s, initially clearing land and establishing farms. Historically, New Zealand's roots, for both Maori and Pakeha (non-Maori) peoples are agricultural.

This concern for the land, its development and its ownership, was addressed in the Treaty of Waitangi, which was signed in 1840 between Maori and the Crown. This Treaty established the constitutional framework within which both Maori and Pakeha would live and assured the rightful place of each in New Zealand. The principles inherent in the Treaty that govern the relationship between Maori and the Crown are partnership, participation, protection and equity. The partnership is understood to be mutually defined and negotiated on an equal basis, with full participation of both partners and ensuring the protection of each (Ramsden 1990). Despite ongoing disputes between Maori and the Crown in relation to land rights and access to resources under the Treaty, the concept of partnership is now culturally embedded in New Zealand society (Guilliland & Pairman 1995). 'Partnership' is a word often used to describe a variety of social, economic and cultural relationships and is part of everyday language in New Zealand. The development of the maternity services and of the midwifery profession have reflected this social and cultural context of varied geography, extensive population spread and broad cultural mix.

THE DEVELOPMENT OF MIDWIFERY

INDEPENDENT PRACTICE

New Zealand has had a regulated midwifery workforce since 1904 but over the last century the scope of practice of midwives has changed significantly as a result of increasing hospitalisation and medicalisation of childbirth. From working as autonomous practitioners in the early 1900s, midwives gradually became 'assistants' to doctors. From working in the community, midwives began to work mostly in hospitals and within specific areas such as antenatal clinics, the labour ward or postnatal wards, as pregnancy and childbirth became fragmented and 'specialised' (Donley 1986). Through this process many midwives lost their understanding of childbirth as a normal life event and of themselves as 'guardians' of the normal birth process. Instead, they experienced highly interventionist and medicalised maternity care, directed by the doctor and the hospital. Legislative changes over the years also decreased the scope of midwifery autonomy and midwives were required to work under the supervision of a doctor. Thus it was that when midwifery autonomy and the full scope of midwifery practice were finally regained in 1990 (through changes in legislation) it was necessary to re-educate the midwifery workforce to believe in and to be able to provide a service for normal birth.

In New Zealand it was primarily women who rebelled against the hospital-directed model of childbirth and demanded the return of the 'traditional' midwife–one who would be alongside them throughout the whole experience, from early pregnancy through to 6 weeks after the birth of the baby. They wanted midwives who would believe in their abilities to give birth without medical intervention and who would support them in reclaiming childbirth as a normal life event. New Zealand women wanted to take back control of their birthing experiences and to take their rightful place at the centre of events rather than be passive bystanders at their own birthing experiences. In the 1980s midwives joined with women in their fight to reinstate the autonomy of midwifery and together they carried out a very successful political campaign that culminated in legislation in 1990 that secured the professional autonomy of midwives.

The model of midwifery that has developed in the decade since that legislation was passed is one of independent practice and partnership between the midwife and the woman. Contrary to practice in countries such as the United Kingdom and Australia, independent midwifery in New Zealand is not related to income, employment or place of practice, but to *how* a midwife practises. 'Independence' is intended to mean autonomous midwifery practice in which the midwife carries her own caseload of clients with responsibility for all their care from early pregnancy through to 4–6 weeks after the birth. When problems arise midwives consult with obstetricians, who provide any necessary obstetric care. Just under half of all New Zealand midwives now choose to work in this way, as independent practitioners (New Zealand Health Information Services 2001). The midwife is not independent of the public health system (as in the UK where an independent midwife charges the woman a fee privately for care), rather the midwife is independent in her practice and is able to make autonomous and professional midwifery decisions. Neither is independence about employment status. In New Zealand independent midwives may be self-employed (paid directly by government) or employed (paid by a hospital) and may care for women in any setting, including home, small (primary) maternity units and secondary and tertiary hospitals. The defining characteristic of all these midwives that makes them 'independent' is that they independently manage their own caseload of clients throughout the entire childbirth experience.

Although the midwife is professionally independent, she does not work in isolation. Generally midwives work in partnership with other midwives and in collaboration with any other health professionals the woman requires, such as doctors or social workers. Most importantly, the midwife is never independent of the woman and in fact works in a unique partnership model with women. We will discuss this partnership relationship shortly. At any one time, an independent midwife (employed or self-employed) may have clients expecting to birth at home, in a small unit or in a base maternity hospital and midwives move in and out of these settings as their clients' needs dictate. All maternity care, except private obstetric care, is free to women.

Over the last ten years the maternity services have changed dramatically as a result of midwifery autonomy and the reshaping of the structures of the maternity service that arose in response to this new group of maternity care providers. The reshaped maternity service is ideally suited to the role and scope of practice of midwives, as they are able to provide all aspects of the maternity service specifications. General practitioner and obstetrician LMCs, on the other hand, do not traditionally provide labour care or postnatal care and they are required to make documented arrangements with a midwife for the provision of this care. Midwives have embraced the opportunity to work within the full scope of midwifery practice with enthusiasm. Nearly 50% of the midwifery workforce now works independently. The majority of these midwives are now community-based and self-employed in that they claim directly from a centralised funding mechanism. The rest are employed in hospitals but practice independently as LMCs in the independent midwifery services that have been set up in most base maternity hospitals throughout New Zealand.

This development of employed midwife LMCs was driven by three separate factors. Firstly, hospital midwives demanded that they should be able to work within the full scope of midwifery practice. Secondly, the provision of this type of midwifery care gave the hospitals access to another funding source–as well as their funding for secondary maternity services, the provision of an independent midwifery service meant that hospitals could also claim from the primary maternity budget on behalf of their employed LMC midwives. Thirdly, hospitals were required to rethink how midwives worked within their institutions when many of their experienced midwives left to establish themselves as self-employed practitioners in the community. Some hospital managers understood that in order to recruit and retain the staff with the mix of skills required to run a hospital maternity service they had to give their employed midwives the opportunity to practice midwifery in the full sense of the word. It also required them to increase salaries and wages if they were to compete with the self-employed midwives' income potential.

The majority of women today receive care from a midwife throughout pregnancy, birth and the postnatal period; previously, continuity of care was only available in a limited way for those few women who chose to have a home birth (Health Funding Authority 2000). Now, instead of doctor-led care being the only option, some 70% of women choose midwifery-only care (Health Funding Authority 2000). Instead of medically controlled maternity services, women expect, and are legally entitled to, information and the right to make informed decisions about their choice of carer, their style of care and their place of birth. Instead of hospital services based around the needs of the institution and the health professionals, there is an expectation of maternity services based on the needs of women and their families. This means choice and control for women and their families; access to services for families; recognition and support for the primary midwife–woman relationship from the institution; antenatal and postnatal visiting in the woman's home; and short stays in hospital with postnatal follow-up in the community. Increasingly, New Zealand society is regaining its recognition of the midwife as the primary practitioner in normal childbirth.

This development of professional autonomy and the full scope of midwifery practice has required significant support for midwives from the wider midwifery profession. The New Zealand College of Midwives has set standards for practice, a code of ethics and guidelines for practice (NZCOM 2002). NZCOM has offered ongoing education to midwives and has worked closely with the midwifery educational institutions to ensure that a range of appropriate programmes is available, from pre-registration courses through to Masters of Midwifery. A Midwifery Standards Review Process has also been developed by the College.

Midwifery Standards Review

Midwifery Standards Review evolved from a process originally developed by home birth midwives in 1987. It is a confidential, intensive, reflective process that aims to educate and support the midwife to develop her practice in a positive way. It enables LMC midwives to review their practice each year with a panel of two midwifery peers and two consumers. The midwife provides an analysis of her year's work, her statistical outcomes and her self-evaluation against the NZCOM Standards for Practice and the feedback from the consumer questionnaires completed by her clients. The panel provides feedback and support for the midwife. It helps her to draw up a professional development plan for her next year of practice. A unique aspect of this review is the equal participation by consumers in the review process and the mechanisms that have been put in place for consumer feedback from the midwife's clients.

The NZCOM Midwifery Standards Review Process is a central strategy in the professional development of LMC midwives. The College is currently developing a Midwifery Standards Review Process for core midwives who do not have a caseload of clients. The intention is to support all midwives as they develop confidence in their clinical judgement and to emphasise midwifery's specific body of knowledge, so enabling them to feel more secure in their independent midwifery role.

The NZCOM Midwifery Standards Review Process is recognised in the Nursing Council of New Zealand competency-based practising certificate requirements (Nursing Council of New Zealand, 1999). The Nursing Council is currently the regulatory body for midwives although new legislation due to be enacted in 2002 will create a Midwifery Council and finally bring midwifery regulation under the auspices of the midwifery profession itself. The Nursing Council, in partnership with NZCOM, has established a competency-based practising certificate regime that requires all midwives to demonstrate that they continue to meet all the competencies required of an LMC midwife on registration. Midwives can demonstrate these competencies through a portfolio mechanism that is similar to that required for midwives in the United Kingdom. Alternatively, midwives can also meet the competency requirements by undertaking the Midwifery Standards Review Process. Both processes require midwives to demonstrate that they meet the standards of the midwifery profession and that they can provide independent midwifery care, in partnership with women, throughout the whole scope of midwifery practice.

MIDWIFERY PARTNERSHIP

The midwifery model that underpins the New Zealand maternity services today is one of partnership between the midwife and the woman. This conceptual framework mirrors the intentions articulated in the Treaty of Waitangi in that the relationship between the woman and the midwife is seen as an equal one, and one to which both partners make equally valuable, but different contributions. Partnership, and in particular the notion of equality in partnership, is a deceptively simple concept. However, like all human relationships, partnership requires a complex set of conditions to be successful. Cultural, economic and social differences between 'partners' can interfere with their ability to understand each other's perspective. These differences need to be acknowledged and worked through to an agreed position. Communication and negotiation are skills and processes fundamental to partnership.

The midwife brings her professional knowledge, skills and experience of pregnancy and childbirth to the partnership relationship. The woman brings her knowledge of herself and her family, together with her needs and wishes for her pregnancy and birth. Over the period of the pregnancy the woman and the midwife get to know each other and to trust each other. They talk about their expectations of each other, they talk about how the pregnancy is progressing, they talk about options for care and the decisions the woman will need to make. The midwife offers information, a specialised midwifery knowledge base, and support for the woman in making informed decisions about her care. The woman remains in control of her birthing experience, making decisions about how she wants it to be. The midwife stands alongside the woman in a supportive role. She guides the woman and supports her decisions but does not take control. The power balance between them is negotiated and equitable. They share responsibility for what happens and for the decisions they make. This increases the self-determination of both and reinforces the midwife's understanding of her role in the partnership. The relationship is therefore reciprocal.

It is these concepts of reciprocity and equality that have been the most difficult for midwives and women to understand and to implement. Society is still dominated by the view that the health professional is always the expert, that the patient (or woman) is the passive recipient of this expertise and that therefore the relationship between them is always unequal. At the other extreme, the constitutional right of women to informed choice and shared decision-making has at times been used as a reason for health professionals to abdicate responsibility for making professional judgements. For example, the right to choose has, in some cases, led to women choosing to have unnecessary obstetric intervention (e.g. induction or elective caesarean section) in the absence of any clinical indication.

In the midwifery partnership model both the woman and the midwife retain responsibility for their individual decisions and the midwife, as a health professional, is expected to apply her professional knowledge base. For both the woman and the midwife the concept of partnership is premised on their autonomy, their ability and their right to make decisions together and their ability and their right to take responsibility for those decisions. Partnership involves a shift of power from the health professional to the woman in the same way that the midwife's allegiance moves from the hospital or doctor to the woman as she supports her and stands alongside her through the process of pregnancy and childbirth. For the partnership to be successful midwives need to have a real knowledge of their support role. Midwives and women have had to learn about this partnership relationship through experience and reflection on these experiences. Midwives and others have begun to write about partnership and to share this developing understanding and knowledge with the midwifery profession (Guilliland & Pairman 1995, Daellenbach 1999, Pairman 1998, 1999, Skinner 1999).

Midwifery education programmes in New Zealand have paid considerable attention to ensuring that midwives understand partnership. Midwives have a responsibility to ensure that professional autonomy does not mean merely the assumption of the power previously wielded by institutions and medicine over women. Equally, emphasis has been placed on midwives' understanding of informed decision-making–that it does not mean that they can opt out of their professional obligations and their responsibility to utilise their midwifery knowledge in practice (Pairman 1998, Tully et al 1998).

Midwifery curricula teach that the aim of the midwife is to support each woman in reaching her full potential and in experiencing a positive, safe and fulfilling childbirth. The underlying philosophy of this midwifery education is that if women have control over their birthing experience they will have more confidence in themselves as mothers and that this, in turn, will have a positive effect on children, on families and on society at large (Otago Polytechnic 1999).

This midwife–woman partnership is now the basis for midwifery services in New Zealand. For New Zealand midwives, partnership with women defines their professional status. Significantly, this partnership model extends beyond the individual midwife–woman relationship, and partnership is embedded culturally, both within the agencies of government and the overall structures of the health service. This meant that when the maternity service was restructured in the mid 1990s there was an understanding at both government and health-provider levels that the service would need to be based around women and their families, and recognition of their right to be involved in their own maternity service.

FUNDING FRAMEWORK FOR MATERNITY SERVICES

The maternity service in New Zealand consists not only of the care provided to women and babies but also the locations in which that care takes place. The unique funding mechanism for the maternity service has directly influenced service development in relation to practitioners and to place of birth.

Since 1938 New Zealand has had a state-funded social security health system that includes a fully funded maternity service that is free to women. This funding is centralised and, initially, a set of fees was established on the Maternity Benefit Schedule for each consultation with a general practitioner or obstetrician. (Private obstetricians were the only practitioners able to make charges on top of these set fees).

The Nurses Amendment Act 1990 reinstated the midwife as an autonomous practitioner who no longer required the supervision of a doctor. It enabled midwives to claim fees from the Maternity Benefit Schedule on the same fee-for-service basis as doctors and at the same rate. It also brought a new element of choice and competition to maternity service provision in that women could now choose between a midwife, a general practitioner or an obstetrician for their maternity care.

The neo-liberal economic influence on government policy in the 1990s was the impetus for extensive health reforms carried out through those years (Gauld 2001). With the underlying emphasis on competition, profit making and contracting for services, the health reforms presented midwifery and the wider maternity service with both opportunities and problems. The Government used the new context of competition between midwives and doctors that resulted from Nurses Amendment Act 1990 to initiate reforms to the Maternity Benefit Schedule. Midwives were new players, providing a different maternity service from that provided by doctors, and could be used as a lever to change the overall funding mechanisms. While supportive of choices for women, the Government's primary aim was economic in that it wanted to move from fee-for-service payments on demand, to a capped budget for a specified set of services. It also understood, however, that if any change was to be successful in the prevailing social context, it would need to reorganise the maternity services around a woman-centred base.

The New Zealand College of Midwives, with its consumer partners, recognised that the way in which maternity services were funded was the key to realising the opportunities that the Nurses Amendment Act 1990 gave for autonomous practice. While this legislation had given midwives equity of pay with doctors and had enabled them to claim from the Maternity Benefit Schedule, it was just the first step. Initially, only a few midwives left hospital employment and many of these were obliged to provide 'shared care' with doctors, as general practitioners were still perceived as the gatekeepers to the maternity services. Most midwives remained employed by hospitals, where their main role in primary care was providing labour and postnatal midwifery services for clients of general practitioners–much as the role of the hospital midwife had always been. The reshaping of the maternity services funding mechanism provided an unprecedented opportunity not only to develop and reclaim the midwife's role in the provision of primary maternity services but also to reinstate pregnancy and childbirth as a community-based life event. Equally, without strong midwifery representation from NZCOM and consumer lobbying, the role of the midwife could have been subsumed into medical and hospital contracts and the opportunity for radical change lost forever.

The College spent 3 years, from 1993 to 1996, in negotiations with combined regional health authorities and the New Zealand Medical Association (NZMA) that resulted in the drawing up of a national framework for the provision of maternity services. Primary maternity service funding and service specifications were set out under Section 51 of the Health and Disability Services Act 1993 (commonly referred to as 'Section 51'). Section 88 of the Public Health and Hospitals Services Act 2001 later replaced this. There was also a national framework for the funding of secondary and tertiary (complicated) maternity services, allocated on a population base, and a separate national framework for the funding of the maternity facilities in which birth takes place. This is available for primary facilities (birthing units), secondary facilities (maternity hospitals) and tertiary facilities (maternity hospitals with high-technology facilities). Home birth is funded through the primary maternity services funding framework.

PRIMARY MATERNITY SERVICE FUNDING

Section 51 of the Health and Disability Services Act (and later, Section 88 of the Public Health and Hospitals Services Act 2001) set out the mechanisms for funding primary health services such as the general medical services provided by general practitioners and primary maternity services provided by midwives, general practitioners and private obstetricians. In New Zealand 'primary health' refers to the first level of contact within the health system. It is universally accessible and involves community participation. It covers a broad range of services, including health improvement and preventive services; first-level generalist services such as general practice and pharmacy; and first-level services in more specialised areas such as maternity, family planning, dentistry and sexual health (King 2001).

The placement of the maternity services within a primary health framework has led to the recognition that pregnancy and childbirth are parts of one life event and continuity of care is the cornerstone of the new system. Moving on from a maternity service that was fragmented, with antenatal care in general practice clinics and birth and postnatal care in hospital, with a variety of carers, the new structure integrates all aspects of the maternity system in order to meet each woman's individual needs. This integration of service provision between primary and secondary care has required that the historical boundaries of service funding be revisited as the distinctions between primary and secondary services have become increasingly blurred. The new model of women-centred continuity of care requires that practitioners cross the traditional boundaries between the community and hospitals as they seek to ensure that the woman has access to all aspects of the primary and secondary maternity services that she requires.

Under Section 51 (and now Section 88) primary maternity funding is attached to four modules of care with the expectation that all four modules will be provided by the same carer. Fee-for-service payments remain for care provided in the first trimester and for consultations with obstetricians and other specialists. Modular payments are made for the second trimester, the third trimester, labour and birth and for the postnatal period (up to 4–6 weeks). The woman must choose a lead maternity carer and this person is then responsible for providing and/or coordinating all necessary care throughout the whole experience. The LMC is the constant in the system, as the provision of continuity of care requires the LMC to move with the woman, facilitating her access to any additional services that may be required.

Midwife LMCs work in the community, visiting women in their homes or in clinics during the antenatal period. During labour and birth the LMC attends the woman in the place of her choice–home, primary birthing facility or larger hospital–and provides her labour and birth care. In the postnatal period the LMC midwife provides care through to 4 to 6 weeks, either totally in the woman's home or initially with hospital visits if the woman has chosen a hospital birth and postnatal stay in hospital. At any stage the LMC midwife may consult with an obstetrician if required and the obstetrician may provide intervention if necessary. The woman may therefore need to access secondary maternity services on an episodic basis, although the LMC remains involved with the woman's care and responsibility for the woman's care is transferred back to the LMC when the need for secondary services is over.

This integrated service has meant that midwife LMCs provide care to a whole range of women with varying risk factors–they do not only provide care to low-risk women. Instead, they are available to all women, recognising that some women will require additional involvement from a specialist. This woman-centred and continuity model has required all maternity providers to re-examine their relationships and their traditional boundaries. New ways of working have had to develop. The funders of maternity services and the managers of maternity facilities have also had to work through the implications of this new model and the traditional boundaries between primary and secondary services have had to be challenged.

Primary maternity facility funding

New Zealand's primary maternity facilities accommodate approximately 10% of the total annual births (Ministry of Health 2001). A primary maternity facility is defined as one that provides 'inpatient services during labour and birth and the immediate postpartum period until discharge home. They may also be referred to as level 0 or level 1 facilities.' (Health Funding Authority 1999b). The primary facilities have no access to on-site medical and obstetric specialists. Historically, these facilities were known as 'general practitioner units' or 'cottage hospitals'. In line with overseas trends there has been an exodus of general practitioners from obstetric services and these facilities have now become midwife units (Guilliland 1998). In some rural and provincial areas general practitioners still provide a back-up service for medical emergencies, but in most rural areas midwives provide the only maternity service available to women. Only six primary facilities are actually called 'birthing units' and these do not provide inpatient postnatal care, being opened up by the midwife when a woman arrives for labour and birth and closed again once the woman transfers back home (Health Funding Authority 1999b).

Primary maternity facilities in New Zealand resemble what are known in other countries as 'stand-alone birth centres'. However, there are no specific booking criteria and practitioners make decisions with women on an individual basis on their suitability for birthing in these facilities, in accordance with generic guidelines for referral to specialist services (Ministry of Health 2002).

There are 52 primary maternity facilities in New Zealand, some of which are stand-alone and some of which are attached to community hospitals. There are no birthing centres attached to secondary or tertiary hospitals in New Zealand. For the most part, primary maternity facilities are located in provincial and rural areas as most major centres lost their primary maternity facilities in the drive for centralisation of obstetric services to the main teaching hospitals that occurred in the 1970s and 1980s (Donley 1986). Only two of our major cities have primary maternity facilities that survived: Auckland City has three units and Christchurch has retained five, in part due to a strong consumer lobby lasting over many decades. The survival of primary maternity facilities in provincial and rural

New Zealand, particularly in the South Island, is mainly due to geographical factors and the difficulty in ensuring access to main centre hospitals.

In the mid-1990s the competitive funding and contractual culture created an opportunity to establish new primary maternity facilities. For a short time, funding for health services became contestable and available outside the traditional hospital-controlled contracts. A few innovative midwives took up this opportunity. Midwife-run birthing facilities were established in the cities of Hamilton (Riveridge) and Christchurch (Avonlea) and in rural Alexandra (the Charlotte Jean Birthing Unit). These midwives were able to access maternity facility funding for their buildings through the national primary facility contract and their LMC midwifery services were funded through Sections 51 and 88. As will be discussed later, the funding of these midwife-led facilities is now under threat unless alternative sources of funding can be found.

Despite geographical difficulties and the distance of the primary facilities from specialist services (commonly 1 to 2 hours away), there is no evidence that maternity care in primary maternity units is detrimental to the outcomes for women and babies (Ministry of Health 2001). The average normal birth rate in primary facilities is 92%, with the majority achieving over 96% (Ministry of Health 2001). The antenatal assessment and referral system is well developed and facilitated by a set of specialist referral guidelines negotiated in conjunction with the Section 51 structures of 1996 and again in 1999 (Ministry of Health 2002). New Zealand's neonatal and maternal outcomes are in line with most western countries, which suggests that LMC referral patterns from the relatively isolated primary facilities to the secondary services are both appropriate and timely (Ministry of Health 1999, 2001). For example, it is known that in-utero transfer rates of over 90% are associated with improved neonatal outcomes for preterm labour before 32 weeks gestation–LMCs using New Zealand's primary facilities achieve a 97% in-utero transfer rate for this group (Ministry of Health 2001). Overall, New Zealand's preterm labour rates have decreased since 1990, as have admissions to neonatal units (Ministry of Health 1999).

Despite the accessibility and safety of primary maternity facilities, the number of women choosing to birth in many of these units is decreasing. Part of this decrease may be explained by a 6% rise in home birth rates, but there are probably a number of interrelated reasons. These include declining birth rates overall and a population drift from rural to urban centres. This is compounded by the exit of general practitioners from obstetric services and denial of access to facilities for some midwife LMCs by hospital managers who still believe that there must be a doctor present at every birth. LMC midwives may also be faced with inconsistent obstetric opinions when they ask for a second opinion or consultation from obstetricians, many of whom view birth in primary facilities as unsafe and recommend that the woman birth in a secondary facility.

General practitioners, obstetricians, midwives and the women themselves are all influenced by an increasing climate of fear of birth in society. The medical profession is increasingly citing medico-legal risk as a reason for denying women the choice of non-interventionist birth in a place of their choosing (Cunningham and Dovey 2000). This reasoning lacks support from any New Zealand case law as New Zealand is in the enviable position of having accident compensation insurance for all members of the public. In return for this insurance New Zealanders do not have the right to sue their health practitioner (New Zealand Government 1998). Finally, midwives themselves, for reasons similar to those of the doctors, often bypass primary facilities and take their clients to secondary facilities to birth.

From a midwifery perspective this decline in the use of primary maternity facilities is disappointing, given that these units enhance opportunities for independent decision-making, continuity of care and normal birthing. Because primary facilities rely completely on midwives to provide the service, it is imperative that the midwifery profession encourage midwives and

their clients to support these units if they are to survive. In rural areas primary maternity facilities can fulfil several functions in the community. They are part of the traditional health services and many communities have incorporated other services within the facility such as care of the elderly and child health services.

Proponents of home birth argue that primary facilities offer no more guarantees of safety than birth at home. This is true. However, they may provide 'psychological' security for some women. In urban areas in particular, primary maternity facilities can provide an extremely important 'half-way position' for women and midwives who have experienced generations of highly medicalised maternity services. The move from secondary facilities to home birth is too great for most women and for most midwives used to a medicalised service. It is for these reasons that the New Zealand College of Midwives has begun to investigate the possibility of developing stand-alone birth centres in urban areas where there are no primary facilities. It is also working on strategies to increase the usage of the primary care facilities already in existence (NZCOM, Quality plan 2001–2003, unpublished, 2001).

Home birth

For LMC midwives who are grounded in normal birth philosophy, home is the ideal place for women to give birth. The new maternity structure under Section 51 (Section 88) has provided very favourable conditions for women to give birth at home. Home birth is now a mainstream option, offered and funded alongside all other birth options. Funding has been designated, in recognition of the savings made to facility funding by home birth. LMCs are required to provide a specified maternity service but this requirement is not linked to place of birth. Midwife LMCs can therefore provide care to women in all settings and many have begun to offer home birth services. Since women have been able to choose this option the home birth rate has risen to approximately 6% of the annual birth rate, a figure not too dissimilar to the 10% achieved by primary birth facilities (Health Funding Authority 1999b, Ministry of

Health 2001). For some rural midwives the choice of home birth by women may pose a dilemma as it may threaten the viability of the primary facility–these facilities are mostly funded on a per capita basis. In some areas where primary birthing facilities have closed, such as the central North Island, it is interesting to note that home birth rates are as high as 12% (Midland Region Health Funding Authority 1998). This may reflect the presence of a high Maori population in this area as Maori women generally are more likely to experience normal birth and tend to view birth at home more favourably than Pakeha women (Ministry of Health 2001).

Birth at home and birth in primary maternity facilities are two strategies that are easily available to midwives in their bid to reduce the escalating obstetric intervention rates that are typical of the secondary facilities.

SECONDARY SERVICE AND FACILITY FUNDING

Section 51 primarily funds the LMC continuity service for all women. It also funds private specialist consultations. There is separate funding for hospital-based secondary services, including hospital specialist consultations. This is intended to ensure that there is no financial disincentive for LMCs to delay consultation or referral to obstetric services if necessary. Secondary maternity services provide 'additional care during antenatal, labour and birth and postnatal periods for mothers and babies who experience complications and have a clinical need for referral to the secondary maternity service' (Health Funding Authority 1999b). Secondary maternity hospitals are also referred to as 'level 2 hospitals' and they provide access to obstetricians, anaesthetists, paediatricians and other medical specialists employed by the hospital and a core midwifery service. The core midwife has become important in the development of the partnership model of midwifery practice as she facilitates communication between the primary and the secondary services for both the woman and the midwife LMC.

With the implementation of the LMC model, the majority of women who choose to birth in

hospital arrive with their own midwife who provides their labour and birth care and who is on call 24 hours a day for their postnatal care. This has led to a change in the way that hospitals staff their maternity units and redefinition of the role of those midwives who choose to be employed in the various areas of the maternity hospital on a rostered basis. The rostered midwife staff numbers have decreased significantly, particularly in labour wards. The main role of these core midwives in primary birth is to provide midwifery services for general practitioner or obstetrician LMCs and, in most hospitals, to facilitate the midwife LMC/woman relationship by supporting the midwife LMC in the hospital environment (Campbell 2000). In labour they provide a welcome second pair of hands, relieve LMC midwives for breaks during a long labour and are available to the LMC for discussion and midwifery peer support. All core midwives also provide a secondary midwifery service when LMC midwives have transferred care for an episode of intervention. In antenatal and postnatal areas core midwives work with the LMC and the woman in developing the woman's care plan and deciding who will provide particular aspects of the care.

When a woman requires secondary care and the services of an obstetrician or other specialist, the LMC midwife is still paid from Section 51 (88) for the midwifery service. She is therefore able to provide continuity of care to all her clients, regardless of their risk status. However, if the midwife feels that the woman's care is outside her scope of practice she is able to transfer that woman's care to the core midwife in the hospital, although she may choose to stay on as a support person and work with the core midwife. Generally, the woman's care is transferred back to the LMC midwife once the need for additional services or obstetric intervention has passed.

Secondary hospital facilities

Most of New Zealand's secondary care maternity hospitals were built in the 1960s and reflect the fragmented, interventionist maternity care model of the time, with separate antenatal, labour and postnatal wards. The labour wards were also separated into rooms for labour and theatres for birth. During the 1980s, as a result of consumer pressure, cosmetic changes were made in an effort to make the facilities more 'home-like'. During the 1990s the new focus on continuity of care provided the impetus for most facilities to reorganise their labour wards as a series of birthing rooms. In many areas these birthing rooms are fitted out in a similar way to birth centres in other countries. They are large enough to accommodate families, emergency equipment is hidden and many have 'normal' beds and other furniture. Most hospitals have some form of water immersion available for women who choose to labour in water and increasing numbers of hospitals are installing birth pools.

Most secondary maternity facilities are old and scheduled for rebuilding. New maternity facilities are now being purpose-built to reflect the new maternity service model, with few antenatal and postnatal beds and with large family birthing rooms. The difference between these large family birthing rooms in New Zealand's maternity hospitals and those in birth centres in other places is that these rooms are available to all women, regardless of risk status. There are no booking criteria. The facilities in new maternity hospitals are designed to accommodate women and their families during labour and to fit in with the women-centred and continuity of care model of maternity care available to all women in New Zealand.

THREATS AND OPPORTUNITIES

For a short period of time in the competitive climate of the mid-1990s it was possible to contract outside of the national Section 51 maternity framework. This policy shift was based on the market model ideology, that competition between health providers will result in cheaper health services and will also shift responsibility for these services from the state to the individual health provider (Gauld 2001). The medical profession saw this competitive contracting arrangement as an opportunity to become the budget-holder for the total primary health budget and therefore the gatekeeper to all health services. Individual general practitioners rapidly grouped to form medical independent practitioner associations (IPAs). The government of the day funded and encouraged the IPAs to bid for health service contracts on behalf of their members in areas such as laboratory and pharmaceutical services and well child and sexual health service provision. The ability of IPAs to cost-shift within these many and varied contracts gave them a major financial advantage when it came to maternity funding.

Several IPAs were successful in gaining contracts for maternity services that were outside the Section 51 framework. These contracts created a number of potential threats for midwifery and the wider maternity service. Firstly, they pitted midwives against each other as some midwives joined the medical IPA maternity contracts and doctors were able to obtain midwifery services for 'shared care' arrangements at a cheaper price than they would through Section 51 arrangements. Secondly, they undermined the LMC model of maternity care as the IPA arrangements invariably replicated the doctor-dominated model that had existed prior to 1990 in which care was given by a number of providers, leading to reduced continuity for the woman. Thirdly, they threatened the financial stability of individual midwife LMCs as these contracts were funded by surplus money that would normally have been channelled into Section 51. Over time, Section 51 became significantly underfunded in comparison. Fourthly, these contracts were awarded with no requirement for reporting maternity outcomes data into the national maternity dataset. The first national data available on maternity services outcomes in New Zealand therefore do not include some 30% of births that came under these alternative contracts (Ministry of Health 2001).

During this period of competition it was difficult for the midwifery profession to know whether Section 51 would survive as a national funding mechanism or whether maternity funding would eventually be split into a number of smaller contracts. The New Zealand College of Midwives strongly favoured the continuation of a national funding mechanism because it ensured a consistent fee for midwifery services throughout the country and, more importantly, because the national framework and LMC model supported midwifery autonomy.

The College developed two main strategies in response to this competitive environment. The first was a pragmatic approach. If the national Section 51 framework were to disappear, midwives would need another mechanism by which to contract for maternity services and so NZCOM also sought a contract outside of Section 51 and formed its own service-contracting organisation, the Midwifery and Maternity Provider Organisation (MMPO). This organisation provided a payment mechanism for its midwife members, receiving contract money for its maternity service and passing this on to the midwife members. Initially, only midwives working in the South Island of New Zealand were able to use MMPO and its operation remained quite small, while most midwives were able to continue to claim from Section 51. Its main purpose, however, was to provide an alternative that could be used by midwives if Section 51 were to be removed as a national funding framework in the future.

The College's second strategy was to mount a concerted campaign to re-establish the national funding framework for maternity care and to increase the level of its funding. The College was supported in this strategy by various women's groups who, like the midwives, believed that standardisation of funding would lead to more equitable access for women. The College argued that all contracts outside Section 51 should be cancelled and that all maternity funding should return to the national framework, with any additional monies being used to increase the overall level of funding within Section 51. The College realised that this would require the cancellation of its own contract through MMPO as well as medical IPA contracts. Other potential casualties were the few midwifery groups that had negotiated primary facility funding to establish midwife-led birthing units or midwifery-led service contracts.

This strategy has been successful and the Ministry of Health is currently in the process of bringing all contracts back into the Section 51 (Section 88) national framework, which has also received a significant increase in overall funding.

However, for the fourth time since 1983, the New Zealand health system is undergoing another major restructuring (Gauld 2002). This time, 21 District Health Boards (DHBs), made up of both appointed and community-elected representatives, will be responsible for the provision and funding of integrated health services within their regions. The centralised maternity funding mechanism will eventually be devolved to these DHBs and, once again, the maternity system risks fragmentation and regional variation in services. The newly evolving DHB system poses either another threat or an opportunity for the midwifery profession. Midwifery will be able to retain control of its own services through a more powerful national MMPO, which will contract with each of the 21 DHBs to provide midwifery services for primary health. If the DHBs do not take up this opportunity but defer to IPAs or other primary health organisation structures, midwifery again faces a considerable risk of losing its professional independence. Women would also return to the kind of fragmented, multi-provider system that existed before 1990.

Even in its short lifetime the College of Midwives has already experienced a similar threat. The rapid demise of the national Section 51 contract in the mid 1990s and its replacement by non-uniform provision, dominated by medicine, was a salutary reminder to midwives that their position would always be vulnerable if they did not remain collective in their political actions and in their funding negotiations. The overriding philosophical understanding of NZCOM is that the entire midwifery profession needs to be in a position of strength, rather than just a few of its individual members. Putting midwives into a position of having to compete against each other is detrimental to the profession as a whole and also results in inequitable provision of services to women. A consistent level of funding for all midwives is more likely to achieve an egalitarian service for women.

With this in mind, NZCOM has refocused on the Midwifery and Maternity Provider Organisation. The MMPO can provide a national structure to which midwives can belong and to which the DHBs can contract in order to access midwifery services for their regions. A national approach strengthens the midwifery profession and is more likely to ensure consistency in the funding and provision of midwifery and maternity services throughout New Zealand. As well as providing a collective negotiating tool for midwives, MMPO offers a practice management system that will be available to all midwives throughout New Zealand and will encourage a collective approach to financial and business management for self-employed midwives. The development of this strategy to maximise the opportunities and minimise the threats of this current health system restructuring is a priority for the College.

Alongside this strategy is the recognition by midwifery that primary birthing facilities provide an important focus for normal birthing and independent midwifery services. While New Zealand has not had to develop birth centres as a way to achieve midwifery autonomy and normal birth services for women, the time is now right to work on developing birth centres (primary maternity facilities) in order to protect and strengthen midwifery autonomy and the women-centred services that already exist. Midwives and women need locations for birth that are not dominated by the medical model philosophy of birth. They need to strengthen their understandings of birth as a normal physiological process and they need to reduce their reliance on technological intervention for routine screening and pain relief. It is only by relearning about normal birth and understanding the impact that medicalisation has had on their attitudes and practice that midwives and women will be able to bring about any reduction in obstetric intervention rates. And it is through women and their families that fundamental changes in society's understanding of childbirth will occur. The place for this relearning is in the home and in primary maternity facilities or birthing centres. It is time for the New Zealand maternity service to actively promote both home and primary facilities/birthing centres as the most appropriate places for the majority of women to give birth.

CONCLUSION

This chapter has attempted to trace the history of midwifery and the place of birth in New Zealand within the context of repeated changes in the country's health system. There is no single factor that guarantees the realisation of the ideal maternity or midwifery service. When midwives in New Zealand regained autonomy in 1990 they thought that a midwifery-led service would be relatively easy to achieve. What they failed to recognise was the energy and political acumen that would be required to maintain the midwife's position within the maternity service. The midwife's position is really only important to midwives and to the women who have experienced the difference a midwife can make. The maternity system is much more strongly influenced by the wider health system and by external factors such as economic and political priorities. Maternity services are only a small part of the overall health system and changes in the wider system may have unexpected consequences for midwifery and maternity. The New Zealand midwifery profession has realised that in order to maintain a stable midwifery and maternity service it needs to become embedded in the political system. It must remain constantly vigilant, recognising opportunities and threats as they arise.

Historically, New Zealand has looked overseas for models of health that have worked and New Zealand midwifery has adapted a largely British model. Its biggest adaptation has been in its workforce development, working towards a self-employed business model of autonomous midwifery practice. It is this ability to be both self-employed and autonomous in her practice that has allowed the New Zealand midwife to tailor her service to individual women. She is able to care for all women, regardless of their risk status, and can work with women in all settings. Under the funding mechanisms that exist in this country, the New Zealand midwife is in a unique position in that she holds the contract of service with each and every woman she attends. The funding mechanism lends itself to and reinforces the philosophical position of midwifery as a partnership between the woman and the midwife. This, we believe, is the strength of the New Zealand maternity system. Maintaining these achievements for midwifery and for women through changes in future health policy direction and possible changes to this funding mechanism will require new strategies, including the establishment of mechanisms for collective midwifery action and the development of birth centres and primary maternity facilities as preferred locations for birth.

REFERENCES

Campbell N 2000 Core midwives–the challenge! 6th National Conference of New Zealand College of Midwives 2000 September 28–30, Cambridge New Zealand College of Midwives, Christchurch, p 187–193

Cunningham W, Dovey S 2000 The effect on medical practice of disciplinary complaints: potentially negative for patient care. The New Zealand Medical Journal 113 (1121): 464–467

Daellenbach R 1999 Midwifery partnership: a consumer's perspective. New Zealand College of Midwives Journal 21: 22–23

Donley J 1986 Save the midwife. New Woman's Press, Auckland

Gauld R 2001 Revolving doors: New Zealand's health reforms. Victoria University of Wellington, Wellington

Guilliland K, Pairman S 1995 The midwifery partnership: a model for practice. Victoria University of Wellington, Wellington

Guilliland K 1998 A demographic profile of independent (self employed) midwives in New Zealand Aotearoa. (Masters thesis) Victoria University of Wellington, Wellington

Health Funding Authority 2000 Maternity services: a reference document. Health Funding Authority, Government Printing Office, Wellington

Health Funding Authority 1999a Consumer perceptions of maternity care: results of the 1999 National Survey. Health Funding Authority, Government Printing Office, Wellington

Health Funding Authority 1999b New Zealand mothers and babies: an analysis of national maternity data. Health Funding Authority, Government Printing Office, Wellington

King A 2001 The primary healthcare strategy. Ministry of Health, Wellington

Midland Region Health Funding Authority 1998 Pregnancy and childbirth in the Midland Region. Health Funding Authority Midland Office, Hamilton

Ministry of Health 1999 Obstetric procedures 1988/89–1997/98. Ministry of Health, Wellington

Ministry of Health 2001 Report on Maternity 1999. Ministry of Health, Wellington

Ministry of Health 2002 Maternity services notice pursuant to Section 88 of the New Zealand Public Health and Disability Act, Ministry of Health, Wellington

National Health Committee 1999 Review of maternity services in New Zealand. National Health Committee, Wellington

New Zealand College of Midwives 2002 Midwives handbook for practice. New Zealand College of Midwives, Christchurch

New Zealand Government 1998 Accident Insurance Act. New Zealand Government Printer, Wellington

New Zealand Health Information Services 2002 New Zealand workforce statistics 2001: nurses and midwives. Available at: *http://www.nzhis.govt.nz/stats/nurses.html*

Nursing Council of New Zealand 1999 Guidelines for competence-based practising certificates for registered midwives. Nursing Council of New Zealand, Wellington

Otago Polytechnic 1999 Bachelor of Midwifery curriculum document. Otago Polytechnic, Dunedin

Pairman S 1998 The midwifery partnership: an exploration of the midwife/woman relationship. (Masters thesis) Victoria University of Wellington, Wellington

Pairman S 1999 Partnership revisited: towards midwifery theory. New Zealand College of Midwives Journal 21: 6–12

Ramsden I 1990 Kawa Whakaruruhau: cultural safety in nursing education in Aotearoa. Ministry of Education, Wellington

Skinner J 1999 Midwifery partnership: individualism, contracturalism or feminist praxis? New Zealand College of Midwives Journal 21: 14–17

Tracy M, Guilliland K, Tracy M (in press)

Tully E, Daellenbach R, Guilliland K 1998 Feminism, partnership and midwifery. In: Du Plessis R, Alice L (eds) Feminist thought in Aotearoa New Zealand. Oxford University Press, Auckland, p 245–253

22

Autonomy, clinical freedom and responsibility

Marion Hunter

INTRODUCTION

The material presented in this chapter is based on research carried out in New Zealand from 1999 to 2000. A group of independent midwives agreed to be interviewed, and their experiences are discussed. Independent midwives are better able to practise what they call 'real midwifery', with greater autonomy and more clinical freedom, in small maternity units than they can in large obstetric hospitals. Midwives also related the feeling of having to 'carry the can' on occasions, however, and the additional responsibility can be a worry in the small maternity unit. The paradox for midwives practising in small units is that while these provide an excellent setting for natural birth and for 'letting birth be', the midwives need to have the foresight and confidence to avert or manage any problems that might arise.

BACKGROUND TO THE STUDY

There were no studies in the literature that addressed the differences between providing intrapartum care in small maternity units and large obstetric hospitals. The research question posed was: 'How is the provision of intrapartum care by independent midwives different in a small maternity unit as compared with a large obstetric hospital?' A qualitative study using Van Manen's method of hermeneutic thematic analysis was designed and deemed appropriate to answer the research question (Van Manen 1990). The aims of the study were:

- to describe the experiences of independent midwives providing intrapartum care in a small maternity unit and in a large obstetric hospital
- to highlight the differences in providing labour care in the different settings
- to identify issues that influence independent midwives' choice of environment for provision of intrapartum care.

Since 1970 the number of small maternity units in New Zealand has steadily decreased. Rosenblatt et al reported that approximately one-third of rural maternity units in New Zealand were closed between 1970 and 1983 (Rosenblatt et al, report for the New Zealand Government, unpublished, 1984). Initially, small units were closed because of concerns about the quality of care provided, while in later years cost saving was the driving force for closure. The remaining small maternity units tend to be used primarily as postnatal facilities for women who have given birth in large obstetric hospitals. According to the Health Funding Authority (1999) only 8% of births in New Zealand during 1997 occurred in small (stand-alone) maternity units. The small number of births in these units is probably associated with the fact that lead maternity carers (LMCs), including independent midwives, are not using these facilities for intrapartum care and with the closure of so many small units.

Rosenblatt et al (report for the New Zealand Government, unpublished, 1984) commented that indigenous Maori women were particularly affected by the closure of remote small hospitals. A number of other authors (Donley 1986, Mikaere 2000, Rimene et al 1999) emphasised the need for Maori women to have access to a birth environment that does not alienate them from traditional customs. The friendly, home-like ambience of small maternity units might be less alienating than the busy, crowded environment of many large obstetric hospitals.

Since legislative changes made in 1990, independent midwives have been able to contract to individual clients and are legally able to be the sole maternity provider. They can book women for birth at home, in a small unit or in a large hospital, so gaining experience in all these settings over the same period of time. Independent midwives are paid by the government for their service and are not employees of any particular maternity unit. The impact of the maternity unit on them is the impact of its culture, values and priorities as opposed to the impact of staff shortages or other issues which would be experienced as an employee.

The small maternity units referred to in this study are low-technology units with no facilities for inductions, Syntocinon augmentation, epidurals, or caesarean operations and no neonatal facilities. These units are government-funded and are located in different towns (rural and urban) from the large obstetric hospital. The travelling time from the most distant small unit to the large base hospital is approximately 1 hour. Independent midwives book women into small units, attend the women during labour and visit periodically during the postpartum period. All of the participants in this study provide continuity of care to women throughout the childbirth experience.

THE RESEARCH METHOD

Ethical approval for this study was gained from two authorities in New Zealand, the Massey University Human Ethics Committee and the Auckland Health Ethics Committees. Letters were sent to independent midwives who used one of three small maternity units in the greater Auckland area. Ten participants responded to the information sheet and subsequently consented to be interviewed. Each participant had provided intrapartum care to women in both small and large maternity units within the previous 2 years, and had been qualified for at least 3 years. Anonymity (when desired) was assured by the use of a pseudonym chosen by the midwife.

In keeping with a qualitative study, the sample size was kept small in order to gather the richness of each participant's experience.

Interviews were audiotaped and lasted between 60 and 90 minutes. Data was transcribed and the process of data analysis occurred over 10 months. Van Manen's 'wholistic (*sic*) reading approach' and 'selective reading approach' guided data analysis (Van Manen 1990). Sandelowski (1995) emphasised the need for the researcher to get a feeling of each individual interview before comparisons were made *across* interviews. The process of re-reading and writing assisted my interpretation of the data, the development of themes and the uncovering of a deeper meaning in the midwives' stories. This process also revealed new meanings within specific areas that, in turn, modified the overall meaning.

Rigour was established by detailing every step of the research process and by eliciting feedback on data analysis from my supervisor, an academic colleague and two of the participants. Koch (1994) said that consulting with participants concerning the researcher's analysis establishes credibility and Van Manen (1990) suggested that themes (from the data) might become items of reflection for the researcher and the interviewees.

STUDY FINDINGS

There was unanimous preference for providing labour care in small maternity units and the midwives described practising in this setting as 'real midwifery'. Real midwifery is seen as doing normal midwifery and attending to women, as opposed to attending to machines. This theme gave rise to several subthemes that further elucidated the notion of real midwifery. The subthemes included: practising more autonomously, having time, giving time, and tolerating noise.

The notion of real midwifery is introduced by the following account:

At [the small maternity unit] it's like real midwifery in a way, because you're not interfering. ... When you are using the synto and the epidural, a lot of it's taken away from the woman and, in a lot of respects, probably taken away from you a little bit as well. ...I think with real midwifery, a lot of it is not doing, in a way letting it happen, being there, but you're

still there and you still want to make sure that things are happening as they should. ...And I think real midwifery can be not being that overpowering person there (Elizabeth).

Leap (2000) used the phrase, 'the less we do the more we give' to illustrate that midwives' work might be 'sitting in the corner of the room in watchful anticipation during labour, but on the whole [being] quiet and very non-directive'. Leap claimed that this type of practice shifts the power to the woman, as indicated in this present study by Elizabeth, who did not want to be 'that overpowering person there', preferring to be 'quietly assistive without taking the main focal position' (VandeVusse 1997). Leap (2000) suggested, 'Our expertise as midwives rests in our ability to watch, to listen and to respond to any given situation with all of our senses'. The midwife has the knowledge and the skills to know when to act or seek help, and when to be still and withdraw.

Grace described the midwifery skills required when providing labour care in the small maternity unit like this:

You've actually got to use gut feelings and perhaps just really listening to what the women are saying, and adjusting your thoughts and practices to what the needs of the women are. That's a huge shift to working in a big hospital where you've got machines and technicians interfering with that basic in-built knowledge that you've got. You turn off, I'm sure you switch off at [the large obstetric hospital], because you're too busy, too busy watching all those other things instead of listening to the women.

Buus-Frank (1999) indicated that there is a tendency to use technology because it is available rather than because it is necessary. However, the skilled midwife's senses provide irreplaceable ongoing assessment. The following participants supported this view:

I actually find that part of midwifery at [the large obstetric hospital] almost easier, because it's all black and white, and the woman's lying there with her epidural and you're watching machines. Whereas this way, when I'm at [the small unit] it's more hands-on. You know, it's sort of like watching and waiting, and I think it's more enjoyable, but it can be more emotionally draining perhaps, that you are getting it right from reading it. (Bronnie)

You need your eyes and your hands more than any equipment. That will tell you more than any monitors. (Cluain Meala)

Bronnie's statement, that 'watching and waiting can be more emotionally draining', is echoed by Kirkham (2000), who described the work of the midwife as 'emotional labour'. This emotional labour is undervalued in a culture that values interventions, where the midwife focuses on monitoring and abnormality. This focus on detecting abnormality is more likely to cause apprehension and panic, which is then transmitted to the woman. Siddiqui (1999) revealed through her qualitative research that midwives referred to 'tuning in' or 'keying in' to the labour itself, knowing intuitively if a labour was going all right or if it was deviating from the normal and that this was quite distinct from exercising the technical skills of monitoring. In order to do this 'keying in', midwives need to be in touch with their own being. Sutton (1996) and Hodnett (1996) suggested that midwives have sacrificed their own assessment skills to the technology of obstetrics.

There appears to be a paradox in that technology is purported to make birth safer for women, yet all the midwives in this study indicated that using technology takes the midwife's focus away from the woman and so might make it less safe. Being able to practise 'real midwifery' was associated with the culture of small maternity units. One may ask the question, 'What prevents real midwifery from happening at the large hospital?' Perhaps it is the dominance of the medical model that prevails in large hospitals, with its focus on protocols and fetocentric care (Sandelowski 2000).

There are a number of situations in which midwives seemed to feel constrained in the large obstetric hospital and this will be explored further through examination of the subtheme of practising more autonomously in small units.

PRACTISING MORE AUTONOMOUSLY

The ability to be able to practise more autonomously is rated highly by independent midwives and this influences their preference of providing labour care in small maternity units.

Midwives often referred to 'them' or 'they', who seemed to interfere with their practice in the large hospital. One may ask, 'Who are "they"?' Heidegger (1927/1962) said that our 'being' is affected by the 'other' and what 'they' might say. 'They' seem to be undefined, nameless faces. The independent midwives tend to practise at the large hospital in accordance with what 'they' expect. The following accounts illustrate this theme:

[At the large obstetric hospital] you've got to do a CTG [cardiotocograph]. They like you to do a 20-minute CTG. Completely unnecessary in the majority of cases. You see I have a suspicion that they leave me alone. They might well comment on what I do afterwards or what I don't do, as the case may be. I don't feel compelled to give ecbolics like I used to, and I don't. (Mary)

Kirsty spoke of a difference between the two units:

When you are looking after women in those small units, there is this expectation of going with the flow and the normal. Nobody's knocking on my door or asking if there are any problems. Women are treated as normal, therefore there isn't the intervention automatically, and there isn't CTGs as soon as you walk in the door. There are no routines and, as an autonomous practitioner, I do what I feel is appropriate at the time without having to really discuss it with anybody.

Elizabeth related her experience of beginning to use small units:

I really enjoyed it at the beginning [at the small maternity unit]. It was like–now I can do what I want to do here. There were no CTGs and, in fact, sometimes you feel like a bit of a rebel as well. . . . maybe I felt that I could push my wings out a little bit more or whatever. . . . I now find myself going into [the large obstetric hospital] and not routinely doing what I class as [large hospital] stuff, which I was doing in the early days of independent practice. I would still routinely do those things, like the routine half-an-hour CTG at [the large hospital], even though I don't do it at [the small unit]. And I started questioning myself, 'Well, is it just a routine? Why am I doing it? Is it the place that's dictating to me?' So, I guess now it's just finding what I find, so that I can dictate to myself.

Elizabeth described 'pushing her wings out', as if to test her own ability, as a bird tests itself prior to launching into flight. She also describes feelings of being 'a bit of a rebel'. The use of technology is frequently associated with claims of safety (Tew 1990)–not using technology might therefore be perceived as rebellious and associated with lack of safety. Garcia and Garforth (1989) stressed the importance of midwives being able to use personal judgement when providing labour care, as opposed to having to follow formal policies, and Walsh (2000) commented that the clinical freedom to practise as one wishes is more possible in a birthing unit. Some practitioners might question why independent midwives feel obliged to follow protocols at the large obstetric hospital. The participants in this study indicated that they felt an atmosphere of surveillance at the large hospital, and that they feared that if a problem arose that requires medical consultation their practice would be viewed judgementally.

HAVING TIME

It would appear that for a midwife to be able to practise 'real midwifery' she should have a feeling of 'having time'. A recurrent theme was the sense of not having time at the large obstetric hospital, compared to having ample time at the small maternity unit. Friedman (1954) claimed to have redefined labour in terms of setting time limits and demonstrating what may be expected of a normal labour. However, Friedman does not address the fact that in his initial study only 29% of the women had a spontaneous birth. This cannot be representative of normal labour.

Friedman's research ushered in the use of the partograph and the imposition of time-frames on labour. The modern obstetric hospital has a large amount of technology, used to hurry things on if there is any deviation from so-called acceptable progress of labour (Leap & Hunter 1993), including protocols such as artificial rupture of membranes and the use of Syntocinon augmentation if the woman's labour is not progressing at the rate of 1 cm per hour (Enkin et al 2000).

Rosemary reflected on the sense of a time-frame in large hospitals:

When you go into a big base hospital, it is based on a policy of mass production, where it is important to have the woman come in, have her delivered and

have her out again. ... It was quite revolting to have to treat people so aggressively in the system, all because it wasn't better for their outcomes or whatever their birthing experience was going to be–it was going to be better for the hospital. That is the difference between working in a major base hospital, and working in a smaller unit–you don't have that heavier focus of sort of shunting these women along on a conveyor belt and getting the job done as quickly as possible.

Rosemary likened the large base hospital to a factory, saying that women are 'shunted along on a conveyer belt', because of the pressure of time. Davis Floyd (1992) and Walsh (2000) wrote of an 'assembly-line production' adopted by modern obstetrics. Hunt and Symonds (1995) confirmed that the analogy of hospital births to a factory assembly line was almost a cliché of discontentment of consumers and midwives in the 1980s.

Mary provided an unusual example of providing care to a woman in labour during a busy time at the large obstetric hospital:

There's always a sense of urgency [at the large hospital] because so many people are coming and going. At [the small maternity unit], to a greater extent, you can allow the woman to labour at her own pace. I probably would be one of the few people who actually transferred a woman from a base hospital to a small unit for delivery. Like the example would be, say, in the base hospital, with a perfectly normal gravida 2, who was labouring quietly but well, but I was taking up a room and too much time, and people kept coming and saying to me, 'Is she going to deliver soon? Is she going to deliver soon? Have you ruptured her membranes?' I didn't want to do any of that and it got on my nerves.

I went to the woman and said, 'Look, how about we move to [the small unit] now?' So I went and rang [the small unit] and said, 'I know this is an unusual request, but can I take a woman over there for delivery? I'm at [the large obstetric hospital].' They said, 'Yes, of course you can', so we went to [the small unit] and delivered in her own time and had a lovely normal delivery. ... So I think that probably will illustrate the difference. The difference is when you get to the small units, OK you take your safety parameters with you, but you're not pressured, and the mother is not pressured because, if you're pressured, it rubs off on the mother.

Mary did not intervene to reduce the length of time the woman was in labour and when they transferred to the small maternity unit the woman was able to birth 'in her own time'. This example is unusual as, although women may be transferred into a large hospital during labour, they are almost never transferred out until after the birth. It could have been embarrassing if this woman had required transfer back into the large hospital because of unforeseen problems. Mary's actions show courage and a determination to allow this woman to labour in her own time. Katz Rothman (1983) highlighted the issue of time constraints in institutions where the tempo of individual births is matched to the limitations of space and staff. Policies such as active management of labour are adopted by large hospitals in order to manage time and space, as opposed to meeting the individual needs of women.

GIVING TIME

'Giving time' refers to midwifery practice in which midwives are able to allow time for women to settle into the small maternity unit. In contrast, midwives feel a need to examine women soon after arrival at the large hospital, to confirm labour. Hunt and Symonds (1995) observed from their ethnographic study that midwives undertook a vaginal examination on each woman admitted to a large hospital. This ensured that the woman was in established labour and would not 'block' a labour ward bed that might be required for women arriving in advanced labour. The following examples describe the experience of midwives who were able to assess women in a watchful patient manner. Joyce explained how she preferred not to undertake vaginal examinations unless requested to do so by the woman (although this depended on the setting):

I guess in a situation where I was pretty sure of the presentation and the engagement, if the woman was contracting really well and hadn't been in labour too long, ... and had a good fetal heart, I wouldn't examine her right away, unless she was really keen to know what dilatation she was. Maybe 3 or 4 hours later, if I didn't feel that she was making the progress I expected, I would ask her if she wanted to know.

It would probably be about a third of the labours I go to, I don't do an internal examination when I arrive. At the large obstetric hospital I probably would feel more that I would need to do everything by the book. I suppose the feeling is that it is more medical over there.

Nettie felt that a vaginal examination (VE) at the large obstetric hospital became a major focus:

Well, I don't always do VEs on arrival [in small units]. ... I give women time to settle in ... a vaginal examination is just one part of the whole picture. I think probably when you're practising in [the large obstetric hospital] it becomes the major part of the picture because it's something concrete. You can say, 'She's this or she's that', but I'm saying it's not that accurate necessarily... . On two occasions it has happened where a specialist has examined the woman and said, 'Oh no, 6 cm, you need an epidural'. The epidural just gets in and then they're ready to push. I really hate that, because I feel like we could have hung in there a bit longer.

Gould (2000) and Stuart (2000) agree that vaginal assessments should not become the sole focus of assessments and that the midwife should be adept at recognising descent of the head by abdominal palpation and have the confidence in practice wisdom to make an assessment of the progress of labour. Duff (1998) encouraged midwives to record the changes they observed in women that they use to assess progress of labour. The changes in the woman's behaviour should be documented alongside any abdominal and vaginal assessments. In contrast, Enkin et al (2000) claim that the vaginal assessment is the most reliable measure of the progress of labour. This reflects a medicalised view of childbirth in which something that is measurable is considered the most accurate tool for assessing progress of labour and estimating time of delivery.

TOLERATING NOISE

Unexpectedly, all the independent midwives talked about noise, and whether or not noise during labour was tolerable. Midwives articulated the difference between acceptable noise levels in the small unit and what was considered acceptable in the large obstetric hospital. The following accounts suggest that midwives may resort to the use of epidural analgesia in a large hospital to control noise from women:

When you're at [the large obstetric hospital] the expectation is that when things get too hard to handle, we get an epidural in. The pressure is on, subtle pressure. You can feel that your woman is making all this noise in there [and people are thinking,] 'What's going on?' ... Whereas, in [the small maternity unit] people are making the noise that they want to make and, if the whole ward is hearing them, then the whole ward is supporting them. (Rosemary)

The woman's making a noise, nobody wants women to make a noise–'Can't you either give her some pethidine or give her an epidural?' They're the kind of things that irritate you. (Mary)

Bronnie corroborated the ready availability of epidurals at the large obstetric hospital:

The women are not allowed to make a noise at [the large obstetric hospital]. ... The only time you really hear a lot of people making a noise at [the large hospital] is when they are in transition, pushing, or when the anaesthetist is a bit late with the epidural. It's acceptable then. I think it's an unspoken rule. It's a feeling. [There] was a woman who had had a previous caesarean. It was her third baby, she was from Romania, and she does make a lot of noise, and the Charge Midwife said, 'Are you all right?', sort of thing. And it's off-putting for the woman. At [the small maternity unit] I don't think that anybody worries too much about noise.

These midwives spoke of 'subtle pressure' and 'an unspoken rule' as indicating a lower tolerance of noise in the large hospital. There is an inference that good midwives do not have noisy women during labour. It is possible that the culture of the large hospital imposes a noise limit on the labour ward and that the midwife in turn imposes an epidural or other forms of pain relief on the woman. McKay and Roberts (1990) conducted a grounded theory study of the meaning of maternal sounds during the second stage of labour. They commented, 'The hospital culture holds strong norms about what is and is not appropriate behaviour for those who work in it or come to it for its services'. The authors suggested that maternal behaviour, including the suppression of noise, is shaped to conform to these core institutional beliefs, often with the help of medication.

'CARRYING THE CAN'

During the course of the interviews the independent midwives talked about some of the difficult situations they had been in, when they had been concerned for the mother or baby. The feeling of 'carrying the can' arises when independent midwives experience a challenging situation, or when 'others' challenge their practice. Joyce introduced the subject with the following account:

We had a primip who was in second stage and past the point of being able to be transferred because the head was on view, and we suddenly got very thick fresh meconium, and it was five in the morning... I suppose, because the distress had only been very short-lived, that the baby wasn't affected by it and he cried right away and didn't have any problem. But you go through in your mind, situations where maybe the baby isn't going to get out very quickly and it's past the time when it's safe to move. It is quite lonely because you think, well, I've got another midwife here, but maybe she's got no more experience than me, so really I'm going to carry the can if there is any problem. So you do live with that, but I think you balance that by believing that, in most cases, the outcome is going to be good.

On reflection, Joyce wondered how the baby's well-being might have been affected if the baby had not been born so quickly. Joyce spoke of it being 'past the time when it's safe to move'. Moving may mean that the baby is born in the ambulance, and that is less satisfactory than being born in the small maternity unit where, although facilities are limited, resuscitation equipment is available. Joyce described this reality with her comment, 'I'm going to carry the can if there is a problem'. However, the risk of a poor outcome is balanced by a belief that, in most cases, (and as in this case), 'the outcome is going to be good'.

Kirsty emphasised the midwife's feeling of responsibility and of being alone:

I've had one major flat baby... I phoned [the large obstetric hospital]... and it wasn't very helpful... . And so at that point, it was very distressing and I felt like I might as well be in the desert as being in the small unit. I'm bagging the baby, and I just carry on bagging, whilst my brain is working overtime... my adrenaline is obviously working overtime at this point.

Kirsty recalled that the response from the team at the large hospital was not helpful. Her feeling of 'being in the desert' reflects a sense of isolation, a feeling of being solely responsible and possibly a vulnerability and sense of fear associated with the distance from help.

Reflecting on one's practice can raise issues that were not previously considered, as illustrated by Cluain Meala:

I think working in a small unit...your senses have to be a lot more acute I suppose. You are solely responsible if something does happen. You have to know what you have to do then, just right then, like 'A, B, C'. I suppose, you're usually totally aware of that all the time, even though it doesn't come to the fore all the time.

In a small maternity unit the midwife's senses need to be more acute, there is an awareness that she is 'solely responsible' if anything goes wrong. This sense of alertness never leaves the midwife–though it may be in the background, it is always there. Smythe (2000) described the following qualities as belonging to the safe practitioner: watching and alertness, anticipation and a concerned mindfulness.

Tyrrell illustrated confidence in her practice:

My hands never shake when I am doing things, and I just think if there is going to be a problem, we will deal with it. Some problems happen in labour, and you have to deal with them. You always have to be aware in those small places, if you are going to transfer someone, or things are not progressing, the transfer can take, like, 3 hours before you actually get the woman seen. You have to take that into consideration, so that is difficult. But no, if you know what could happen, you just think–when it happens, I will know what to do.

Tyrrell revealed a calm and competent approach to dealing with the problems that might arise in a small unit. The midwife needs to recognise and respond to the abnormal–ahead of time–in order to provide safe care. The difference for a midwife working in the large obstetric hospital is that assistance is closer to hand, perhaps only minutes away. In small maternity units it may take several hours to transfer a woman and have her seen by an obstetrician.

The distance from the large hospital and therefore the time needed to get assistance is inextricably linked to the midwife's use of foresight:

I can honestly say I was nervous about the labour...there is a part of you that thinks, what's going to happen when I get to [the large obstetric hospital]? Am I going to be told, 'You should have come two hours ago'? I mean, that happens. Or if you ring, 'Well does she really need to come?' (Bronnie)

Smith (1998) conducted a quantitative study of the referral of labouring women to consultant hospitals and reported that 27% of doctors and midwives, predominantly from the consultant hospital, felt that transfers were either too early or too late although, with the benefit of hindsight, practitioners might tend to make more critical judgements as to whether or not the transfer of a woman occurred at an appropriate time. Participants in this study showed how difficult it can be to judge the optimum time to transfer a woman.

The midwives who practise only in the large hospital do not need to concern themselves with the complexities of transferring women in labour–they are already deemed to be in the safest place, from the standpoint of a medical model of childbirth. When receiving a woman who has been transferred, Waldenström, et al (1997) advised practitioners in a large hospital to respond seriously and to respect the decision of a midwife to transfer a woman as a safe decision. They recommended that the consultant unit assess women who have been transferred promptly, and that attention be paid to the history given by the accompanying midwife.

CONCLUSION

The key finding from this study (Hunter 2000) is the importance of being able to practise 'real midwifery' in small maternity units where midwives feel autonomous, free of time constraints and free of technology that may interfere with the woman's labour. The participants acknowledged, however, their feeling of being solely responsible or 'carrying the can' on the rare occasions when emergencies occur and when transferring women to the large hospital. The paradox of having the freedom to practise in the small unit is that when problems manifest themselves, this very freedom can become a burden of responsibility. Findings from this study also suggest that the medicalised environment of the large hospital is so pervasive that midwives are influenced by the expectation that admission cardiotocographs and time-frames should be imposed on labouring women. Therefore, it appears that independent midwives do practise differently in different contexts.

Small maternity units are an important historical feature of maternity care in New Zealand and in many other countries. Midwives practising in small maternity units are meeting the needs of women who do not wish to, or need to, birth in large obstetric hospitals. If the majority of births continue to occur in large obstetric hospitals, with technological interventions, some midwives will become increasingly removed from the art of real midwifery, with its belief in natural childbirth, and the opportunity for midwives to feel affirmed as they practise normal, low-intervention midwifery will be diminished.

REFERENCES

Buus-Frank M 1999 Nurse versus machine: slaves or masters of technology? Journal of Obstetric Gynecologic and Neonatal Nursing 28 (4): 433–441

Davis-Floyd R 1992 Birth as an American rite of passage. University of California Press, Berkeley

Donley J 1986 Save the Midwife. New Women's Press, Auckland

Duff M 1998 Labour behaviours: a journey in assessing labour progress. 5th National Conference of the New Zealand College of Midwives, Auckland.

Enkin M et al 2000 A guide to effective care in pregnancy and childbirth, 3rd edn. Oxford University Press, New York

Friedman E 1954 The graphic analysis of labor. American Journal of Obstetrics and Gynecology 68 (6): 1568–1575

Garcia J, Garforth S 1989 Labour and delivery routines in English consultant maternity units. Midwifery 5 (4): 155–162

Gould D 2000 Normal labour: a concept analysis. Journal of Advanced Nursing 31 (2): 418–427

Health Funding Authority 1999 New Zealand mothers and babies: an analysis of national maternity data. Government Printing Office, Wellington

Heidegger M 1927 Being and Time. McQuarrie J, Robinson E, trans. 1962 Basil Blackwell, Oxford

Hodnett E 1996 Nursing support of the labouring woman. Journal of Obstetric Gynecologic and Neonatal Nursing 25 (3): 257–264

Hunt S, Symonds A 1995 The social meaning of midwifery. Macmillan Press, London

Hunter M 2000 Autonomy, clinical freedom and responsibility: the paradoxes of providing intrapartum midwifery care in a small maternity unit as compared with a large obstetric hospital. (MA thesis) Massey University, Palmerston North

Katz Rothman B 1983 Midwives in transition: the structure of a clinical revolution. Social Problems 30 (3): 262–271

Kirkham M 2000 How can we relate? In: Kirkham M (ed.) The midwife-mother relationship. Macmillan Press, London, 227–254

Koch T 1994 Establishing rigour in qualitative research: the decision trail. Journal of Advanced Nursing 19: 976–986

Leap N 2000 The less we do, the more we give. In: Kirkham M (ed.) The midwife-mother relationship. Macmillan Press, London, 1–18

Leap N, Hunter B 1993 The midwife's tale. Scarlet Press, London

McKay S, Roberts J 1990 Obstetrics by ear. Journal of nurse-midwifery 35 (5): 266–273

Mikaere A 2000 Mai te Kore ki te Ao Marama: Maori women as Whare Tangata. 6th New Zealand College of Midwives Conference, September 28–30, Cambridge, New Zealand

Rimene C, Hassan C, Broughton J 1999 Ukaipo: the place of nurturing Maori women and childbirth. University of Otago, Dunedin

Sandelowski M 1995 Qualitative analysis: what it is and how to begin. Research in nursing and health 18: 371–375

Sandelowski M 2000 'This most dangerous instrument': propriety, power, and the vaginal speculum. Journal of Obstetric Gynecologic and Neonatal Nursing 29 (1): 73–82

Siddiqui J 1999 The therapeutic relationship in midwifery. British Journal of Midwifery 7 (2): 111–114

Smith L 1998 Referral of labouring women from community to consultant unit. British Journal of Midwifery 6 (1): 47–52

Smythe L 2000 'Being safe' in childbirth: what does it mean? New Zealand College of Midwives Journal 22: 18–21

Stuart C 2000 Invasive actions in labour: where have the 'old tricks' gone? The Practising Midwife 3 (8): 30–33

Sutton H 1996 Childbearing and the ethics of technology: a feminist approach. In: Barclay L and Jones L (eds.) Midwifery: trends and practices in Australia Pearson Professional, Melbourne, 35–52

Tew M 1990 Safer childbirth: a critical history of maternity care. Chapman & Hall, London

Van Manen M 1990 Researching lived experience. The Althouse Press, Ontario

VandeVusse L 1997 Sculpting a nurse-midwifery philosophy: Ernestine Wiedenbach's influence. Journal of nurse-midwifery 42 (1): 43–48

Waldenström U, Nilsson C-A, Winbladh B 1997 The Stockholm Birth Centre trial: maternal and infant outcome. British Journal of Obstetrics and Gynaecology 104 (4): 410–418

Walsh D 2000 Evidence-based care Part three: assessing women's progress in labour. British Journal of Midwifery 8 (7): 449–457

23

Birth centres as an enabling culture

Mavis Kirkham

INTRODUCTION

The birth centres described in this book came into being in different ways and at different times. Forty years ago small and very small maternity units were common. They all must originally have been set up to 'fill a hole in the health care delivery system' (Andrea McGlynn, Ch. 18), whether the hole was recognised by midwife/entrepreneurs or by those who plan the provision of state-funded maternity services. Some of the units described in this book would have been set up as an alternative to home birth in poverty-stricken homes. The Local Government Board Annual Report for 1917–1918 emphasised 'the need for maternity homes for women who cannot safely or conveniently be confined in their own homes'. It was recommended that these maternity homes should be built on the outskirts of towns and have gardens, thus providing better circumstances than those found in most homes at that time (Campbell & Macfarlane 1994). Until the 1960s English towns and cities usually had several maternity homes in their suburbs. Though such maternity homes have almost all been closed, poor housing still exists and locally 'poor and overcrowded living conditions' contrast with the 'good home environment' of the Edgware Birth Centre today (Jean Beney, Ch. 10).

Birth centres also create a base for midwives in sparsely populated areas, or where there are few midwives. Gladys Milton, a 'granny midwife' and 'national treasure' in a rural area of Florida

(Gaskin 1993), built a birth centre behind her home in the 1970s. Her supervisor, Nurse Kirkland, 'was so happy for me to have the birthing centre. She knew it would be safer for the babies to be born in a more controlled atmosphere, where things could be kept clean' (Bovard & Milton 1993). She also rejoiced that, 'after being on the road for seventeen years', as the only midwife in her community, 'I only had to walk through the den and into the clinic'. As more medical and technical maternity services became available, however, authoritative opinion turned against birth centres almost everywhere. The health authority which had supported Gladys Milton, and which had originally recruited and trained her as a midwife, went on to persecute her and endeavoured to close her birth centre.

Of the 55 birth centres in England (Hall 2001 and Ch. 1), some are remnants of an era when small, low-technology maternity units were normal. The longest established have resisted both the pressures to centralise maternity services and the 'technocrat imperative' (Davis-Floyd 1994). Such successful resistance is rare and is rooted in several factors. Local geography is important–many of the older rural birth centres are in places that are easily cut off by snow, or where the distance to the nearest consultant unit is unacceptably long. The support of the local community matters greatly: local people and organisations have rallied to the defence of the Darley Maternity Unit in Derbyshire on the many occasions I can remember when its future was threatened. Key friends are also important, as demonstrated by Wiltshire, which has been influenced by particular geographical factors (see Ch. 3) and which has a consultant obstetrician, Rick Porter, who supports birth centres. A local political situation can also be exploited, as when birth centres have been set up as a by-product of centralisation, when a local consultant maternity unit is closed. Examples of this include Edgware (see Ch. 6), Grantham (see Ch. 4) and the birth centre described in Chapter 2.

There is also a realisation, by increasing numbers of childbearing women and by midwives, that birth centre care can offer advantages over hospital care. Gladys Milton started in the 1950s as a lay midwife, serving poor black women. By the early 1980s she noted that 'the background of my patients was changing': increasingly, they were well educated and 94% of them were white (Bovard & Milton 1993). Such women are increasingly seeking out birth centre care where it exists.

Groups of mothers and midwives are lobbying for birth centres in many parts of England. Networks exist to support the cause of birth centres in England (*http://groups.yahoo.com.group.birthcentres*), Europe (*www.birthcenter-europe.net*) and the USA (*http://www.birthcenters.org*).

WHAT IS A BIRTH CENTRE?

The birth centres described in this book are all different from each other and some call themselves by different titles. Most are separate from maternity hospitals but some are in the same building or even form part of a consultant unit labour ward. Birth centres differ in whether they are 'open', and staffed by midwives round the clock, or 'closed', with midwives present only when caring for a woman in labour or immediately after birth (see Ch. 2 for examples).

Some birth centres provide postnatal care only for a brief period for women who deliver there. Others have postnatal beds and accept transfers of local women after complicated births in the local consultant unit. The midwives working in these birth centres pride themselves on providing excellent postnatal care.

Yet, for all their differences, the philosophy of birth centres is usually centred on 'the concept of midwifery being at the heart of a social (rather than medical) model of care', with midwives providing skilled support 'within which women can achieve normal, physiological birth' (Ch. 2). The Birth Centres Network in this country has a similar philosophy:

Birth centres are known for providing friendly, individualised woman- and family-centred maternity care, with a strong emphasis on skilled, sensitive and respectful midwifery care. Women's voices are at the heart of the organisation and their influence on care is apparent. (Birth Centres Network UK)

The Birth Centres Network is based on 'Ten steps to normal birth' (Birth Centres Network UK 2001), with every birth centre seeking to promote normality in childbirth by:

1. providing care from a small group of midwives and others who are kind, compassionate, gentle, friendly, and skilled in their work
2. using as a basis for all policies, guidelines, and clinical decision-making, a profound understanding of the anatomy and physiology of pregnancy, birth and breastfeeding
3. offering to women only those interventions for which there is clear evidence that they do more good than harm
4. creating a physical environment which protects and promotes the natural hormonal releases which are needed for normal labour and birth
5. honouring a woman's preference for place of birth and birth companion, and ensuring she has skilled, one-to-one support during labour
6. adopting the 'Ten steps to successful breastfeeding', with a special emphasis on skin-to-skin contact straight after birth
7. recognising the wider context of women's lives and seeking, through support groups and inter-agency working, to acknowledge and address problems such as a history of abuse, violent relationships, poverty, mental illness and poor housing
8. explaining clearly and honestly to women the advantages and disadvantages of the available screening tests, and being equally accepting of acceptance or refusal of such tests
9. encouraging and providing a range of minimally invasive measures to support women through the pain of labour, such as: birth pools, TENS, birth balls, massage etc. Neither epidurals nor pethidine are consistent with normal birth
10. offering an antenatal programme which is empowering and which prepares women for the physical, mental and spiritual dimensions of birth and parenthood.

Similar philosophies are found in birth centres throughout the world. The first of the ten steps is echoed and developed by the midwife proprietress of a Japanese Birth House: 'When all women are treated with this degree of care, their confidence in every aspect of their lives will grow, and they in turn will treat others, including their babies, with equal care' (Turner 2002).

Underlying beliefs recur throughout this book: women as active in birth; care adapted to women and families; the importance of relationships, trust and a nurturing environment, all on a scale where individuals matter and relationships can be developed. The small scale and separate identity of birth centres is important. It is probably true to say that where a separate location from a consultant unit is chosen, rather than determined by geography, this is done to protect the small, safe place within which a philosophy, very different from that of a consultant obstetric unit, is held in common by staff and clients.

Criteria for birth centre booking vary but they aim to select women who are at low risk of needing medical facilities which are not available in a birth centre. Sometimes this risk is lumped together with other obstetric risks which can cause confusion (see Ch. 1). In some places booking criteria are precise; in others they are very relaxed. In New Zealand there are no specific booking criteria, each decision being made with the woman 'in accordance with generic guidelines' (Ch. 21). Several authors in this book state that women who fulfil the criteria for booking a home birth would be appropriate candidates to deliver in a birth centre (though women cannot insist on a birth centre birth if they do not fit the criteria in the way that some women resolve to stay at home). It is interesting that in Wiltshire, definitions are laid down for women who need review by a consultant or who should deliver under consultant care, all others being eligible for birth centre care if they wish. The aim of the different birth centre criteria is, however, the same–to book low-risk women and promote normal childbearing.

BIRTH CENTRE CARE IS EFFECTIVE CARE

A number of studies have demonstrated that, when evaluated against obstetric outcomes of safety, birth for low-risk women is at least as safe in small low-risk maternity units as it is in hospitals (Albers & Katz 1991, Campbell et al 1999, Fullerton & Severino 1992, Rooks et al 1989, 1992a, 1992b, 1992c, von Schwarzenfeld et al 1999, Young 1987). There are two key factors here: place of birth and professional carer. Surveying the data on birth outside hospitals (home births and birth centre births) led Rona Campbell and Alison Macfarlane (1994) to the conclusion that, 'There is no evidence to support the claim that the safest policy is for all women to give birth in hospital.' Ole Olensen's meta-analysis of the safety of home births echoes these findings and goes on to state: '...the analyses also reveal significantly and consistently increased morbidity and intervention rates in the hospital group' (Olensen 1997).

Birth out of hospital may be safe for low-risk women because the gains of high-tech obstetrics are offset by the risks that come in their wake. Or, it may be that the very different philosophy and skills of all those involved in birth out of hospital may make a positive difference. These two factors are closely related and probably impossible to separate.

Debate that focused on the place of birth rather than on the carers 'made midwives almost invisible' (Campbell & Macfarlane 1994) yet midwives have always delivered most of the babies born in England. Studies looking specifically at midwife-led care have consistently demonstrated safe outcomes (Campbell et al 1999, MacVicar et al 1993), as have studies of units led by general practitioners (Young 1987), though in traditional GP units, care was largely provided by midwives. Such evidence supports the argument for birth centres but conceals the considerable variation in midwifery care that exists between different centres, as described by Marion Hunter (Ch. 22).

Economic evaluation of health care is notoriously difficult, especially within the National Health Service (Campbell & Macfarlane 1994). Studies comparing costs by place of delivery usually find home births to be cheapest (see Ch. 13). The relative costs of birth centre and hospital care, however, differ in different studies using different costing methods. Free-standing small units have higher overhead costs because of their relatively low number of clients, though an increase in the number of clients can dramatically reduce costs (see Ch. 5). Where birth centres share a site and services with other NHS facilities, their cost-effectiveness can be effected by the economics of these facilities. John Stilwell's 1979 study of the cost of normal delivery by place found that service costs were lowest for home birth and that GP maternity unit births were less costly than those in consultant units. Unusually, he also measured costs to the family and found these to be lowest for GP unit births. Wider savings to the NHS, such as those resulting from increased breastfeeding rates or improved maternal mental health, have not been studied. Surveying the evidence, Rona Campbell and Alison Macfarlane (1994) concluded:

The continuing closure of small units and centralisation of maternity care are not based on good evidence about the cost-effectiveness of this policy.... Closure of small units on grounds of rationalisation may simply represent a transfer of costs between sectors of the economy, in particular from NHS to individual families or to social services and social security. Districts may lose unmeasured resources, as voluntary support for community hospitals may not be transferred to the district hospital on closure of the small units.

As well as safe clinical outcomes, birth centre care is linked to high satisfaction ratings. This was evident with regard to maternal satisfaction in the Edgware (see Ch. 12) and Stockholm (see Ch. 14) birth centres. In a small study of women who had used Japanese birth houses, the women reported that they were satisfied with their care and described their experiences as 'spiritually rewarding' (Misago et al 2000). It is noteworthy that satisfaction is also reported by socially marginalised women from several cultures (Esposito 1999). Fathers expressed satisfaction with the support and respect which they received in the birth centre in Stockholm (Waldenström 1999) which reflects the focus of birth centre care on the family rather than only on the birth. It is interesting that the feeling of being 'treated with respect' is a parameter used in these evaluations, particularly with regard to people who do not often report such treatment (Esposito 1999, Waldenström 1999). Such perceptions of respect echo the emphasis which birth centre midwives place on facilitating supportive relationships around birth. In enhancing the satisfaction of families, birth centre midwives are clearly doing something positive and empowering and not just avoiding iatrogenesis.

Midwives, too, report satisfaction with working in birth centres (see Ch. 14 and Saunders et al 2000) despite, or perhaps because of, the differences from working in a hospital and the greater responsibility.

The evaluation of the Edgware Birth Centre (Saunders et al 2000) breaks down the different elements of satisfaction in a way which enables us to examine what constitutes satisfaction for women using birth centres, local midwives and local GPs. Respondents were asked to classify a series of statements about birth centre care as attractions or drawbacks–the postnatal women were asked if each feature added to or took away from their experience. There was a high level of agreement between the mothers who had used the service and GPs and midwives in that area of London on the advantages of the birth centre in terms of its 'homely and relaxed atmosphere' and women's freedom to do 'what feels right' for them during labour and delivery.

Where the statements involved medical issues, views diverged: not being 'attached to any monitor or high-tech equipment' and being 'looked after by midwives and no doctors were involved' were rated as positive features by the vast majority of women and midwives but by less than half of the GPs, a substantial minority of whom identified these issues as drawbacks. Not being able to have an epidural at the birth centre was simply accepted by most of the mothers, with few seeing it as having affected their experience, yet half of the midwives and

three-quarters of the GPs saw this as a drawback. Only a minority of the women saw the possibility of having to transfer to another hospital if a problem developed, having limited specialist equipment at the birth centre in case of emergency and there being no doctor at the birth centre in case of emergency as drawbacks, whereas the vast majority of the midwives and GPs saw these features in a negative light. One might expect these differences in views to spring from the apprehension of GPs and midwives about emergencies, yet the core midwives who actually worked at the birth centre and dealt with the emergencies that arose there held views much closer to those of their clients. They saw the birth centre as a safe alternative to hospital birth and had confidence in their ability to cope with emergencies:

We have the ability to deal with every situation that arises, even if that is by calling an ambulance and doing whatever we have to in the time between. We have got the necessary equipment that we would need to deal with any situation and we have our guidelines as to dealing with different emergencies and situations. (Saunders et al 2000)

These contrasting perceptions say much about the values of those concerned.

Given the good clinical outcomes and the high levels of satisfaction of the families using birth centres and of their staff, one would expect birth centre care to be widely available for the majority of low-risk childbearing women.

THE WOMEN WHO USE BIRTH CENTRES

There are considerable pressures to maintain the status quo in maternity services, with service providers (Kirkham & Stapleton 2001) and service users tending to assume that 'what is, must be best' (Porter & Macintyre 1984). Maternity care has become increasingly centralised and technical in recent years and intrinsic in the provision and funding of new technical services are assumptions about the value of the complete care package and 'an expectation of compliant behaviour' on the part of service users

(Robins 2002). Women learn about maternity services from their own experience or from that of friends or family and expectations of the service and standards of good care are inevitably drawn from past care experience, which may make women reserved about using new services.

When new birth centres are opened, users of the new service are likely to be a special group. Ulla Waldenström compared women who had chosen to use the new Stockholm Birth Centre and a matched group of pregnant women who had chosen not to use the centre. The women choosing the birth centre were older, better educated and more likely to work in health- or culture-related jobs.

Women in the [birth centre] group had more positive attitudes to and expectations of the approaching birth and a greater interest in not being separated from the newborn and the rest of the family immediately after birth. They were also more interested in being actively involved in their own care. ...[and] were more concerned about the psychological aspects of childbirth. (Ch. 14)

These women, and their partners, were similar to women booking home births in their thoughtful, self-confident approach and their wide definitions of safety for birth, which included family well-being (N Edwards, unpublished PhD thesis, 2002). They fitted well the social model of birth in birth centres. Such women were described in the Edgware evaluation as 'clinically and self-selected for non-intervention in pregnancy', and in the birth centre 'their own aspirations for natural childbirth were supported by the midwives' (Ch. 12). Expectations influence outcomes (Green et al 1988) and the whole ethos of birth centres is one of expectation of normality. Such positive expectations should be nurtured in preference to the medical approach to childbearing, which is increasingly centred upon 'expecting trouble' (Strong 2000).

In Stockholm, the women who initially chose care in the birth centre were then randomised to receive either birth centre or hospital care. Intervention rates in the control group in hospital were generally lower than the national rates, 'which may be explained by the selection of low-risk women in early pregnancy but also by the

selection of rather outspoken women who were able to get what they wanted, even within the standard system of care' (Ch. 14). Such women are frequently seen as deviant within the wider medical definition of birth and often do not get what they want from maternity services in England (Kirkham & Stapleton 2001).

Though women who book in newly established birth centres are a special group, one of the most exciting aspects of birth centre care is how its availability changes local expectations. Once women have friends or neighbours who have delivered in a birth centre and are highly satisfied with their care, more women consider this option. Established birth centres become accepted as a local option for childbirth (Esposito 1999), or may be the only option for those who wish to give birth locally in some rural areas. The women I meet at Darley Maternity Unit are a much more mixed group than those who initially chose the Stockholm Birth Centre. Most want to give birth locally; a few travel considerable distances for what the birth centre offers. The existence of the unit has undoubtedly changed local expectations.

Examples of what is possible lead to change locally. The example of Edgware Birth Centre has led to changes in nearby maternity units: midwife-led care has developed at Northwick Park Hospital and a birth centre has opened at the Central Middlesex Hospital (Ch. 9). The Crowborough Birth Centre guidelines are now used in the local consultant unit (Ch. 5).

THE MIDWIVES WHO WORK IN BIRTH CENTRES

Midwives who choose to work in new birth centres are also a special group, seeking to work within an accepting and positive culture. In hospital maternity care midwives are subject to considerable pressures to conform, which are often reinforced by hierarchical disapproval or horizontal violence (Kirkham 1999, Kirkham & Stapleton 2001). Such a culture can stifle creativity and clinical judgement. It is therefore not surprising that when the Edgware birth centre was set up it was not able to recruit midwives locally, even with the job security of secondment, yet national advertisement brought a flood of applicants willing to relocate for jobs with short-term contracts.

In evaluating the birth centre in Edgware it was noted that :

...the birth centre has attracted and selected a group of midwives who share a common philosophy of midwifery care and an enthusiasm for putting it into practice. In their commitment to the Birth Centre, they have forged a dedicated and cohesive team. It is the philosophy that they share and the commitment that they have made to it that define the character of the Birth Centre and evoke the praise and loyalty of their clients. (Saunders et al 2000)

The small scale of a birth centre has a real influence on the relationships within it. This is especially true of the relationships between midwives and women. The opportunity to develop relationships with women changes the midwife's professional allegiances (Brodie 1996a, 1996b, Coyle et al 2001). It can create a shift in power similar to that achieved by the New Zealand midwifery partnership model, where 'partnership involves a shift of power from the health professional to the woman in the same way that the midwife's allegiance moves from the hospital or doctor to the woman as she supports her and stands alongside her through the process of pregnancy and childbirth' (Ch. 21).

The philosophy and the small scale of birth centres make it possible to develop the skills and confidence of the midwives who choose to work there. Olive Jones (2000) described how group reflection on practice was set up at Edgware:

It took time for midwives to become confident in group reflection, to accept critical enquiry as non-judgmental and to trust each other in terms of confidentiality and support.

[One midwife said,]

'It would be unrealistic to say that nobody's feelings are ever hurt because this sometimes causes inevitable pain. We all care deeply that what we do is right, so realising there could be a better way causes us discomfort...these are growing pains and far preferable to the anaesthetised routine that has

always been good enough.' Once trust was established midwives valued reflective sessions.

While the midwives who choose to work in birth centres go there in order to practice in a more autonomous and woman-centred manner, it is the philosophy and organisation of birth centres that enable them to safely develop their skills to that end: 'By challenging traditions in practice through critical enquiry, they emerged as competent practitioners with confidence in physiology using guidelines underpinned by research in making evidence-based decisions. Self-development is high on the agenda' (Jones 2000).

The special groups of women and of midwives who choose birth centres have common aims and grow in confidence and skill as trust develops between them. 'Confident midwives who extend the boundaries of their knowledge and practice assist women in making informed choices about their care' (Jones 2000); 'women learn to expect choice' and to exercise choice (Ch. 20). The 'focus on childbirth as something normal' led midwives to be 'more guided by the woman's own needs than by established routines' (see Ch. 14). This mutual development led Olive Jones to speak of 'the cycle of empowerment' and positive feedback for staff and families in birth centres: 'As long as the cycle of empowerment remains unbroken, it is self-perpetuating' (Jones 2000).

Expectations are therefore changed and skills developed. Confident midwives transmit confidence to women and expectations rise, are confirmed and are fed back into the local community.

Midwives who grow and develop in this way may be less vulnerable to burn-out because they experience fewer of the alienating work experiences reported by those who leave midwifery (Ball et al 2002) and are protected by their relative autonomy and relationships of respect with colleagues and with clients. Birth centres have waiting lists of midwives wanting jobs, despite the overall national shortage of midwives. This demonstrates how, for midwives as well as for women, the availability of the birth centre option changes expectations.

Birth centre practice is therefore important for midwifery because it demonstrates what is possible. In this there are parallels with independent midwifery practice in demonstrating to the mainstream what midwifery can be.

MIDWIFERY SKILLS IN BIRTH CENTRES

In birth centres, '[care] is no longer provided on an "industrialised" basis, with the inevitable protocols of routine' (Ch. 15). Nor is there evidence of the 'resigned docility' (Weil 1965) of the production line which is so often evidenced in women who form the work objects and the majority of the workers in large maternity hospitals (Kirkham 1987, Kirkham & Stapleton 2001). With the reduction in scale, from industrial to craft, 'all points of reference change' (Ch. 15) and different skills develop.

Birth centres work within a social rather than a medical model of birth: the small scale and the absence of the major technologies which operate in large maternity hospitals necessitate this and it was noted long before the philosophy of birth centres was developed (Kirkham 1987). Although doctors may see this absence as a drawback of care in small units, birth centre midwives see it as a strength. Throughout this book, birth centre midwives speak of the freedom from technology which enables them to give more attention to women and families. This philosophy is in stark contrast to obstetrics, with its technological imperatives and with the increasing number of technical skills and competencies which are required of midwives.

Birth centre midwives identify the absence of such equipment as electronic fetal heart monitors as freeing them to attend to the woman rather than the machine. To respond to her as an individual and to 'wait on' the process of labour and birth, in the sense of giving it their full attention (Weil 1951). Such levels of attention, and the skill that is subsequently developed, cannot be achieved in the presence of distractions such as attending to machines, doctors or more than one woman in labour. This everyday balancing act is tellingly portrayed in Valerie Levy's picture of the midwife on a tightrope (Levy 1999). In hospital, women wait as patients

(Ch. 16) and midwives strive precariously for balance; in birth centres, women labour and birth and midwives wait upon that process and that family.

Midwifery care in birth centres is personalised and is given in response to the individual needs of women and their families. Kate Griew sees the birth centre environment as one in which it is possible for midwives to 'truly listen' (Ch. 20). From this listening there follows a different use of language, with less jargon, less instruction and a focus on support for the woman, rather than the use of language which protects the midwife. Birth centres are noted for their excellent communication, both within and outwith the unit (NHS Management Executive 1993).

Marion Hunter draws from her research a list of the 'additional skills' required by midwives providing intrapartum care in small units (Hunter 2000):

- being confident to provide intrapartum care in a low-technology setting
- being comfortable to use embodied knowledge and skills to assess a woman and her baby as opposed to using technology
- being able to let labour 'be' and not interfere unnecessarily
- being confident to avert or manage problems that might arise
- being willing to employ other options to manage pain, without access to epidurals
- being solely responsible for outcomes without access to on-site specialist assistance
- being confident to trust the process of labour and be flexible with respect to time
- being a midwife who enjoys practising what the participants call 'real midwifery'.

This list is strikingly different from the usual lists of midwifery skills or competencies, though one competency includes the emergency skills which are so necessary for isolated practice. These are the fundamental, but invisible midwifery accomplishments. The skills on this list are all states of 'being', statements regarding the midwife's self and her use of self, rather than tightly defined manual or intellectual skills. These are skills for relationships, not for narrowly defined tasks. While is it unusual to see skills described as concerned with 'being', I have never before encountered a list of midwifery skills which contains the word 'enjoy'–yet how appropriate for midwives who have chosen to work in such settings.

Trust is highly significant here. The woman learns 'to trust her body' and the midwife to 'trust her own judgement' (Ch. 20), as well as trust for each other and the process of labour. Trust is infectious, and the midwife's trust is conveyed to the woman. Indeed, it must be one of the key reasons for the midwife being 'with women' historically: to convey by her calm presence that all is well and that what the woman experiences, whilst painful, is normal and can be coped with as women have coped before. This is the opposite of the self-fulfilling prophesy of needing to have intervention ready, 'just in case'.

Being able to 'let labour be' also contrasts with medicalised practice. Obstetrics is geared towards action and there are immense pressures to act. To be seen to have done everything that could be done is widely seen as good, if defensive, practice. The sins for which midwives and obstetricians are criticised are almost always those of omission–yet it is midwives' ability to *not* act that enables women to be active (Leap 2000). This is particularly important in labour, when, in the absence of epidural anaesthesia, women must cope with pain, and several chapters in this book have examined midwives' skills in supporting women as they 'work with' the pain of labour.

BIRTH CENTRES AS A THREAT

Relationships and core beliefs within birth centres are very different from those of mainstream maternity care. 'A birth centre seeks to preserve the possibility of birth not being exclusively medical' (Ch. 16). Madame de Béarn and many other birth centre midwives in this book do not reject medical knowledge or medical services. They see the resources of obstetrics as backing up and supporting, not replacing, women's knowledge and efforts and midwifery care.

Their practice is rooted in 'a vigilant attention to physiology' and the view that 'the majority of births do not need obstetric intervention' (Ch. 16).

As many chapters in this book have illustrated, birth centres can fit well within a continuum of maternity services, ranging from intensive obstetrics to home birth. To see birth centres in such a continuum requires an overall view which is not always taken. It requires an understanding of both the nature of birth and the ways it can be undertaken which is not restricted to the beliefs and practice of mainstream obstetrics. In this sense, birth centres and their philosophy deviate from the medicalised view of birth, which is now the social norm in western countries. Though few in number, their existence demonstrates other ways of doing birth and this alternative, can be perceived as a threat.

'Physicians fear losing control, clients and power', states Verene Schmid in Chapter 15. Few obstetricians actively support birth centres, though where they do, as in Wiltshire, the birth centre's service can be accepted as part of the range of maternity services. In private practice, birth centres may directly compete with obstetricians for clients and therefore fees (see Ch. 19). Within health services, the situation is even more complex. Overall, it is not unusual for professional opinion to be 'mostly antipathetic, and at times hostile' to birth centres (Ch. 7).

The perception of threat is not confined to obstetricians. Hospital midwives can be extremely unsupportive towards colleagues, especially those who practice differently from the hospital norm (Kirkham & Stapleton 2001). As a midwife, Verene Schmid reports that, in Italy, it is frequently the case that colleagues prove to be the greatest obstacle to the creation of birth centres (Ch. 15).

In order for women and families to play the key roles in birth, professionals need to acknowledge that their role is a supporting one. This does not fit well with the image of active professionals rescuing needy women from pain or risk, combating emergencies and delivering babies. The birth centre midwife's role is one of prevention and vigilance–states of calmness and readiness, not of activity. Many birth centre babies are simply born, often in water, and do not require 'delivering'. While birth centre midwives see this work as 'real midwifery' (Ch. 22) in a long tradition of being 'with woman', the lack of opportunity for heroic activity may be perceived as a threat to professional identity by those who are orientated to providing obstetric services.

Birth centres provide a conspicuous geographical focus for a different way of doing birth. This cannot be provided by home birth because of its essentially private nature. Birth centres are much visited. I really enjoy taking visitors to see the Darley Maternity Unit, where the furnishings and absence of a bed in the birth room speak louder than words. Even when empty, that room conveys the power of the women who birth there and the support of the local community who provided its pleasant furnishings. Verene Schmid, speaks of 'feminine power' embodied in birth centres being perceived as a threat by local politicians in Italy (Ch. 15).

There are real differences in how power is exercised in birth centres and in hospitals. The potential for 'sharing power' (Ch. 17) and for the mutual empowerment of mothers and midwives within birth centres is described many times over in this book. However, midwives in hospitals (at least in England and Wales) feel very unsupported (Kirkham & Stapleton 2000) and the 'positive spiral' of mutual support (Jones 2000) is very rare. Mutual empowerment does not fit with hierarchical structures. There is no hospital hierarchy to be found in birth centres and this freedom, as well as the freedom from technology, enables midwives to truly listen to women and be flexible in their responses.

These fundamental differences between birth centres and hospitals, and the satisfaction and loyalty of the families who use birth centres, can be seen as implied criticism of the overall maternity services, rather than as features of a centre of excellence and a source of pride and education. I have so often heard it said that a service cannot afford a birth centre because of its excellence: 'a deluxe service for a few is inequitable' is a phase often used by managers intending to close a birth centre down, irrespective of its achievements in terms of outcomes, satisfaction and costs. Maternity services sometimes become so rigid as to exhibit a fear of excellence. Where diversity cannot be tolerated, the social model of birth is likely to be seen as a threat to mainstream services. Ironically, this is where birth centres are most needed.

BIRTH CENTRES AS THREATENED

It is not only where birth centres compete with obstetricians for fees that birth centres are threatened. With the ubiquitous centralisation of maternity services and constant pressures to cut costs, existing publicly funded birth centres are vulnerable to threats of closure. This climate also makes it very difficult to open new birth centres in spite of good supporting evidence and vigorous local campaigns.

Most of the birth centres described in this book have been repeatedly threatened with closure, with no economic or clinical justification. This is extremely wearying for all those involved. The 'goldfish bowl' feeling of being watched in a hostile manner is very difficult for staff. Threat of closure undermines the morale of staff and service users and can lead to a decline in bookings (see Ch. 5), which can then be used to support the argument for closure. Such a vicious circle takes much campaigning energy to break.

The very nature of small units makes them vulnerable. They can easily be identified as centres of a model of practice that is very different from that of obstetric hospitals and as areas of potential savings if cut. The pressure to provide the full range of clinical services (which usually comes from those who provide such services as paediatrics or anaesthetics) has led to the closure of units with less than 300 births per year in France and 500 births per year in Italy. The belief that such services are needed for *all* women, 'just in case', is the opposite of the positive outlook of the social model of birth. Yet, like much public policy on birth historically, this medical model of birth is accepted as the one that is obviously 'right' because it is supported by authoritative experts. Like the 'obvious economics' of centralisation, it usually goes unquestioned.

In some places small maternity units have almost been wiped out. Yet they tend to reappear. It is significant that the one remaining French birth centre is owned and organised by parents (see Ch. 16) and parents are in the forefront of campaigns to save or create birth centres in many places.

PARTNERSHIP AND COOPERATION

One thread which runs through this book concerns the high levels of collaborative working described in the setting up and running of birth centres. Working in centres on this small scale, where relationships are allowed to develop, professionals come to feel accountable to individuals rather than to the system. This builds confidence in all concerned. Ironically, midwives and clients who gain confidence in birth centres are the groups least likely to develop confidence or autonomy in hospitals, where they are at the bottom of a hierarchy which tends to pass blame downwards.

Women and families play an important part in the creation, sustenance and successful development of birth centres. Without their efforts there would be very few birth centres. Childbearing women and families are central to all the relationships described. Service users were originally, and still are, 'in the driving seat' at Edgware (see Ch. 6). The only remaining French birth centre is run by parents, and residents of an Austrian village recently designed and built their own birth centre (Dörfler & Saal 2002). Where families and professionals work together in setting up and continuing to develop a birth centre, high levels of cooperation are forged which continue to be of mutual support and benefit.

The words 'value' and 'respect' are used repeatedly in this book with regard to relationships with colleagues and clients. This is not usual in books about health care. 'Valuing everyone's contribution' (see Ch. 11) is an attitude of generosity which is part of the positive spiral. Such generosity is manifest where individuals feel confident, not threatened, and their own value is demonstrated to them in their working relationships. Excellent role modelling is vital, as is the small scale of birth centres, so that relationships with individual colleagues and clients can develop, and these two factors together create another positive spiral.

Reflective meetings and having opportunities to review incidents are described as developing individual practice and a supportive team spirit in Edgware and Crowborough birth centres. The way these meetings are facilitated, and the safe setting for learning which they provide, have been very important. Joint discussions with management and supervisors are also described as improving morale in Crowborough Birth Centre (see Ch. 5).

Jane Walker sees the success of the midwifery assistants' role at Edgware Birth Centre as grounded in an ethos of partnership and mutual respect rather than fear of role confusion (Ch. 11). The doula aspects of the midwifery assistant role have been fostered by the midwives and valued by families. Yet, elsewhere in England midwives find the concept of doulas to be threatening (Mander 2001).

The confidence and skills which midwives develop in birth centres seem to equip them well to collaborate with other professionals as equals. This is very different from the culture of deference and 'passing the buck' which is common in hospital hierarchies. The planning of new birth centres requires extensive multiprofessional support and the Edgware birth centre is a good example of how the many different agencies and interests can be mobilised. Collaboration is important in sustaining birth centres too. A 1993 study of midwife- and GP-led maternity care concluded:

Successful schemes displayed high levels of interdisciplinary working.... Informal exchanges of advice allow continuity of care and avoid unnecessary transfers. Willing collaboration and mutual respect among professional groups, unhindered by professional differences, resulted in and helped to sustain jointly owned guidelines. (NHS Management Executive 1993)

Despite the skills in communication and collaboration which are nurtured within birth centres, other professionals are unfortunately not always willing to collaborate.

AN ENABLING CULTURE

Thus it is that the small scale of birth centres and their integration into their local communities make it possible for them to achieve so many of the aims of modern maternity care which often remain mere rhetoric elsewhere (Kirkham & Stapleton 2001). Choice, control and continuity for childbearing women are described as the reality of women's experience in this book. Partnership is described in detail, together with high levels of interprofessional collaboration. Sophisticated communication skills are fostered and developed at a time when failures in communication lie behind so many complaints and litigation about health care. Midwives enjoy their work and families feel cherished, at a time when midwives are leaving the profession because of dissatisfaction with midwifery (Ball et al 2002) and professionals live in fear of litigation.

In some ways birth centres represent a move back in time in terms of the organisation of care, but they also combine 'modern ideas and old fashioned values' (Ch. 10) and provide a safe 'place for relearning' midwifery skills (Ch. 22). A focus for resistance to the unremitting centralisation of maternity services is needed, and only small units and their networks can provide that focus. It would be possible, but probably fruitless, to debate how much the achievements of birth centres spring from their small scale and how much from their philosophy. I saw what has since been developed as the philosophy of birth centre care in practice in small GP units back in 1981 (Kirkham 1987). Now that this philosophy has been articulated, it is logical and efficient to apply it, in order to achieve the safety that lies 'within the social model of midwifery' (Ch. 2).

Birth centres provide a focus for midwives, a safe haven for the practice of 'real midwifery', a place where like-minded midwives can turn the rhetoric of modern maternity care into reality, without feeling vulnerable and deviant. Separation from obstetric units is necessary for midwives to be able to attend to families without the fragmentation of their attention which, like fragmented care, results from industrialised obstetrics. Theoretically, obstetric care could change, though that would be extremely difficult, and other initiatives may lead to change, such as one-to-one care or extending home birth. Meanwhile, birth centres develop the transferable skills without which humane care is impossible. I read this in a national newspaper:

The medical establishment has failed new mothers by refusing to embrace more natural and confidence-building methods of supporting women in childbirth when the research strongly suggests that they work. There is also a shameful erosion of midwifery skills. (Figes 2002)

While statements such as this remain true, midwives have a duty to maintain and develop new birth centres.

Birth centres demonstrate what is possible in maternity care. They are a positive model for change in the scale of services and for change within neighbouring maternity hospitals. There are networks of support and tools (RCM 2002) for those who work to extend birth centres. There is still much resistance to this model of care, yet its existence establishes an alternative to a single, industrialised model of birth and so ensures the debate that is essential if maternity services are to improve.

REFERENCES

Albers L, Katz V 1991 Birth setting for low-risk pregnancies: an analysis of the current literature. Journal of nurse-midwifery 36: 215–222

Ball L, Curtis P, Kirkham M 2002 Why do midwives leave? Royal College of Midwives, London

Birth Centres Network UK. Available at: http://groups.yahoo.com/group/birthcentres

Bovard W, Milton G 1993 Why not me? The story of Gladys Milton, midwife. The Book Publishing Company, Summertown, Tennessee

Brodie P 1996a Australian team midwives in transition. Proceedings of the 24th Triennial Congress of the International Confederation of Midwives, May 26–31 1996, Oslo

Brodie P 1996b Being with women: the experience of Australian team midwives. (Masters thesis), University of Technology, Sydney

Campbell R M, Macfarlane A 1994 Where to be born? The debate and the evidence. National Perinatal Epidemiology Unit, Oxford

Campbell R M et al 1999 Evaluation of midwifery-led care provided at the Royal Bournemouth Hospital. Midwifery 15: 1–10

Coyle K et al 2001 Ongoing relationships with a personal focus: mothers' perceptions of birth centre versus hospital care. Midwifery 17: 171–181

Davis-Floyd R 1994 Culture and birth: the technocrat imperative. International Journal of Childbirth Education 9 (2): 6–7

Dörfler S, Saal 2002 The Geburtshaus Isis Noreia. A love space. (Ab. in programme) 26th Triennial Congress of the International Confederation of Midwives, April 14–18 2002, Vienna

Edwards N 2002 Views and experiences of women planning home birth. (PhD thesis), University of Sheffield, Sheffield

Esposito N W 1999 Marginalised women's comparisons of their hospital and free-standing birth centre experiences: a contrast of inner-city birthing systems. Health Care for Women International 20 (2): 111–126

Figes K 2002 A distress not to be borne. Guardian, 24 June 2002, p 18

Fullerton J, Severino R 1992 In-hospital care for low-risk childbirth: comparison with results from the National Birth Centre Study. Journal of nurse-midwifery 37 (5): 331–340

Gaskin I M 1993 Foreword to: Bovard W and Milton G 1993 Why not me? The story of Gladys Milton, midwife. The Book Publishing Company, Summertown, Tennessee

Green J M, Coupland V A, Kitzinger J V 1988 Great Expectations: a prospective study of women's expectations and experiences of childbirth. Child Care and Development Unit, University of Cambridge, Cambridge

Hall J 2001 Directory of free-standing low-risk maternity units in England. Available from: Local Supervising Authority Midwifery Officer, Yorkshire Consortium of LSAs at Leeds Health Authority, Leeds

Hunter M 2000 Autonomy, clinical freedom and responsibility: the paradoxes of providing intrapartum midwifery care in a small maternity unit as compared with a large obstetric hospital. (MA thesis) Massey University, Palmerston North, New Zealand

Jones O 2000 Supervision in a midwife-managed birth centre. In: Kirkham M (ed.) Developments in the Supervision of Midwives. Books for Midwives Press, Hale

Kirkham M 1987 Basic supportive care in labour. (PhD thesis) University of Manchester, Manchester

Kirkham M 1999 The culture of midwifery in the NHS in England. Journal of Advanced Nursing 30 (3): 732–739

Kirkham M, Stapleton H 2000 Midwives' support needs as childbirth changes. Journal of Advanced Nursing 32 (2): 465–472

Kirkham M, Stapleton H 2001 (eds) Informed choice in maternity care: an evaluation of evidence-based leaflets. NHS Centre for Reviews and Dissemination, York

Leap N 2000 The less we do the more we give. In: Kirkham M (ed.) The midwife-mother relationship. Macmillan, London

Levy V 1999 Protective steering: a grounded theory study of the processes involved when midwives facilitate informed choice in pregnancy. Journal of Advanced Nursing 29 (1): 104–112

Local Government Board 1918 47th Annual Report of the Local Government Board, 1917–18. Part 1. Cd 9157. The Stationery Office Books, London

MacVicar J et al 1993 Simulated home delivery in hospital: a randomised controlled trial. British Journal of Obstetrics and Gynaecology 93: 183–187

Mander R 2001 Supportive care and midwifery. Blackwell Science, Oxford

Misago C et al 2000 Satisfying birthing experiences in Japan. Lancet 355: 2256

NHS Management Executive 1992 A Study of midwife- and GP-led maternity units. Department of Health, London

Olensen O 1997 Meta-analysis of the safety of home birth. Birth 24 (1): 4–16

Porter M and Macintyre S 1984 What is, must be best: a research note on conservative or deferential response to antenatal care provision. Social Science and Medicine 19(11): 1197–1200

Robins J B 2002 Compliant behaviour in the antenatal setting. Electronic letter to British Medical Journal, 20 March 2002. Available at: *BMJ.com/cgi/eletters/324/7338/639*

Rooks J et al 1989 Outcomes of care in birth centres. The National Birth Centre Study. New England Journal of Medicine 321 (26): 1804–1811

Rooks J P, Weatherby N L, Ernst E K M 1992a The national birth center study: Part I–Methodology and prenatal care and referrals. Journal of nurse-midwifery 37 (6): 361–397

Rooks J P, Weatherby N L, Ernst E K M 1992b The national birth center study: Part II–Intrapartum and immediate postpartum and neonatal care. Journal of nurse-midwifery 37 (6): 361–397

Rooks J P, Weatherby N L, Ernst E K M 1992c The national birth center study: Part III–Intrapartum and immediate postpartum and neonatal complications and transfers, postpartum and neonatal care, outcomes, and client satisfaction. Journal of nurse-midwifery 37 (6): 361–397

Royal College of Midwives 2002 Vision 2000 into Practice Toolkits 1-7. RCM, London

Saunders D et al 2000 Evaluation of the Edgware Birth Centre. Barnet Health Authority, London

Stilwell J A 1979 Relative costs of home and hospital confinements. British Medical Journal 2: 257–259

Strong T H 2000 Expecting trouble: the myth of prenatal care in America. New York University Press, New York

Turner S 2002 Midwifery in Tokyo. The Practising Midwife 5 (4): 34–35

von Schwarzenfeld D M, Dimer J, Kentenich H 1999 Perinatal outcomes in hospital and birth centre obstetric care. International Journal of Gynaecology and Obstetrics 65(2): 149–155

Waldenström U 1999 Effects of birth centre care on fathers' satisfaction with care, experience of the birth and adaptation to fatherhood. Journal of Reproductive and Infant Psychology 17: 357–368

Weil S 1951 Waiting on God. Crawford E (trans.) Fontana, London

Weil S 1965 Simone Weil: seventy letters. Rees R (arr. trans.) Oxford University Press, London

Young G 1987 Are isolated maternity units run by general practitioners dangerous? British Medical Journal 294: 744–746

Index